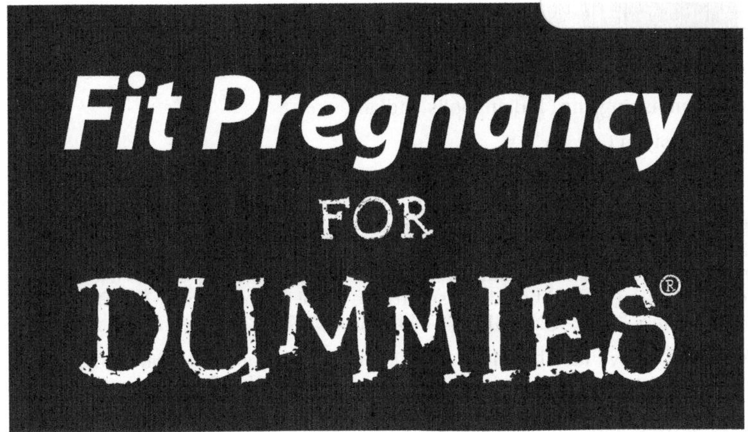

Fit Pregnancy For Dummies®

by Catherine Cram and Tere Stouffer Drenth

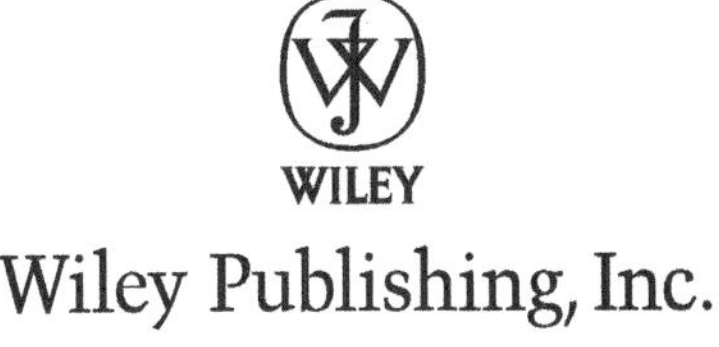

Wiley Publishing, Inc.

Fit Pregnancy For Dummies®

Published by
Wiley Publishing, Inc.
111 River St.
Hoboken, NJ 07030-5774
www.wiley.com

Published by Wiley Publishing, Inc., Indianapolis, Indiana

Published simultaneously in Canada

For general information on our other products and services or to obtain technical support, please contact our Customer Care Department within the U.S. at 800-762-2974, outside the U.S. at 317-572-3993, or fax 317-572-4002.

Wiley also publishes its books in a variety of electronic formats. Some content that appears in print may not be available in electronic books.

Library of Congress Control Number: 2004103166

ISBN: 0-7645-5829-3

Manufactured in the United States of America

10 9 8 7 6 5 4 3 2 1

1B/RV/QW/QU/IN

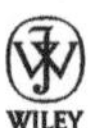

About the Authors

Catherine Cram is an exercise physiologist who specializes in prenatal and postpartum fitness. Her consulting company, Comprehensive Fitness Consulting, LLC, provides maternal fitness certificate training courses for health and fitness professionals. She's an expert advisor to and writes for *Baby Years, Pregnancy, Women's Health and Fitness,* and iparenting.com. Catherine has been featured in prenatal fitness articles for *Fit Pregnancy, Parenting, Glamour, Babytalk,* and *The American Journal of Medicine and Sports,* and is a contributing author of *Women's Health Care in Physical Therapy: Principles and Practices for Rehabilitation Specialists* (Lippincott Williams & Wilkins). You can contact her at `compfc@aol.com`.

Tere Stouffer Drenth is both a full-time writer and a semiprofessional runner who works, trains, hikes, and lives in northern Michigan. A former cross-country All-American, Tere (which rhymes with Mary) writes about fitness and the outdoors in the hope that people of all ages and backgrounds will challenge themselves physically and reap the many rewards of exercise. She is the author of *Marathon Training For Dummies* (Wiley) and several other books. You can reach her at `tdrenth@earthlink.net`.

Dedication

From Cathy: To the many women who have generously shared their unique and enlightening insights on pregnancy and motherhood with me through the years. Also to Beverly and Ramon Cram for their consistent support and encouragement. And in loving remembrance of Bertina Mikkelson.

From Tere: To all women who bravely undertake motherhood and dare to become and stay fit during those physically demanding 40 weeks of pregnancy.

Authors' Acknowledgments

Writing a book requires an entire team of professionals, and we're fortunate to have worked with the best. Natasha Graf, acquisitions editor at Wiley, first championed the idea of publishing this book and shared her vision with Joyce Pepple, acquisitions director, and Diane Steele, publisher, who gave their stamp of approval. Chrissy Guthrie, project editor, then took over the reins and skillfully drove this project to completion, despite some bumps in the road. Copy editor Kristin DeMint made the text flow smoothly and sound so much better. And Barbara Moore, production coordinator, managed the layout and proofreading of this project.

Special thanks to Ellen Houston, Natalie Hagen, Ann Wilson, Karen Dettinger, Joan Bonazza, Tina Lemon, Lorie Cahn, and Lana Turner for their assistance and for providing a humorous and honest view into the real world of motherhood.

We also want to send many thanks to our models — Barbara and Rachel Boulden, Lisa and Annika Sanborn, Jennifer Folmer, and Sheila Erbach McGinn — and our photographer, John Urban. Thanks to the University of Wisconsin Health Sports Medicine Center in Madison, Wisconsin, for the use of its facility and assistance of its staff during our photo shoot.

Publisher's Acknowledgments

We're proud of this book; please send us your comments through our Dummies online registration form located at `www.dummies.com/register/`.

Some of the people who helped bring this book to market include the following:

Acquisitions, Editorial, and Media Development

Project Editor: Christina Guthrie

Acquisitions Editor: Natasha Graf

Copy Editor: Kristin DeMint

Technical Editor: John F. Wagner, MD, FACOG

Editorial Manager: Christine Meloy Beck

Editorial Assistants: Courtney Allen, Elizabeth Rea, Melissa Bennett

Cover Photo: © Corbis

Cartoons: Rich Tennant, `www.the5thwave.com`

Composition

Project Coordinator: Barbara Moore

Layout and Graphics: Amanda Carter, Brian Drumm, Denny Hager, Shelley Norris, Barry Offringa, Heather Ryan, Brent Savage, Julie Trippetti

Special Art: Interior photos by John Urban; illustrations by Lisa S. Reed

Proofreaders: TECHBOOKS Production Services

Indexer: TECHBOOKS Production Services

Publishing and Editorial for Consumer Dummies

Diane Graves Steele, Vice President and Publisher, Consumer Dummies

Joyce Pepple, Acquisitions Director, Consumer Dummies

Kristin A. Cocks, Product Development Director, Consumer Dummies

Michael Spring, Vice President and Publisher, Travel

Brice Gosnell, Associate Publisher, Travel

Kelly Regan, Editorial Director, Travel

Publishing for Technology Dummies

Andy Cummings, Vice President and Publisher, Dummies Technology/General User

Composition Services

Gerry Fahey, Vice President of Production Services

Debbie Stailey, Director of Composition Services

Contents at a Glance

Table of Contents

Introduction

Are you intrigued by the idea of working out during pregnancy, but think it can't be safe? Are you unsure how the words *fit* and *pregnancy* actually make sense in the same sentence? If so, you've come to the right place. *Fit Pregnancy For Dummies* is your guidebook to a fit and healthy pregnancy, showing you how you can be fit *and* pregnant, whether you're new to exercise or have been working out for years, and whether you're in your 2nd week of pregnancy or your 32nd.

About This Book

Whether you've never exercised before or are a competitive athlete, this book helps you find the right type of exercise during your pregnancy and explains how to set up a workout routine that works for you. You find out which activities tend to work best for pregnant women and have a chance to read about activities you may not have tried before. You also get tips on eating enough to gain weight regularly, but not so much that you're faced with a completely different body after you deliver. And you find out how to take care of your body after you deliver your baby, how to keep your workout routine going, and how to help your child grow up healthy and fit.

If you're a first-time exerciser, you find chapters and sections just for you — ones that help you understand common fitness terminology and basic concepts about setting up an exercise program. You get the lowdown on getting started and staying motivated, and you'll never feel as though this fitness stuff is over your head.

If you're an old pro, you don't have to wade through the basics; go ahead and skip chapters and sections that don't apply to you. You do, however, find plenty of information about how to modify your existing workout routine so that you make sure your pregnancy progresses properly but that you still maintain much of your old fitness level.

Conventions Used in This Book

Like all *For Dummies* books, this book doesn't use a lot of strange conventions that cause you to scratch your head in wonder. Instead, we keep the conventions and definitions simple, as follows:

- When we introduce pregnancy terminology or fitness jargon, we *italicize* the term.
- On those rare occasions when we suggest typing a term into an Internet search engine, like Google, we type that term in **boldface.**
- For those times that we direct you to a Web site for information or workout gear, the Web address is set in a special typeface, such as `www.dummies.com`.
- When talking about fitness, we use the term *activity* to mean the sport or other type of exercise in which you're choosing to participate.
- The total time that you exercise in a day is called a *workout,* and a workout usually includes a warm-up, an activity (or more than one activity, if you're cross-training — see Chapter 17), and a cool-down.

  Note that *workout* is a noun — a thing. When we're talking about the verb form of that work — for example, when we say, "In order to *work out,* you have to first warm up" — the term is actually two words. Yeah, we admit that's a little confusing, but our grammar- and spelling-conscious editors wouldn't have it any other way.
- Often, we refer to your overall workout plan as an *exercise routine* or *workout routine,* and it includes all that you do over the course of weeks, months, and years to keep yourself fit.
- We frequently recommend that you talk to a *healthcare provider* or *healthcare practitioner,* and by that, we mean a doctor — an obstetrician and gynecologist (OB/GYN), medical doctor (MD), or osteopath (DO) — a certified nurse-midwife (CNM), a nurse practitioner (NP), a physician's assistant (PA), or any other qualified medical professional who's assisting you with your pregnancy.

Foolish Assumptions

What foolish assumptions do we make about you, dear reader? Just two:

- You're pregnant (or are thinking of becoming pregnant).
- You want to be as fit and healthy as you can be — whatever your current fitness level — without in any way jeopardizing your health or the health of your baby.

If this sounds like you, you've picked up the right book. But if you're not pregnant, pick up *Fitness For Dummies,* by Suzanne Schlosberg and Liz Neporent (Wiley), which is your guide to general fitness. And if you're looking for all-purpose advice on your pregnancy — not pregnancy workout advice — check out *Pregnancy For Dummies,* 2nd Edition, by Joanne Stone, MD, Keith Eddleman, MD, and Mary Duenwald (also published by Wiley).

How This Book Is Organized

This book is organized into six parts, each with chapters that relate to specific areas of pregnancy fitness.

Part I: Fit Pregnancy: Isn't That an Oxymoron?

Striving for a fit pregnancy may sound like an oxymoron, but the fact that many women don't try to become fit or even continue their current fitness levels during pregnancy isn't physical, but cultural. Up until the past decade, most healthcare providers discouraged pregnant women from doing any exercise during their pregnancies for fear that exercise would cause problems like premature labor and very low-birthweight babies. Recent research shows that moderate exercise has a wonderful positive impact on pregnancy and doesn't cause any additional health problems for you or your baby. Even so, many women are unsure whether exercising during pregnancy is a good idea, and few women know how to go about pursuing a fit pregnancy.

This part comes to the rescue, answering your most pressing fitness questions, helping you recognize the many benefits that a fit pregnancy brings to you and your baby, putting together a workout routine that fits your goals and lifestyle, and discovering the best activities to do while pregnant.

Part II: Getting Up and Moving: Fit Pregnancy Basics

Before you start working out, you need to think about a few basics. If you're an exercise novice, the first chapter in this part helps you with the very basic basics, like what to wear while exercising and how to get started with a workout program. In fact, this part also includes an entire chapter on finding clothing and other workout gear for whatever activity you choose to pursue. And you also find out how to warm up and stretch so that you increase flexibility and keep yourself injury free.

If you've already spent time exercising, this part offers a special chapter that helps you decide whether to continue your current activity, discusses activities that you may be able to substitute and still maintain a high level of fitness, and gives advice on how to modify your current training program to maintain your and your baby's health.

Part III: Eating Well for Nine Months — and for Life

Pregnancy is certainly a time for weight gain, but you want the gain to be only the amount your healthcare provider recommends — no more, no less — and you want to eat the foods that best nourish your body. In this part, you find out which foods are most nutritious, get a report on the latest carbohydrate versus fat controversy, find out which vitamins you need and how to get them from foods, and hydrate yourself with water and other beverages. You also get tips and tricks for keeping food down (if you're struggling with nausea) and find out how to *not* give in to certain cravings.

Part IV: Fun and Healthy Activities for Pregnancy and Beyond

This part introduces you to a variety of activities that tend to be comfortable and safe for pregnant women. You're introduced to the tools of the trade (the gear and equipment needed for each activity), get a few tips on the best technique to use, and discover ways to come up with a workout plan that works for you. This part also includes a chapter on cross-training to help you figure out how to incorporate two or more activities into a workout routine.

Part V: The Tenth Month and Later: Staying Fit for Life

Although the focus of this book is on your fitness routine while you're pregnant, we would be remiss if we didn't give you some tips for continuing your workout routine after you deliver your baby. In this part, you find chapters on how (and whether) to exercise in the days following your baby's birth, how to continue exercising in spite of the demands of motherhood, and how to help your child grow up fit and healthy. This material could be a book all in itself, so you're just getting a taste here, but we give you enough information to keep you working out throughout the rest of your life.

Part VI: The Part of Tens

Like all *For Dummies* books, this one has a Part of Tens — the last part in this book — that gives you quick, fun lists of ten: ten effective ways to exercise indoors, ten ideas for getting your family hooked on fitness, and ten great resources for pregnancy workout gear.

Icons Used in This Book

You know those roadside signs that you see during highway construction projects that inform you of lane closures, slowdowns, and other critical information? Because your fit pregnancy is a work in progress much like a construction site, this book offers *icons* that are structured like informational road signs, only they appear in the margins of the book instead of in six-foot-tall neon signs. Here's what they mean:

This icon gives you tips, tricks, and techniques that, with time, you'd surely figure out on your own. But instead of spending years and years finding out the hard way, you get the benefit of our nearly 50 years of combined experiences as athletes and fitness advisors by reading these tips.

This icon highlights information that you want to tattoo on your brain. Keep these reminders in the forefront as you work out during your pregnancy.

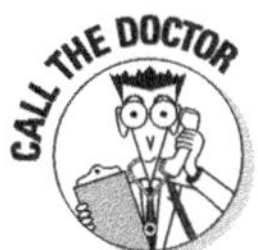

Although this icon is called "Call the Doctor," it really means that you should call whichever healthcare professional is guiding you through your pregnancy. "Call the Healthcare Professional" just doesn't have the same ring to it, so we chose the word "doctor," although we have no intention of suggesting that a doctor is a more appropriate pregnancy medical professional than the other options, such as a certified nurse-midwife, a nurse practitioner, or a physician's assistant. This icon alerts you to signs, signals, and symptoms that may mean that you need to cut back on your workout program. Only your healthcare provider can help you decide whether your pregnancy is proceeding as it should, so contact him or her as soon as possible if you experience any of the warning signs flagged by these icons.

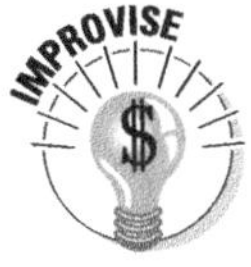

Are you tightening your budget as you get ready for your new little roommate? Or are you already saving for your baby's college education? If so, this icon points out ways to save a bit of money on the many "essential" pieces of clothing, other gear, and equipment that the fitness industry tries to convince you to buy.

Where to Go from Here

Most authors expect you to read their books from cover to cover, and although you're free to do that with this book and will gain a great deal of information by doing so, don't feel as though you have to read the entire book or read it in any sort of order. You're invited to skip around, using the Index and Table of Contents to find what you need, or rely on pure chance by flipping this book up in the air and reading whatever page is open when it lands.

If you're brand new to exercise, think about reading Chapter 5 first — it's meant just for you and includes a lot of pointers about how to get started. If you're not yet ready to commit to exercising during pregnancy, read Chapter 2 for a look at the many benefits. Chapter 3 tells you how to devise an exercise plan that fits your goals, lifestyle, and current fitness level. And if you're not sure which activities are best to take up while pregnant, visit Chapter 4 for a listing, and read how to get started in and/or continue doing these activities in Chapters 11 through 16. Also, visit Chapters 18 and 19 for postnatal fitness advice.

Part I

Fit Pregnancy: Isn't That an Oxymoron?

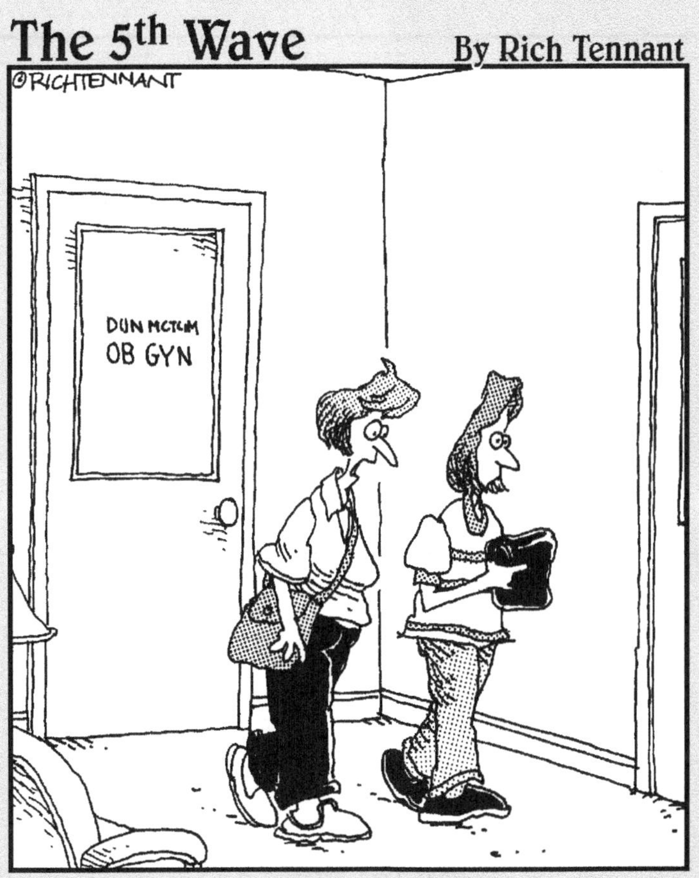

"I can exercise as long as I avoid becoming light headed, flush, or short of breath. Of course, if I could have avoided those symptoms a few months ago I wouldn't be pregnant in the first place."

In this part . . .

You find out that having a fit pregnancy is not only possible — but it's also the preferred approach to pregnancy. And it's so much healthier for you and your baby than sitting in front of the TV for nine months!

This part answers your most important fitness questions and helps you better understand the multitude of benefits that a fit pregnancy brings your way. You discover how to design a workout program throughout each trimester and find out which signs and symptoms to watch for as you exercise. You also get a quick glance at which activities tend to work best for pregnant women.

Chapter 1

Making Your Pregnancy a Fit Pregnancy

In This Chapter

- Knowing what a fit pregnancy is all about
- Understanding the benefits of staying fit while pregnant
- Discovering how your workouts need to change throughout your pregnancy
- Narrowing your fitness goals

Congratulations on your pregnancy! With a healthy lifestyle and good advice from your healthcare provider, in a few months, you're going to deliver a healthy, happy baby.

To make you and your child even healthier, you're thinking about starting or continuing an exercise program, but you may not know where to begin. Perhaps your healthcare provider doesn't have a lot of experience with pregnant women who want to work out, and maybe your partner (or your mom) isn't so sure that exercising while pregnant is a good idea. The truth is, staying fit during a healthy pregnancy is a *very* good idea, one that's safe for you and your baby and brings both of you all sorts of benefits.

To figure out what sort of exercise routine works for you, this chapter is a good place to begin. It introduces you to some of the basic concepts of a fit pregnancy and answers some of your most important questions.

What Does "Fit Pregnancy" Mean?

In a nutshell, a *fit pregnancy* means that during the nine months between the time you conceive and the time you go into labor, you're doing the following:

- **You're setting yourself up for an easier labor and delivery.** This is what you've been waiting to hear, isn't it? Women who exercise during pregnancy deliver their babies about five days earlier, spend less time in labor, experience fewer complications during labor and delivery, have fewer inductions and cesarean sections, and need fewer drugs to relieve pain than women who don't exercise.

- **You're establishing cardiovascular fitness.** Getting fit while you're pregnant means that your heart and lungs (your *cardiovascular system*) get stronger, healthier, and more efficient. This means that you'll not only be a mother, but also you'll likely live to be a great-great-grandmother!
- **You're developing strength.** You tone your arms, chest, abdomen, butt, hips, and legs. You may never look like a bodybuilder (and probably don't want to), but you can make yourself strong. This strength comes in handy with all the bending and lifting you'll be doing in a few months.
- **You're improving your flexibility.** By stretching after your workout and on your days off, you'll become far more flexible, which means that you experience fewer injuries and are far less limited in what your body can do throughout the rest of your lifetime. (Chapter 8 is all about stretching.)
- **You're balancing exercise with proper nutrition.** Exercise and nutrition go hand in hand; the food you eat fuels your body (doing so either efficiently or inefficiently), and the exercise you do changes the amount of food you need to eat to maintain your weight. This is why you see articles about food in workout magazines and articles about workouts in health-food magazines. The two are inseparably linked. So, this book includes a part (Part III) on eating in a way that complements your exercise routine as well as your pregnancy.

Being fit during pregnancy doesn't mean training for a triathlon or getting certified as a fitness instructor (although if those ideas become future goals of yours, that's terrific). And you don't have to start eating macrobiotic food or anything like that. Instead, a fit pregnancy is about normal people taking seriously the advice of physicians and researchers to get in shape and stay that way.

Weighing In on the Benefits

One of the most significant benefits of a fit pregnancy is that you gain less fat than nonexercisers do during their pregnancies. And for the weight you do gain (keeping in mind that weight gain during pregnancy is healthy and absolutely necessary), if you're a fit woman, you'll have an easier time shedding your weight after you deliver.

If you're tempted to think of these 40 weeks as a time to throw caution to the wind and eat whatever you want, you'll probably gain far more weight than you need to and will have a difficult time getting back to your pre-pregnancy size. To stay fit during your pregnancy, you have to approach your pregnancy with a different mindset: not throwing caution to the wind, but using common sense in every decision. You do so by incorporating healthy eating habits and burning additional calories as you work out. (Chapter 9 covers healthy foods for you and your baby. Chapter 10 discusses how many extra calories you need during your pregnancy, what those calories mean in terms of everyday foods, and how many *more* calories you can eat without gaining more weight than your doctor recommends, based on the fitness activities you choose.)

Besides the benefit of managing your weight gain and loss before and after you deliver your baby, a fit pregnancy brings other incredible benefits, from making your pregnancy more comfortable to improving your mood to helping your body get back to normal after you deliver. Even your baby benefits from your workouts. (Chapter 2 is chock-full of the benefits of a fit pregnancy that you and your baby can enjoy.)

Finding the Right Activities for You

If you've talked to your mother or to girlfriends about exercising during your pregnancy, you've probably been inundated with advice about what activities you can do, how long you should do them, and when you should work out, such as

- "You shouldn't run while you're pregnant."
- "Don't exercise for more than 20 minutes at a time."
- "Never exercise first thing in the morning."
- "Don't do any outdoor activities."
- "A gym's room temperature is too hot for a pregnant woman."

So what's the real story? The truth is that every one of the preceding bullets is false but has a grain of truth in it. For example:

- If you've been running and your pregnancy is going well, you're free to keep up this activity during pregnancy. Many newcomers to fitness, however, find running to be too demanding during pregnancy. See Chapter 12.
- Pregnant women exercise for as much as an hour a day and see fantastic benefits, but if you experience any problems during your pregnancy, your healthcare provider may ask you to reduce your duration or to stop exercising altogether. See Chapter 3.
- Plenty of pregnant women exercise first thing in the morning and love the energy it gives them and the flexibility it gives to the rest of the day. If you're experiencing severe morning sickness, however, you may not have any desire to exercise until later in the day, when you feel less nauseated. See Chapter 5.

- Although some outdoor activities are just fine for pregnant women, you may need to modify your outdoor exercise if your activity becomes uncomfortable, especially if the discomfort's due to outdoor weather extremes.
- You shouldn't allow yourself to become overheated while exercising, but many gyms are air-conditioned, making them ideal for working out during your pregnancy.

You'll get advice from all corners, but the bottom line is this: Do an activity that you like, that makes sense given your current fitness level, and that your healthcare provider approves, and then do this activity in a place and at a time of day that's convenient for you and healthy for your baby.

Getting started with a fitness routine

If you're pregnant and are just getting started with a fitness routine, you're probably feeling a bit overwhelmed about which activities you can do and how you get started: what to wear, when to work out, how often to exercise, how much to work out during each session, and how to listen to your body to determine whether you're overdoing it.

If so, Chapter 5 is designed just for you! That chapter clears the air and helps you get started in your new workout routine — today, if you're so inclined. You also want to take a peek at Chapter 3, which discusses some safety issues, and Chapter 7, which gives you a good look at the various types of workout gear that make you the most comfortable. Then flip to the individual chapter in Part IV that discusses the activity (or activities) you're interested in pursuing.

Modifying your routine if you're an exercise pro

If you've been exercising and aren't sure what you can and can't continue during your pregnancy, take a hike over to Chapter 6 and read all about the ways that you'll need to change your workouts to keep your baby healthy. Chances are you can keep doing your current activity, but with some modification for the length of time you're working out, the pace at which you're exercising, and so on.

Also take a peek at Chapter 3, which discusses the basics of pregnancy workouts. If you're at all gung-ho about exercise and tend to dislike slowing down for any reason, you want to stay especially aware of the warning signs listed in Chapter 3 that let you know you or your baby may be stressed.

Working out throughout your trimesters

Throughout each of your three *trimesters* (roughly three-month time periods by which the length of your pregnancy is measured), your healthcare provider may ask you to modify your workouts in one or more of the five following ways, listed in order from most likely to least likely (see Chapter 3 for details).

- Move an activity from outdoors to indoors (for example, going from cycling outdoors to riding a stationary bike inside) to minimize the risk of falling; the effects of sun exposure, heat, humidity, or bitter cold weather; and the inhalation of traffic fumes.
- Change the activity you've been doing to one that offers less risk of falling or is a little easier on your body (for example, from skiing to walking).
- Reduce the *intensity* with which you're working out — that is, how hard you work out.
- Reduce the amount of time you're working out (the number of days per week and/or the number of minutes in each session).
- Stop working out completely and/or go on bed rest in the event of a medical problem.

In addition, each activity has its own guidelines for ways that you may want to modify your chosen activity as your pregnancy progresses through each of the three trimesters. The chapters in Part IV not only introduce you to each type of activity and explain the technique you want to use, but they also describe some common modifications that pregnant women make as they go through each trimester.

Turning Your Fit Pregnancy into Fit Motherhood

After you deliver your baby, you may feel overwhelmed by the responsibilities you face: taking care of your baby, eating right, sneaking in naps in order to get enough rest — plus taking time to work out. If you're not diligent, your workout routine may fall by the wayside as you struggle to keep up with your baby's needs, and as a result, you may lose some of the great fitness gains you've made. You can plan now, though, to not let that happen to you.

Although the subject of *postnatal fitness* (that is, the time after you deliver your baby) could be a book all its own, the chapters in Part V of this book help you find ways to keep fitness a priority in your life, even after your baby is born. In Chapter 18, you find out how to let your body heal from labor (or from a cesarean section) and do some gentle workouts in the days following your delivery. Chapter 19 gives you tips for squeezing fitness into your newly demanding lifestyle. And Chapter 20 shows you some techniques for keeping your kids fit and healthy — after all, with the loads of news reports on growing rates of childhood obesity, you want your kids to fall in love with fitness at a young age.

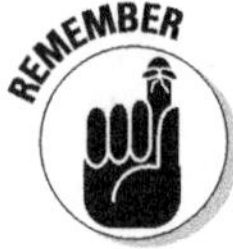

The power of exercise and healthy eating can't be underestimated. When you start exercising — even for just 15 or 20 minutes, 4 or 5 days per week — you soon begin to realize tremendous benefits, from having more energy to seeing muscle definition to protecting yourself from serious diseases.

Chapter 2

Recognizing the Benefits of a Fit Pregnancy

In This Chapter

- Recognizing physical changes throughout the next nine months
- Making labor a lot easier
- Giving your baby a great start
- Looking forward to life after pregnancy

In this chapter, you discover how staying fit during your pregnancy makes your entire 40-week marathon easier to manage, both physically and emotionally. From helping you sleep better to improving your mood to making labor easier, staying fit during your pregnancy brings you and your baby phenomenal benefits. You also find out how staying fit during your pregnancy helps you get back to your pre-pregnancy weight and size after your baby is born.

Coping with the Changes Your Body Is Experiencing

Your body undergoes dramatic changes during pregnancy, and these physical changes can make women downright uncomfortable for much of the 40-week duration. These changes range from how your heart and lungs operate to how you process the food you eat to how your muscles and joints change.

- **Weight gain:** During pregnancy, you need to gain weight regularly so that your baby grows properly and is well nourished. (Chapter 10 tells you how much weight most women gain and in which areas of the body.) Exercising while pregnant helps you gain a healthy amount of weight that tends to come off fairly easily after you deliver. See the "Getting back to your pre-pregnancy weight" section near the end of this chapter for more.

- **Change in posture; low-back discomfort:** As your abdomen increases in size and you gain the weight required to have a healthy baby (see Chapter 10), you'll likely see a shift in your posture (either a greater curve in the low back or a hunched-over appearance in the shoulders — both no-nos that your mother warned you about!). You may also experience some low-back pain as the curvature of your lower spine changes with the added weight of your baby and body fluids. Both of these changes can make workouts more uncomfortable as your pregnancy progresses, but exercise generally improves your posture and helps get rid of low-back pain (see the following section).
- **Shift in your center of gravity:** As your uterus pushes your abdomen up and out, your center of gravity may also change. Because you don't have a lot of time to get used to this shift, you may find that you can't balance as well as you used to be able to, which can result in falling down. This is why, as your pregnancy progresses, many healthcare providers urge you to stay away from activities that require excellent balance.
- **Joint instability:** During pregnancy, your body releases a hormone called *relaxin,* causing your joints to loosen slightly and allowing the joint in front of the pelvis to widen so that your baby's head can pass through that region during birth. Because your ligaments are quite loose, they don't "stop" as they normally do when you jump or lunge or trip over something small. Be cautious with activities that require quick movements or a lot of balance.
- **How much heat you generate:** Throughout your pregnancy, you're like a little furnace, generating far more heat — and, therefore, raising your body temperature faster — than you did before you were pregnant. Both you and your baby can suffer if you overheat, so you need to take extra care during these 40 weeks to stay away from situations that can raise your body temperature too high, like exercising outdoors in high heat or in a hot, unvented gym.
- **Fatigue:** Even if you're able to sleep well (and many pregnant women have trouble getting comfortable in bed during their second and third trimesters), the physical stress of your pregnancy can make you more fatigued. Exercise, however, helps with both nighttime sleep and daytime alertness.

One of the best ways to alleviate the discomfort of many of the changes your body is experiencing is to exercise. That's right: If you exercise during pregnancy, you'll spend nine months being far more comfortable than you would be if you didn't exercise.

Saluting a pregnancy fitness pioneer

Much of the current research on the benefits of fitness during pregnancy comes from fitness pregnancy guru Dr. James Clapp III, MD, who has been researching the effects of exercise on women and their babies since the 1970s. His research and writing led to a revolution in pregnancy fitness; chances are, you wouldn't be reading this book (or even toying with the notion of exercising during pregnancy) had Dr. Clapp not shown the world how beneficial fitness during pregnancy is to moms and babies alike. His groundbreaking book, *Exercising Through Your Pregnancy,* was recently rereleased by Addicus Books.

Easing back pain and soreness

Has your mother been telling you to stand up straight for most of your life? At last, you have a legitimate excuse for poor posture! During pregnancy, your growing baby changes your center of gravity, and muscles in your legs, hips, butt, back, and shoulders either lengthen or shorten because of this shift. Without exercise, these muscle changes can lead to poor posture, which, in turn, leads to back pain, stiffness, and soreness.

Exercising during pregnancy, however, helps get those muscles back into balance and improves your posture. And many types of exercise specifically strengthen your back and abdominal muscles (see Chapter 11).

Fine-tuning your circulatory system

Exercising during pregnancy increases the volume of blood your heart pumps with each beat, increasing the amount of oxygen and nutrients delivered to your baby. This increase in cardiovascular fitness also provides a safety margin for you and your baby by enabling your cardiovascular system to pump out adequate blood flow during times of physical stress.

This extra blood also means that you probably won't experience as many of those not-so-delightful physical changes that pregnancy often brings; you'll likely get fewer varicose veins, fewer leg cramps, and less swelling of your feet and ankles.

Helping you sleep better and giving you more energy

During pregnancy, many women tend to not sleep well at night and experience extreme fatigue during the day. Exercise, however, can lick these problems, making you sleep more soundly at night and feel refreshed throughout the day. It's true! If you lie awake at night or sleep fitfully, set up a regular fitness routine and you'll find yourself dozing faster and more soundly as your body recovers from the paces you're putting it through.

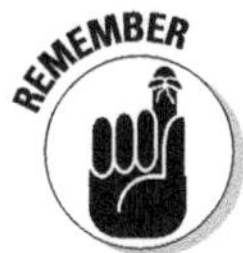

Essentially, exercise creates a system in which you're very alert throughout most of the day, and then you crash at night, sleeping like a log. As long as you exercise in the morning, afternoon, or early evening, you should feel sleepy at your bedtime. However, because of its power to make you alert, if you exercise three or fewer hours before your bedtime, you'll throw off your body clock and be alert at night and dead tired throughout the next day.

Developing muscle tone and flexibility

Exercise at any point in your life builds muscle tone, and if you stretch regularly (see Chapter 8), you'll also improve your flexibility.

If you currently watch your flabby arms wiggle when you brush your teeth, tend to hide your legs under sweat pants, and could barely touch your toes even when you weren't pregnant, exercise can change your life. Imagine being able to lift heavy objects without help and without hurting your back, wear sleeveless shirts and short shorts with pride, and snake yourself under couches and dressers to retrieve lost toys. A whole new world is waiting for you if you just add exercise to your daily routine.

The best news, though, is that you're not only improving your appearance, but you're also getting your body ready for some difficult tasks ahead: labor, delivery, and motherhood.

Weathering gestational diabetes

Gestational diabetes, a form of diabetes that appears during pregnancy and may increase your risk of developing Type II diabetes later in life, often leads to delivering a very large baby and increasing the risk of complications during labor and delivery. But here's the good news: Research shows that pregnant women experiencing gestational diabetes who exercise just three times per week lower their blood sugar.

Getting into a great mood

Have you heard of distance runners getting high on endorphins? That's not an illegal substance they're taking; rather, *endorphins* are natural, pain-relieving chemicals that the brain releases during physical activity, and not just during distance runs. Get on the exercise bandwagon, and you, too, can experience a daily dose of free, safe, mood-enhancing drugs sent throughout your body by your brain. You'll feel relaxed and calm instead of tense and stressed.

Exercise also helps you work through whatever's bothering you. Many women find that by using their 20- to 60-minute workouts to sort out the problems of the day, they tend to get less upset about minor frustrations.

Controlling weight gain

A study by Dr. Clapp showed that women who regularly exercised to the end of their pregnancies gained nearly eight pounds less than nonexercising pregnant women, yet were still well within the normal weight gain limits for a healthy pregnancy.

Preparing Your Body for Labor and Delivery

Anyone who tells you that childbirth is a breeze isn't being very honest with you. Childbirth is hard, and you don't want to approach it without being physically ready. One of the best ways to get yourself ready is by exercising during your pregnancy.

Having a less complicated delivery

Several research studies have shown that women who exercise have fewer complications during delivery, including fewer instances of fetal intervention because of abnormal fetal heart rates, *forceps deliveries* (in which a large tonglike tool helps the baby come out), and *cesarean sections* (in which the baby is surgically removed from the uterus).

Women who exercise during pregnancy also tend to need fewer drugs for pain relief.

Spending less time in labor

As you see in Figure 2-1, a study by Dr. Clapp (a physician who's an expert in pregnancy fitness — see the sidebar, "Saluting a pregnancy fitness pioneer") showed that labor is significantly shorter (by about one-third) for women who exercise regularly during pregnancy than for a control group made up of physically active women who didn't continue exercising during pregnancy.

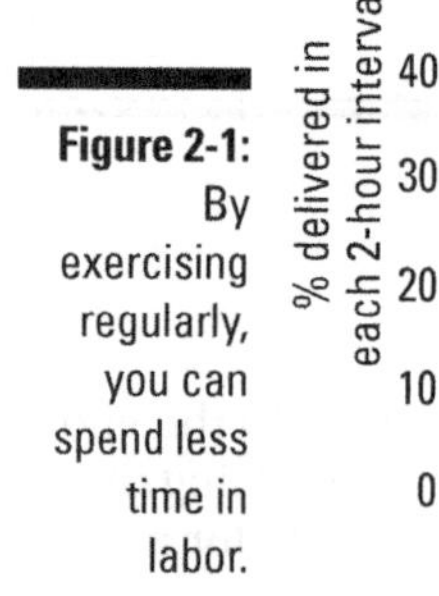

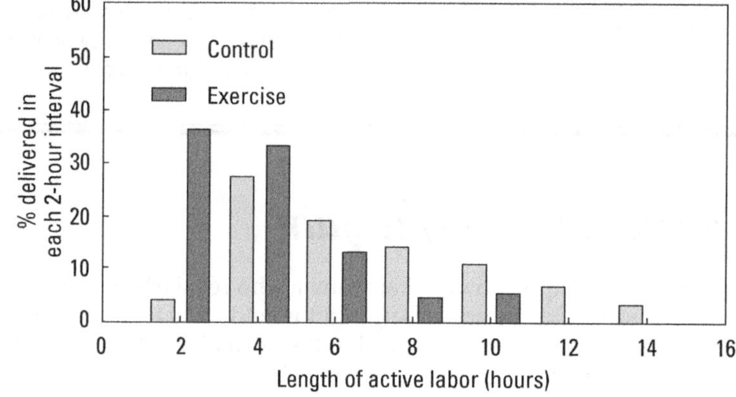

Figure 2-1: By exercising regularly, you can spend less time in labor.

Also, babies of women who exercise regularly throughout pregnancy are born about five days earlier than those of women who don't exercise, making pregnancy that much shorter (and five days is a really big deal when you're in your third trimester).

Passing the Benefits to Your Baby

You're not the only one who benefits from your fit pregnancy — your baby gets in on the action, too! Women who exercise during pregnancy see the following benefits in their babies.

A better-functioning placenta

Okay, so your baby may not thank you for producing a better-functioning placenta the way he would thank you for, say, a car when he turns 16, but a better-functioning placenta is actually better for your baby than any hot rod will ever be!

Can exercise produce a smarter baby?

Recent research published in the *American Journal of Obstetrics and Gynecology* shows a link between women who exercise during pregnancy and babies who are alert and score better on intelligence and coordination tests than babies born to mothers who don't exercise. Although this is good news, keep in mind that other factors could account for this increased intelligence — for example, if women who exercise tend to be better educated than nonexercising women (and studies have shown this to be true), the increase in education, not the exercise, could be the reason for the smarter baby.

Still, this link has been established by the medical community, so if you're exercising, you may want to start a Harvard University college savings account the day your baby is born.

The *placenta* is an organ that develops inside your uterus during your pregnancy. Throughout your pregnancy, the placenta provides the transport of nutrients, oxygen, and waste products between your baby's and your blood supply via his umbilical cord. The better the blood flow to and from the placenta, the healthier the baby. A study by Dr. Clapp (see the sidebar, "Saluting a pregnancy fitness pioneer") has shown that regular exercise during pregnancy leads to a placenta that grows about 30 percent faster in mid-pregnancy and has about 15 percent more blood vessels and surface area at the end of pregnancy. This effect on the placenta may have an added benefit of providing a safety margin for the fetus in times of stress-caused decreases in uterine blood flow.

A leaner child

Dr. Clapp discovered that when women exercise regularly (three to five times per week) during pregnancy, their babies are born with less fat. And though babies of exercisers are leaner, they're not born with low birth weight; in fact, they're well within normal limits — the same size range as babies born to mothers who didn't exercise, in terms of weight, limb lengths, and head and chest circumferences. They're just leaner.

And this leanness continues. Dr. Clapp's studies discovered that by age 5, children of women who exercise while pregnant are still leaner than children born to women who didn't exercise during pregnancy. What a great way to help your baby start her life as a healthy person!

Bouncing Back after Your Baby Is Born

Studies show that women who exercise during pregnancy have a much easier time returning to their pre-pregnancy weight and size than women who don't exercise while pregnant. In addition, having a fit pregnancy also gets you up and around faster after you deliver and helps you not crumple while carrying your ever-growing baby in your arms.

Recovering quickly

Babies don't give you much time to recover from your pregnancy. They have needs, and they want those needs met *now!* In order to do a bang-up job as a new mother, you need to be up and out of bed as quickly as possible, and exercising through your pregnancy is just the way to do that. Not only do women who exercise throughout pregnancy have shorter labors and deliveries, but they also get back to their lives faster than women who haven't exercised.

Getting back to your pre-pregnancy weight

Exercising during pregnancy helps you control the amount of weight you gain to a healthy level. (See Chapter 10 for more on this topic.) Research also shows that women who become or stay fit during pregnancy have less weight to lose after they deliver, and those women find that the weight they do gain comes off more easily and quickly than it does for their nonexercising counterparts. And given that an inability to lose weight is one of the top two complaints of new mothers (the other is lack of sleep), this is welcome news.

Carrying your baby

Have you ever lifted a ten-pound sack of potatoes off the display at the supermarket and were barely able to carry it over to your cart? Your baby's going to weigh almost as much as that sack of potatoes at birth and will quickly exceed that weight as he grows. Exercising now gives you time to strengthen your arms, back, hips, and legs so that you can lug Junior around with ease. (See Chapter 18 for quick advice on carrying your baby.)

Chapter 3

Designing a Safe Prenatal Fitness Program

In This Chapter

- Making your healthcare provider a partner in exercise
- Recognizing the four components of exercise
- Keeping close tabs on your body
- Modifying your routine throughout each trimester
- Knowing when to take a break and when exercise is off-limits

Think of this chapter as the fine print — all the information that you need to know but that exuberant friends, trainers, and fitness book authors may have glossed over. This chapter helps you get your healthcare provider on board with your *prenatal* (another word for pregnancy) fitness goals so that you don't ever put your baby at risk. It also tells you how to continuously monitor — and modify — your and your baby's responses to your exercise routine. You discover some key signals that indicate you should call or visit your physician immediately, and you even find a few exercises that you can do if you're prescribed the dreaded bed rest. Safety may not be the most exciting topic you'll ever read about, but this chapter is jampacked with tips and advice.

Consulting Your Healthcare Provider

Here's the bottom line on your healthcare provider's role in your pregnancy fitness goals: Always consult with him or her before starting an exercise program. Discuss your goals and the type of activity you plan to do, making sure it's safe for you to get started.

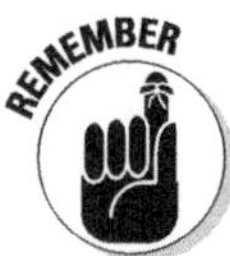

You're reading this book because you want to get fit and/or stay fit while you're pregnant, improving your health and that of your baby (see Chapter 2 for a listing of the benefits of a fit pregnancy). However, your number-one goal for your pregnancy is to deliver a healthy child — that has to take precedence over your fitness goals. If your healthcare provider feels that your exercise routine will put your baby at risk, don't push it. In nine months, you can pick up your fitness regimen and work out wholeheartedly, knowing that you have a healthy baby at home.

Recently, the American College of Obstetricians and Gynecologists (ACOG) revised its guidelines for exercising during pregnancy and after delivery, and that advice serves as the basis for this and every other book on fit pregnancy. Go to `www.acog.com` for info on ordering these guidelines. In addition, ACOG issued a set of *contraindications* (medical conditions and complications) and put them into two categories:

- **Relative contraindications:** These conditions *may* indicate that something's amiss and may mean that you shouldn't start or continue your exercise program. We discuss these contraindications in the "Knowing How Much May Be Too Much" section later in this chapter. That section also includes some potential warning signs that you want to watch for as you exercise. Warning signs are different from contraindications in that warning signs aren't diseases or serious pregnancy complications; they're simply some signs and symptoms that may indicate a problem is developing and that you should stop exercising and check with your healthcare provider.

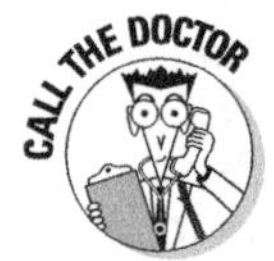

  Keep the relative contraindications in mind whenever you exercise, and if you ever experience any of them, stop exercising and call your healthcare provider right away. Together, you and your healthcare provider can decide whether continuing to exercise is appropriate for you.

- **Absolute contraindications:** We list these contraindications in the "Understanding Conditions That Make Exercise Off-Limits" section at the end of this chapter. If you began your pregnancy with any of these conditions or if they develop during your pregnancy, your healthcare provider will very likely tell you that exercise isn't an option during your pregnancy. And if you are cleared to exercise but begin to develop any of the absolute contraindications, call or visit your healthcare provider as soon as possible.

Healthcare providers who may not have been exposed to patients wanting to exercise while pregnant may feel uncomfortable with the idea of your exercising during pregnancy. If this is the case, show him or her the contraindications and warning signs listed in this chapter and be frank with your healthcare provider about your desire to exercise, letting him or her know about the many benefits of a fit pregnancy. Discuss your exercise program and explain that you'll stop exercising and call immediately if you develop any of the warning signs listed in this chapter if you don't feel terrific or if your baby isn't growing properly.

Review with your healthcare provider the warning signs in the "Knowing How Much May Be Too Much" section later in this chapter, and talk about any other symptoms you may be experiencing (even if they aren't on that list). And if, for whatever reason, you're asked to refrain from exercising or are put on bed rest, ask your healthcare provider whether the very low-key exercises listed at the end of Chapter 4 can work for you, or see whether you can work with a physical therapist who specializes in women's health.

Developing an Exercise Plan

Exercise has four main components, which we discuss in the following four sections. By putting these four components (intensity, duration, frequency, and type) together, you build strength, cardiovascular fitness, and flexibility without injuring yourself or being uncomfortable. All four pieces of the exercise puzzle fit together, though, so you need to think of each as you and your healthcare provider develop a workout plan.

Intensity

The *intensity* of your workout is the effort you put forth as you exercise — hard, moderate, or easy. With some sports, you measure your intensity in miles per hour, revolutions per minute, per-lap time when swimming, and so on so that you know empirically whether you're working harder or easier than the day before. In other sports, you can't measure intensity directly.

Regardless of what the speedometer is telling you, the important measure of intensity is how hard you *think* you're working out, based on how you feel (for example, saying, "Whew, that workout was hard" versus "Today's workout felt easy"). A specific tool, called the Borg Rating of Perceived Exertion (RPE) Scale, lets you assign a number to your response, like this:

6	No effort at all
7	Very, very light
8	
9	Very light
10	
11	Fairly light
12	

13	Somewhat hard
14	
15	Hard
16	
17	Very hard
18	
19	Very, very hard
20	Maximum effort

Borg RPE scale © Gunnar Borg, 1970, 1985, 1994, 1998

Yeah, we know that the scale should start with 1 and not with 6, but we won't argue with the scientist who invented the scale!

You want to feel challenged and slightly winded while exercising, so keep your workouts in the 12 to 14 range. And here's the important point to remember: A rating of 12 on the RPE Scale won't always correlate with the same mile-per-hour rate as you progress through your pregnancy. In other words, one day, you may give a "12" rating when you're walking at a pace of 16 minutes per mile. On another day, later in your pregnancy or as a result of not sleeping well or general fatigue, you may give the same "12" rating when walking at a pace of 20 minutes per mile. Even though you're walking slower, you may feel that the two efforts are equally hard. And that's what's important — how the workout feels to you, not what the clock or speedometer says.

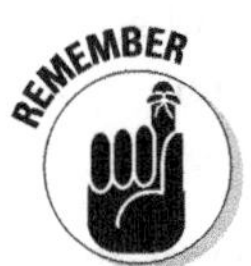

Old wisdom was that your heart rate shouldn't exceed 140 beats per minute while you're pregnant, but because everyone's response to exercise is different, it isn't a good method to determine whether you're overdoing your workouts. That 140-beat-per-minute rate may be way too high for you if your resting pulse rate is quite low, if you're fatigued, or if you're in the last weeks of pregnancy; on the other hand, that rate or an even higher one may not indicate that your workout is unduly intense. Instead of using heart rate, use the RPE Scale, keeping all your workouts between 12 and 14 or at a level that feels moderate to somewhat hard (you can talk while exercising without feeling exceedingly short of breath).

Duration

Duration refers to the amount of time you spend exercising each day. When you're exercising at a 12 to 14 on the RPE Scale (see the preceding section) and you don't feel any discomfort or fatigue, you can begin to gradually increase the duration of each workout from 15 or 20 minutes up to 30 minutes or more.

Duration and intensity are super-glued together: You may be able to exercise without discomfort or fatigue for 45 minutes at a level of 12 on the RPE Scale, but for only 30 minutes when you're exerting yourself at a level of 14. If, during a workout, you have trouble exercising for a longer duration, scale back your intensity from a 14 to a 12. If you still experience fatigue or discomfort at 12, reduce the duration by 5 or 10 minutes.

Frequency

Frequency refers to how often you work out; that is, how many days per week. Most experts agree that exercising for 3 to 6 days per week at a duration of 30 to 60 minutes per workout keeps you in good shape. How many days per week you can comfortably exercise depends on the following:

- **How fit you are right now:** The fitter you are, the more days per week you can work out without experiencing discomfort or fatigue.
- **How your pregnancy is progressing:** Is your baby growing normally? Are you gaining weight normally? Do you feel good? If you answer no to any of those three questions, cut back on the number of days you're working out each week.

  "Feeling good" means not feeling any of the following:

  - Lack of motivation
  - Extreme fatigue
  - Weight loss or failure to gain weight
- **The intensity and duration of your workouts:** If you're working out at a 14 on the RPE Scale for 45 to 60 minutes, you may find that 3 or 4 days per week is a more comfortable frequency than 5 or 6 days per week. And vice versa.

You need one day off per week while you're pregnant, even if you're convinced that you can work out seven days per week. You can, however, stretch your muscles seven days per week — see Chapter 8. And if one of your days is only a strength-training day, seven days is okay. But doing cardiovascular workouts all seven days will cause you to experience too much fatigue. Enjoy that day and the extra time you have as a result of not working out, and you'll be better prepared for the days that you do work out.

Type

The *type* of exercise refers to what activity you choose as your workout. Chapter 4 helps you pin down the activities that tend to work best during pregnancy, and if you're new to exercise, Chapter 5 asks you some questions that may help you decide what sort of exercise routine you're looking for. Ultimately, you want to choose activities that meet the following criteria:

- You enjoy the activity.
- The activity doesn't put your baby at risk (see Chapter 4).
- You can still do the activity as your center of gravity changes throughout your pregnancy (that is, you can still balance well enough to do the activity).
- The activity makes sense as one to do during pregnancy.

If you're doing an activity that you can't easily modify, or if your RPE Scale rating is more than 14 and modifying the duration and frequency doesn't lower the intensity, consider changing to a different type of activity. Part IV gives you the lowdown on a number of activities that many women find comfortable throughout their pregnancies.

Monitoring Your Body

The key to safeguarding your and your baby's health is to monitor your body while you're working out and throughout the rest of your day. This is the time to notice details about your body and to keep tabs on how you feel. Along with your healthcare provider, you need to closely monitor telltale signs:

- Whether your baby is growing normally
- Whether you're gaining weight normally
- Overall, whether you feel good (you have energy and would tell others that you feel "good") or bad (you're tired all the time, seem to be getting sick pretty often, and so on).

Make sure that your healthcare provider is on board with your exercise program. He or she shouldn't have any concerns about you continuing to exercise throughout your pregnancy.

If your baby is growing as scheduled, you're also gaining weight normally, and you feel great, you can continue your workout routine. If any of the preceding three signs are negative, you need to modify your routine until you're feeling good, gaining weight, and helping your baby gain weight again.

In addition, try to stay aware of other body signs, including being aware of pain or discomfort, your weight after a workout, the amount you're sleeping, and the color of your urine. Here are specific tips on what to watch and measure:

- **Hot bod:** When you're pregnant, you produce more heat, so you need to closely monitor whether you're overheating. You can avoid overheating by working out indoors (in an air-conditioned area) during times of high heat and humidity and by staying well hydrated all day long (see

Chapter 9 for tips on taking fluids). If you become lightheaded, feel faint or nauseated, sweat more than usual, or feel uncomfortably hot, stop exercising, hydrate, and rest until you feel better.

- **Finger on the pulse:** Although measuring your heart rate is no longer considered an adequate measure of how intensive your workout is, checking your heart rate is an effective way to determine how rested you are and how your body is handling pregnancy overall. Check your heart rate every morning, before you get out of bed (but not directly after your alarm goes off, when your heart may be racing). Take your pulse on your wrist or on your neck (just below your ears) for one full minute. Jot down a daily record of your pulse, and if you find that one morning it's significantly higher (for example, you go from 70 beats per minute to 90), your body may be fatigued, you may be getting sick, or you may be training too much. Whenever your morning resting pulse is elevated, consider taking that day off from your workout routine.

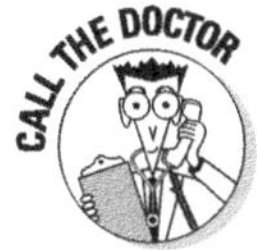

- **No pain:** Although you may feel some initial soreness when you begin an exercise program or increase the duration or intensity of your workouts, you shouldn't feel pain as a result of exercising. The "Knowing How Much May Be Too Much" section later in this chapter explains some common types of pain that may indicate you're overdoing your exercise program. But the general rule is this: If exercise hurts, stop your workouts and call your healthcare provider.
- **Talk time:** Pregnancy isn't the time to exercise to or past the point of exhaustion. You should always be able to carry on a conversation while exercising; if you can't, you need to reduce the intensity or duration of your workout.
- **Toilet test:** If you aren't getting enough fluids, you can get dehydrated, which is bad for you and your baby. If you've never looked at the color of your urine before, try not to get too grossed out by the thought of it — the color of your urine is an excellent indicator of whether you're drinking enough fluids. After you urinate (and before you flush), look into the toilet bowl at the color of the water in the bowl:
    - If your urine is light yellow or nearly clear, you're drinking just the right amount.
    - If the color is orange, dark yellow, or a medium yellow, you need to drink more fluids (see Chapter 9), and you may want to curtail your exercise routine until the color lightens.

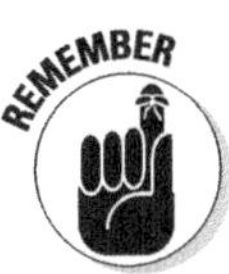

Your urine will usually be medium to dark yellow first thing in the morning, because you've gone eight hours without drinking any fluids. Don't use early-morning urine as a gauge for whether you're getting dehydrated; instead, monitor your urine throughout the rest of the day. Also, some prenatal vitamins can turn urine yellow, so if you're taking prenatal vitamins, ask your healthcare provider whether watching your urine is a good indicator for you.

- **Too tired:** You're bound to feel a little tired as you're exercising, but how do you feel the rest of the day? Do you feel overly tired, fatigued, or downright exhausted? If so, you need to pull back — take a day or more off, reduce the total time you're exercising each week, and/or reduce the intensity of the workout (see the "Intensity" section earlier in this chapter).
- **Weigh better:** Another way to get dehydrated is to work out too intensely during pregnancy or to exercise at a time that's too hot. A great way to determine whether you're losing too much fluid during exercise is to weigh yourself before and after your workout to determine how much sweat you've lost. Be sure to weigh yourself naked both times, and after exercise, drink fluids until you're back up to your pre-workout weight. Weigh yourself after you've fully rehydrated. If you find that you're losing any weight after exercising and drinking as much fluid as you can, modify your workouts by reducing the intensity and/or the duration of each workout and increase your fluid intake. (If you're a beginner to exercise, you probably don't have to worry about the intensity of workouts, but competitive athletes who become pregnant and continue to exercise sometimes have trouble lowering the intensity and duration of their workouts. Check out Chapter 6.)

In addition to weighing yourself before and after exercise, make sure that you're gaining enough weight to support a healthy baby. All pregnant women need to eat about 300 extra calories per day to support their babies, but exercising women need even more to gain enough weight. See Chapter 9 for more information about nutrition for active pregnant women and check out the Cheat Sheet at the front of this book for easy ways to get extra calories. If you're concerned about gaining too much weight during your pregnancy, see Chapter 10.

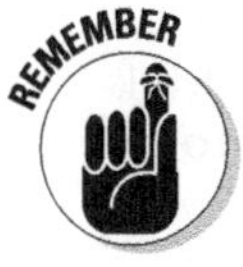

When monitoring your health throughout your fit pregnancy, keep in mind that if your exercise routine feels good to you, you're probably doing everything right. If the routine feels too intense or your body's not responding well after you finish exercising for the day, you need to reduce the intensity and/or duration of your workouts or take a short-term break from exercising. Whenever something just doesn't feel right, contact your healthcare provider for advice.

Protecting yourself from the sun

If you're planning to exercise outdoors, take the following precautions to keep yourself from overheating, becoming dehydrated, or developing skin cancer down the road.

- **Avoid working out between 10 a.m. and 3 p.m.** Don't work out during the hottest hours of summer days, which in most areas are between 10 a.m. and 3 p.m. Instead, schedule your workouts for early in the morning or move your workouts indoors to an air-conditioned or otherwise well-ventilated, cool area. (Don't work out late at night, or you may disrupt your sleep.)

- **Purchase athletic sunglasses.** When you're exercising in the sun, splurge on some athletic sunglasses at your local sporting goods store. Sunglasses meant for running and cycling are usually just barely larger than your eye sockets and sit tightly on your face so they don't jiggle when you're exercising. Those meant for winter sports, such as skiing and snowboarding, tend to be larger and looser, covering more of your face, but also moving around a bit, especially as you sweat. Don't worry too much about what kind of sport the sunglasses are labeled for; just try them all and see what's most comfortable for you.
- **Wear a baseball cap or a wide-brimmed hat.** A $9 baseball cap can save you hundreds of dollars in doctor visits and wrinkle cream. The lowly cap cools you by protecting your head from sunshine, keeps the sun out of your eyes, and captures some sweat so that it doesn't pour down your face. You have a dizzying array of styles to choose from — mesh tops or cloth, adjustable or sized to your head, large brim or small — in dozens of colors and with thousands of logos. You probably have a baseball cap around the house that you can use; if not, stop by your local sporting goods store or athletic outlet store (the Nike Outlet Stores often sell their hats for $7.50 or less) and try a few on.
- **Apply sunscreen.** Before heading out the door, slather on a sunscreen with SPF 15 or higher, preferably one that says it's meant for exercise (which means that it stays on relatively well even as you sweat). Although sunscreen doesn't protect against overheating or dehydration, it's one of the best preventive measures against skin cancer (and premature wrinkling, too). Sunscreen also helps prevent the *mask of pregnancy,* a dark pigmentation on the face that can develop during pregnancy. Flip on ahead to Chapter 7 for information on sun-protective clothing.

Modifying, Modifying, Modifying Your Routine

During pregnancy, you need to modify your exercise routine whenever something isn't quite right. *Modifying* means fine-tuning your exercise program to keep it safe and effective. Your baby's health is your most important priority right now, and if modifying your exercise regimen ensures a safe, healthy baby, that's the only healthy course of action to take. No matter how much you want to continue your current routine, you shouldn't do anything that compromises your baby's health.

You may need to modify your routine monthly, weekly, or even daily according to your body's response to both your pregnancy and your exercise routine. Whatever modifications you need to make are unique to you, your chosen form(s) of exercise, and how you're faring in your pregnancy. However, pregnant women generally make certain modifications throughout each trimester, as the following sections discuss.

First trimester (weeks 1–13)

During the first trimester, you want to continue whatever physical activities you've been doing. If you're new to exercise (see Chapter 5), get into exercise very gently. Either way, consider the following potential modifications and tips during this trimester:

- If your breasts are sore, you experience morning sickness (or nausea/vomiting any time of day), or if you're experiencing extreme fatigue, cut back on your routine or forgo exercise until you feel better.
- The first trimester is a good time to start abdominal and pelvic floor exercises — see Chapter 11 for these core exercises. After 12 weeks, you want to avoid any curl-up exercises that you do while lying on the floor, although pelvic floor exercises can continue throughout your pregnancy.
- If you were exercising before you got pregnant, you can probably wear your sports bras throughout much of the first trimester. You may find, however, that at the end of this trimester, you need a larger size. If you haven't yet invested in a good sports bra, go to a sporting goods store, running store, or fitness store and try on several until you find one that's comfortable. Don't buy too many: You'll quickly outgrow them, and because sports bras are made of fast-drying material, you can quickly wash one or two out, as needed, and wear them over and over.

Second trimester (weeks 14–26)

During the second trimester, you may feel better than at any other time during your pregnancy. (If you don't, that's okay, too.) Continue to monitor your body's reaction to exercise, and if you feel good enough to do so, consider increasing the duration or intensity of your workouts. Also keep the following potential modifications and other tips in mind:

- Sometime during this trimester, you want to shop for a new sports bra, because your existing one is probably getting too tight.
- If you feel unbalanced during these weeks, consider discontinuing any activity that can throw you off balance, like gymnastics, tennis, downhill skiing, skating, horseback riding, trail biking, and hiking in the woods over rutty trails. Replace with swimming, water aerobics, or a stationary bike, which don't require excellent balance.

- Because your baby is growing and becoming more vulnerable if you fall or are hit in the abdomen, during this trimester, your healthcare provider may ask you to stop ball sports (soccer, basketball, racquetball, and so on), contact sports, and outdoor biking. (Note that because of your expanding abdomen, you may find a recumbent bike more comfortable than a traditional stationary bike — see Chapter 15).

  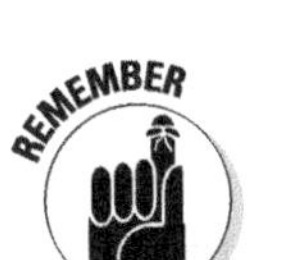

  Outdoor cycling while you're pregnant exposes you and your baby to unwanted exhaust and other fumes as you ride the roads, so if you and your healthcare provider decide that you're able to cycle outdoors, choose low-traffic areas.

- If you're doing step aerobics, make sure that your step is no higher than four inches off the ground, unless you feel absolutely stable and balanced with a higher step.
- If you're rowing, you may find that this super-intense sport is too fatiguing for the rest of your pregnancy. Pay careful attention to how you're feeling and how well you and your baby are gaining weight.
- If you're weightlifting, don't overwork your thigh muscles, because machines that work the thighs also tend to place stress on the ligaments around the pelvis and cause discomfort.
- After the fourth month, avoid lying on your back for long periods, or you run the risk of feeling faint from the pressure your uterus puts on the *vena cava* (the large vein that sends blood from your lower body to your heart). If you feel faint while on your back, roll over on your side to reestablish blood flow. Check out *Pregnancy For Dummies,* 2nd Edition, by Joanne Stone, MD, Keith Eddleman, MD, and Mary Murray (Wiley) to find out how this affects your sleeping habits.
- If you're doing yoga, now's the time to stop doing back bends, any moves that have you lying on your stomach or back, jumps, and inverted poses. (See Chapter 14 for details.)
- Many healthcare providers also recommend that you stop competing in sports events during the second trimester, although this depends on your sport and how you're feeling. If you're in your second trimester and want to continue participating in a competitive sport, ask your healthcare provider for advice.
- Be careful during this trimester (and the next and for about five months after you deliver) not to overstretch or make sudden moves. While you're pregnant, a hormone called *relaxin* gets you ready for childbirth by relaxing all your ligaments and joints. This means that you may be at risk of injuring yourself, because your joints and ligaments won't stop you from overextending yourself as well as they did when you weren't pregnant.
- Check your abdominal separation (diastasis recti) by using the technique described in the "Diastasis recti measurement technique" sidebar.

Diastasis recti measurement technique

The abdominal muscles consist of three muscle groups (*rectus abdominus, transverse,* and *obliques*) that all provide support for the spine and pelvic organs. During pregnancy, hormones cause the fibrous band that attaches the rectus abdominus (or *recti*) muscles to thin and widen the distance between the muscles. This separation is called *diastasis recti,* and although it's a normal process of pregnancy, in some women, the separation can become quite wide and reduce the function of the recti muscles and the support they provide to the low back. You can monitor the width of your muscle separation with this simple technique.

1. **Lie on your back with your knees bent and your feet resting on the floor.**
2. **Take a deep breath and as you exhale, raise your head and neck up until you feel your tummy contract.**

   Do this test quickly and don't remain in the head-raised position for more than ten seconds at a time. You may have to avoid this measurement technique if you become lightheaded while lying on your back.
3. **Place the fingers of one hand down horizontally into your abdomen at the point of your belly button.**

   The back of your hand should be facing your legs. After your fingers are positioned correctly, feel for the two hard sides of your recti muscles and the soft area in the middle. The soft area between the two muscles is the separation, or *diastasis.*

A normal separation is approximately 2½ finger widths or less. If your width measures larger than that, use even more care when standing, lifting, and carrying objects, because your abdominal muscles may not be able to provide proper support for your low back. If your muscle separation is greater than 2½ finger widths, you may benefit from a physical therapy evaluation, especially if the separation doesn't return to normal within three months after you deliver your baby.

Rising up from a lying position, sneezing, coughing, bearing down, and holding your breath can cause outward pressure on your abdominal wall that stresses the weakened area. Apply the lifting and body mechanic techniques covered in Chapter 18 whenever rising from a lying position or lifting objects.

If you notice an increase in back pain, contact your healthcare provider. He or she may be able to provide abdominal bands that help provide support for your low back. To keep your abdominal muscles strong without adding stress to your diastasis and low back the way traditional sit-ups can, try the core strengthening exercises in Chapter 11.

Third trimester (weeks 27–40)

In the third trimester, depending on how you feel, you may need to switch to low-impact activities, such as walking, swimming, and indoor cycling (see Part IV). In fact, some women are so fatigued and have so much difficulty moving around that they aren't able to exercise at all during the third trimester, but if you can, keep it up: Studies show that women who exercise during the third trimester achieve the greatest benefits from that exercise: reduced fat gain, shorter and less complicated labor and delivery, and shorter recovery after delivery from exercise.

As you go through your third trimester, keep the following potential modifications and tips in mind:

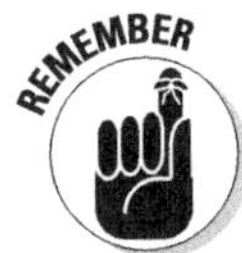

- Keep doing your pelvic floor exercises (discussed in Chapter 11), even if you're not able to do anything else. As you're getting up from the floor, move slowly and carefully to avoid injury.
- As with the second trimester, avoid overstretching. And if you haven't already discontinued outdoor cycling, now is definitely the time to begin cycling indoors.
- In addition to needing a new sports bra, you may need a support belt or belly brace (see Chapter 7). If you've been running, you may decide to stop that activity and walk, instead (see Chapter 12). If you've been doing aerobics, avoid jumps in the last trimester (visit Chapter 14). If you've been cycling indoors on a traditional indoor bike and didn't switch to a recumbent bike in the second trimester, you may need to do so now (see Chapter 15).

Knowing How Much May Be Too Much

In a perfect world, if you were exercising too much or doing anything that could harm you or your baby, a neon sign would begin flashing above your head, alerting you and the world to the dangers before you.

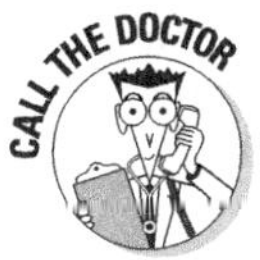

Short of a system like that, the best we can offer is a list of symptoms that *may* mean something's wrong. Only your healthcare provider can determine whether exercise is causing these symptoms and whether the symptoms are anything to worry about. If you experience any of the following, however, stop exercising and call your healthcare provider immediately:

- **Contractions:** Contractions are a positive sign only if you're within a week or two of your due date. Otherwise, contractions may indicate premature labor.
- **Dizziness:** This can be a sign of *anemia* (low red-blood-cell count that results in weakness and fatigue) or other conditions.
- **Shortness of breath not during exercise:** Shortness of breath is normal during exercise but may signal a problem if you experience it when not working out.
- **Headache:** Although many pregnant women report an increase in headaches during their pregnancies (often brought on by fatigue and stress), if you experience a severe headache or a less severe one that doesn't seem to go away, contact your healthcare provider. Headaches can be an early sign of *preeclampsia* (pregnancy-induced high blood pressure).

- **Increased swelling in your legs:** This can be a sign of preeclampsia, which is characterized by high blood pressure and fluid retention in the extremities. It can also indicate *deep-vein thrombosis,* a blood clot that develops in a vein.
- **Muscle weakness:** Muscle weakness can take a couple of different forms: total-body weakness (in which you feel weak all over) or specific muscle weakness (such as your right arm or left side of your body).
- **Vaginal bleeding and/or leaking of amniotic fluid:** Leaking blood or other fluids can be the result of several complications, including *placenta previa* (in which the *placenta,* the organ that grows in your uterus to provide nutrients for the fetus and eliminate its waste, blocks all or part of the cervix), *placenta abruption* (separation of the placenta from the uterus before delivering your baby), premature labor, and miscarriage.
- **You can't feel your baby moving:** If your baby's normal movements (that you usually begin feeling between the 18th and 22nd weeks) have diminished or stopped, your baby may be experiencing problems. Keep in mind, however, that your baby will probably be calm during exercise, but you should start to feel several movements again within 20 to 30 minutes after you stop.

Review this list with your healthcare provider, and ask him or her about any other symptoms you should watch for, based on your own medical history and circumstances.

If you're asked to reduce or completely cut out exercise as a result of one or more of these symptoms, keep in mind that this period of rest may be temporary. Ask your healthcare provider to reevaluate your condition at each prenatal visit and see whether you and your baby are now in a safe condition and can return to some level of exercise.

In addition, the following physical conditions may mean that you won't be able to successfully work out while pregnant. If you've experienced any of the following contraindications, take extra time with your healthcare provider to ensure that exercising during pregnancy is right for you:

- Irregular beating of your heart that hasn't been explained
- *Intrauterine growth retardation* (IUGR), which means that your baby isn't measuring up to what is normal for her gestational age
- History of a sedentary (nonactive) lifestyle
- Orthopedic (bone, muscle, joint, ligament) limitations that exercise may worsen
- History of heavy smoking
- Extremely overweight
- Extremely underweight

- Severe anemia
- Chronic bronchitis
- Type 1 diabetes that isn't well controlled
- *Hypertension* (high blood pressure) that isn't well controlled
- *Hyperthyroidism* (overactive thyroid) that isn't well controlled
- Seizure disorder that isn't well controlled

Note that these conditions are based on the ACOG guidelines, but they're reworded here to make them a bit easier for a nonmedical person to understand.

Understanding Conditions That Make Exercise Off-Limits

A few medical conditions usually — although not always — make exercising during pregnancy an unwise choice. Your healthcare provider is the only one who can verify what conditions make pregnancy workouts off-limits for you, and many physicians ask their patients not to exercise during pregnancy if they're diagnosed with or have a history of any of the following.

- Carrying multiple babies that may be delivered early
- Heart disease that restricts activity
- Incompetent cervix (the cervix dilates prematurely)
- Lung disease that restricts activity
- Persistent vaginal bleeding in the second or third trimesters
- *Placenta previa* (when the placenta partially or completely covers the cervix) after 26 weeks
- Pregnancy-induced hypertension (high blood pressure along with edema and increased urine in protein)
- Premature labor during this pregnancy
- Ruptured amniotic membranes

Chapter 4

Knowing Which Activities Are Best (And Which to Avoid)

In This Chapter

- Examining activities that work for most pregnant women
- Discussing activities that may work for you, depending on your circumstances
- Touching on two out-of-the-question activities
- Considering limited activities even when on bed rest

If you've mentioned to friends and family that you want to start or continue exercising throughout your pregnancy, you've probably already heard a laundry list of what activities you shouldn't do. Although some of that information may be accurate, some may also be old wives' tales. This chapter helps you understand which sports and other activities are well suited to pregnancy and which you want to avoid.

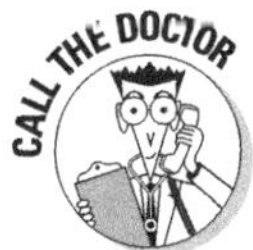

Before beginning any exercise program, talk to your healthcare provider about your plans to make sure that the activities you plan to do are safe for you and your baby. Chapter 3 gives you additional details about having this conversation with your healthcare provider.

Discovering the Best Ways to Stay Fit While Pregnant

Staying fit during pregnancy has never been easier or more fun! Whether you decide to keep your workout indoors or enjoy nature, join a gym or pool or work out at home, take a class or exercise on your own, go with basic clothing and equipment or outfit yourself with the latest and greatest stuff — and whether you're new to working out or are an old pro — you can stay fit throughout your pregnancy in a way that fits your lifestyle and interests.

This section introduces you to the activities that women often find most comfortable and effective during pregnancy. See Chapters 11 through 17 for more detailed information on these activities, along with tips on how to get started and use the best technique.

If you've never exercised before, check out Chapter 5, which helps you get started. That chapter also helps you think about your own interests and personality when choosing an activity.

Using exercise balls, resistance bands, and low-weight bars or hand weights

An excellent way to increase strength and flexibility is to work out with the following, all of which we discuss in Chapter 11:

- **Exercise balls:** You've probably seen these in advertisements or in fitness magazines — they're large balls that you sit on, lie on, or lean against in order to do a variety of exercises. Some are perfectly round, which means that part of the exercise you're doing comes from keeping yourself from rolling off (thereby making the workouts even more challenging); others sit on a flat base, which many pregnant women prefer. As your abdomen grows and your center of gravity changes, staying on a rolling object can seem less and less possible!
- **Resistance bands:** Resistance bands are like extraordinarily large rubber bands, although they usually have special plastic or rubber handles that help you control them. Just as you can hold a rubber band taut and it becomes harder to thwack, when you pull up or out on your resistance bands, they resist your pull the way a heavy weight does. Doing workouts with resistance bands can make a variety of muscles much stronger.
- **Weight bars or hand weights:** Using weights — either individual ones that you hold in your hands or a long, weighted bar that you hold over your head or behind your neck — can quickly improve your strength and muscle tone.

In addition, Chapter 11 discusses several other types of exercise that help get your labor and delivery muscles in shape so that you're ready for the big day.

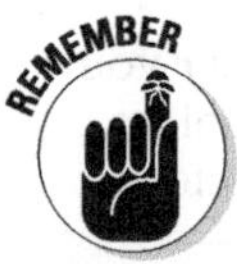

If you combine workouts that improve strength and/or flexibility with workouts that challenge your heart and lungs (called *aerobic* workouts), you turn your body into a finely tuned machine. Check out Chapter 17 for information on combining workouts.

Dancing through the tulips

Not every activity that's healthy has to be considered a sport. Dancing, for example, can be an excellent way to become or stay fit during your pregnancy and after you deliver. Just find a comfortable surface (like carpeting or an exercise mat) in a private place (unless you want the neighbors to be your audience), and then turn on the radio or your CD player with some kickin' tunes.

Gardening is another way to get fit that may not seem like exercise. If you're pulling weeds, hoeing, raking, or shoveling, you're getting an excellent workout. Just be sure to use the lifting and bending techniques presented in Chapter 11 so that you don't injure your growing and changing body.

Fitness walking and running

Fitness walking, discussed in Chapter 12, is an excellent exercise for beginning and experienced exercisers alike, because you can control the intensity, duration, and frequency of your workout — walking faster, longer, and more often as you become fitter.

Running, also discussed in Chapter 12, is another great way to get and stay fit, but is usually reserved for women who were running before getting pregnant and who continue to progress normally in their pregnancies (see Chapter 3). Why? Running is a whole-body activity that can be very physically demanding — more so than you may be up for during your pregnancy. However, if you think running will be the best activity for you during your pregnancy and you haven't been running up 'til now, talk to your healthcare provider about whether running makes sense for you. Keep in mind that you may need to modify your running pace and distance as your pregnancy progresses.

If you like to walk or run but don't like to brave the elements, consider getting a treadmill or joining a gym that has one. Although using a treadmill can be a bit boring, if you can talk to someone on the treadmill next to you or watch TV, the time clicks by pretty quickly.

Swimming and water aerobics

Except for the discomfort you may feel wearing a swimsuit while you're pregnant, you won't find a better pregnancy workout than swimming or water aerobics (which is doing aerobics in a pool, usually in a class setting, while wearing a flotation vest). And you can find comfortable swimsuits to wear while pregnant — see Chapter 7 for information on what to look for in pool workout gear and Chapter 23 for some great places to buy this gear. Also, Chapter 13 discusses water workouts in detail.

In order to swim or do water aerobics, you need access to a pool, not a lake, river, or the ocean, which could introduce infection into your vagina. Check with your local high school or YMCA to see whether a community pool is available in your area that offers convenient times for open swimming or offers water aerobics classes, especially ones designed for pregnant women.

Low-impact aerobics and yoga

Low-impact aerobics (which is similar to high-impact aerobics, but without jumps, kicks, deep bends, step-ups, and so on) is one of the most popular ways to work out while pregnant, and you can probably find a class in your area. Call your local community health agency, high school, gym, and dance studio to see what they may offer; ask, especially, whether they offer prenatal classes so that you can work out with other pregnant women. If you can't find a class in your area, you can set up your own workout area in your home and follow an aerobics videotape or DVD. Chapter 14 has more information on aerobics, including how to find classes and choose a video.

If you're used to doing high-impact or step aerobics, your pregnancy continues to progress normally, you aren't experiencing any discomfort (as discussed in Chapter 3), and your healthcare provider doesn't object, you can continue with higher-impact aerobics throughout your pregnancy. You may be able to modify your routine by reducing the height of the step and the height of your kicks.

Yoga, on the other hand, is a gentle way to work out that strengthens and sculpts your body, and many yoga studios offer special classes for pregnant women. A few yoga poses may not work well for you during pregnancy, but for the most part, yoga and pregnancy go well together. Yoga is also a terrific way to calm your mind, so if you start to feel stressed, give it a try. Like aerobics, if you can't find a class in your area, set up a yoga studio in your own home with a mat and a good video (see Chapter 14).

Pilates is another low-intensity exercise to try. Like yoga, the movements are slow and gentle, but they tend to be a little more rigorous than yoga. See Chapter 14 for details.

Cycling

Because cycling is a seated activity that actively works your heart and a variety of important muscles (legs, butt, back, and so on), it's very popular among pregnant women. As Chapter 15 discusses, you can cycle indoors (on a stationary bike) or out. Whether you can cycle outdoors depends on your experience, how well you're able to balance as your pregnancy progresses, and whether the temperature is moderate (without any excessive heat or humidity). Avoid high-traffic routes to avoid being exposed to excessive amounts of exhaust. Check with your healthcare provider to get additional feedback and advice.

Cycling indoors doesn't have to be a boring experience, especially if you can ride while watching TV and catch up on the news or your favorite show. Riding indoors while lifting light hand weights also works your upper body, creating an incredible total-body workout.

Working out on indoor machines

If you have access to indoor exercise machines, either at home or in a gym, you have an excellent way to exercise indoors, away from the cold, rain, and heat. Whether you choose to use a weight machine, stair-stepper, elliptical machine, cross-country ski machine, or rowing machine, you're going to get an excellent workout in the comfort or your home or a gym. And if the idea of buying such equipment seems ludicrous, keep in mind that some of these machines cost less than $200.

Cross-training

Cross-training is combining two or more types of exercises into one workout; it can also mean working out with one type of exercise on one day and another type of exercise on another day. Cross-training is an effective way to work a variety of muscles and ease boredom that may come from one particular type of workout. Chapter 17 discusses cross-training in detail.

Considering Additional Activities, Depending on Your Background

Traditional wisdom has been that pregnant women should avoid the following activities because of the risk of falling or getting hit and, potentially, harming the baby. Chances are, however, that if you're already doing these activities, you're pretty darned good at them and don't have much risk of falling or otherwise injuring yourself or your baby. So, if you're already participating in these activities *and* you're willing to modify your training regimen if you or your baby aren't responding well to the exercise *and* your healthcare provider is on board, you may be able to continue through part or all of your pregnancy. Remember that your healthcare provider must be aware of *exactly* what type of exercise you plan on doing, especially if it includes one of the following activities. See Chapter 3 for more safety precautions that you need to consider. If you have any concerns about doing any activity, avoid it — pregnancy is only 40 weeks of your life, and your chosen sport can wait that long.

- Downhill skiing, but only if you're an expert skier.
- Figure skating, steering clear of jumps and backward skating.
- Horseback riding, avoiding any jumps or risky riding.
- Mountain biking on flat, stable surfaces.
- Cross-country skiing, avoiding hills and difficult trails.
- Contact sports (soccer, volleyball, basketball, hockey)

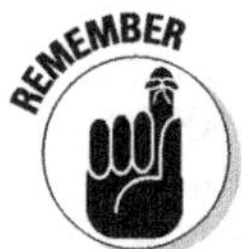

Contact sports are almost always off-limits to pregnant women, because of the risk of falls and other injuries. Be sure that your healthcare provider understands exactly what sort of contact sport you have in mind before taking part in these activities.

If you're new to exercise, don't take up any of the activities listed in this section. They all require either a high fitness level or a superb sense of balance (or both) and aren't for the uninitiated. Instead, choose from the activities listed in the preceding section.

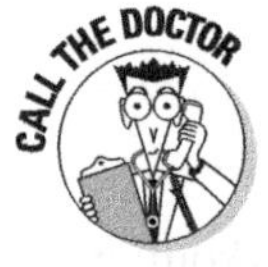

Before taking part in these activities, talk with your healthcare provider. Your skill level, as well as other factors, may determine whether these activities are safe. Always use common sense and err on the side of caution.

Understanding the limitations of altitude

Some pregnancy fitness experts advise you to not train at altitude during your pregnancy, unless you already live in an area of high altitude. Research has confirmed that women who've been training at sea level before pregnancy struggle to train at high altitudes throughout their pregnancies. (Heck, anyone who's been training at sea level — pregnant or not — struggles to train at high altitude!)

If you live at a low elevation, talk to your healthcare provider before exercising at elevation to find out whether it's a good idea for you. If you're cleared to train at altitude, keep a close eye out for the following signs of altitude sickness:

- Lightheadedness
- Nausea
- Dizziness
- Extreme fatigue
- Racing pulse

If you experience any of these symptoms, stop exercising. If the symptoms continue (or even begin to occur) when you're training at a lower elevation, contact your healthcare provider.

Steering Clear of Certain Activities

Two activities are absolutely, positively off-limits to you during your pregnancy, which means that no matter how much you want to continue or try them, you just can't without risking your baby's health. Plan a water vacation next year and try the two activities in this section at that time.

Scuba diving

Scuba diving — deep-sea diving with breathing gear strapped to your back — is absolutely out of the question at any time during your pregnancy. The intense underwater pressure (pressure that you don't necessarily feel because of the equipment you're using) is harmful to your baby.

If you're a die-hard scuba diver, ask your healthcare provider whether you can snorkel during your pregnancy. Snorkeling is done in shallow waters, so your baby doesn't have to withstand the deep-sea water pressure. Snorkeling may also be out of the question, but it doesn't hurt to ask!

Water-skiing

Water-skiing presents two challenges that make it off-limits:

- If you fall while skiing — and many people do — the force of the impact on your abdomen is incredibly high, putting your baby at great risk. In addition, during a fall, a jet of water can enter your vagina at a high force, possibly causing damage.
- You risk infection from contaminated lake or river water entering your vagina. For this same reason, don't swim in a lake, river, or ocean while you're pregnant.

Finding Activities Even When You're on Bed Rest

If a symptom or condition keeps you from exercising — or if your doctor or midwife sees a change in your baby's health during your pregnancy — you may also get a directive from your healthcare provider to spend weeks (or even months) in bed, with little time standing or walking. For an active woman, bed rest may feel like the kiss of death, and you may be concerned that all your fitness gains in the first two trimesters will be wasted during a period of bed rest. However, bed rest doesn't have to mean that you completely stop exercising your muscles and stretching. With the thumbs up from your healthcare provider, the exercises and stretches in this section can help you maintain some of your strength and flexibility.

Don't do any of the exercises listed here if you haven't first shared them with your healthcare provider and received the go-ahead. The purpose of bed rest is to help you and your baby get back to a more normal pregnancy, so unless your doctor or midwife tells you that these bed-rest exercises are acceptable, don't put you or your baby at risk. If you're doing these exercises while on bed rest, your healthcare provider must carefully supervise you. Stop any exercises if you experience warning signs or symptoms, and consult with your healthcare provider immediately.

If you're feeling down in the dumps and could use some support from women who can feel your pain, or if you just want more information about bed rest and high-risk pregnancies, visit `www.sidelines.org`.

Stretching while on bed rest

Gently stretching several times a day improves your circulation and minimizes muscle tightness and discomfort. Do the following stretches up to 3 times per day for 1 or 2 sets of 10 to 12 repetitions (reps), starting off with less than that (1 or 2 sets of 5 to 10 reps once or twice per day) and building up:

- Make circular motions with your ankles, wrists, neck, shoulders (like giant shrugs), and with your arms outstretched to the side. Be gentle. Start with small circles and gradually increase the diameter without going beyond what feels comfortable.
- Bring your chin to your chest, hold for three seconds, and then lift your chin back up. Also do the same stretch to each side of your neck, bending your neck so that your ear nearly meets your shoulder.
- Extend your arms in front of you, bend your elbows, and extend your arms out again.
- Lift each arm all the way up and down.
- Lying on your side or back, stretch your arms as far above your head as you can and push your heels downward (away from your head) as far as you can to get a whole-body stretch.

Strengthening muscles while on bed rest

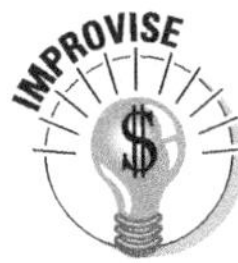

Strength training is not only possible while you're on bed rest, but it's also a great way to keep from losing muscle mass during this time of inactivity. You want to do the following exercises in 1 or 2 sets of 10 to 12 reps, 2 or 3 days per week. Keep some light weights (one to three pounds) or cans of vegetables or soup near your bed so that they're ready when you are. Avoid lifting anything that requires a lot of effort; you should be able to do 10 to 12 reps without straining.

Bicep curls

This exercise works the *biceps,* the muscles on the inside of your arms, above your elbows. The biceps are the muscles you notice the most when you're wearing a tank top — fit celebrities often have biceps you'd kill for.

1. **Sit up with your hands by your side.**
2. **Hold weights in your hands with your palms facing up.**
3. **Take a breath and then exhale as you slowly lift your hands to your chest.**

   Keep your elbows as stationary as possible.
4. **Inhale as you slowly lower your hands to your starting position.**
5. **Repeat.**

Shoulder raise

This exercise strengthens the muscles around your armpits and shoulders (the area that can look a little flabby when you look in the mirror wearing only a sports bra).

1. **Straighten your arms by your sides, holding light weights.**

   You may need to rise up a bit in your bed.
2. **Take a breath, and then exhale as you slowly raise your arms to shoulder level (or as high as you can go).**
3. **Inhale as you slowly lower your arms to your starting position.**
4. **Repeat.**

   Modify this exercise by raising the weights with your arms straight out in front of you.

Chest press

The chest press works your chest and the muscles around your armpits.

1. **Lie on your back with several pillows propping you up so that you're in a semireclining position, and grip a light weight in each hand.**
2. **Put your hands on your chest, facing outward.**

   Make sure the backs of your hands are sitting against your chest.
3. **Take a breath, and then exhale as you slowly press the weights out and away from your chest until your arms are straight.**
4. **Inhale as you slowly lower your hands to your starting position.**
5. **Repeat.**

Triceps extension

This exercise works the *triceps,* the muscles on the outside of your arms, above the elbows. The triceps are notorious for making a lot of women sleeveless-shirt phobic.

1. **Hold a light weight in your right hand.**
2. **Lift your arm above your head so that your bent elbow is next to your ear and your hand is near the back of your shoulder.**

   If you're in a sitting position, lean forward before lifting your arm.
3. **Take a breath and exhale as you slowly straighten your elbow so that your hand is above your head and your arm is straight.**
4. **Inhale as you slowly lower your arm to your starting position.**
5. **Repeat.**
6. **Follow these same steps for the left arm.**

Abdominal press

This exercise helps you maintain abdominal strength during bed rest and also helps get your tummy back into shape after you deliver.

1. **Sit or lie on your side.**
2. **Take a deep breath and exhale, slowly pulling your belly button toward your spine.**
3. **Hold the position for 3 seconds (count elephant-1, elephant-2, elephant-3).**
4. **Inhale and slowly release for a count of 3.**
5. **Repeat, working up to 10 to 12 reps.**

Tummy leg slides

This exercise tightens your tummy and works your leg muscles.

1. **Sit comfortably with pillows supporting your back and with your knees bent and your feet resting on the bed.**
2. **Take a deep breath and as you exhale, tighten your tummy. Keep your tummy tightened as you slide one leg out (knee straight) and then slide your leg back in (knee bent).**

   Use a count of 3 to slide out and then in. Exhale as you slide your leg out and inhale as you slide in.
3. **Repeat.**
4. **Follow these same steps for the other leg.**

Exercising your pelvic floor muscles during a time of bed rest

Chapter 11 shows you the *pelvic floor exercises* (exercises for your pelvic floor muscles) that are essential for pregnant women. You can perform these simple exercises while on bed rest, getting the go-ahead from your healthcare provider in advance, of course.

The muscles of the pelvic floor provide support for the pelvic organs. Keeping these muscles strong helps prevent conditions such as incontinence and prolapsed organs.

Part II
Getting Up and Moving: Fit Pregnancy Basics

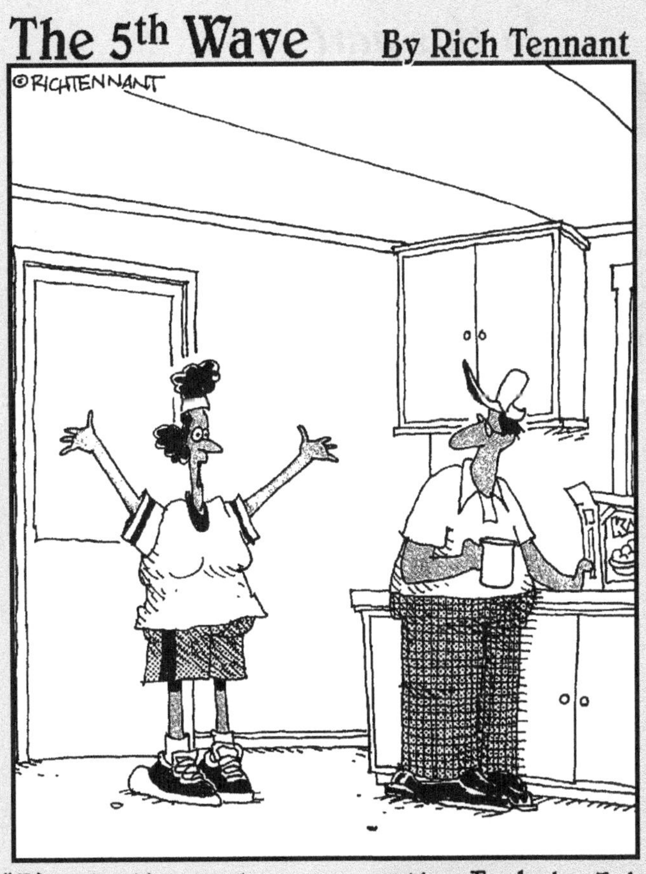

"I'm starting to develop a routine. Each day I do some stretches and aerobics, then follow up with high performance nausea and free style cravings."

In this part . . .

We give you some basic before-you-start advice if you've never exercised before. If you have plenty of fitness experience, you find out how to adjust your current workouts so that you maintain your fitness level and keep your baby safe. You also get the lowdown on finding workout gear that fits your expanding belly but is also comfortable to work out in. And you get to peruse an important chapter on warming up and stretching so that you can improve your flexibility and avoid sustaining an injury.

Chapter 5

Never Exercised Before? No Problem!

In This Chapter

- Finding a fitness activity you enjoy
- Choosing the right workout clothes
- Understanding some basics of exercise
- Getting into a fitness routine

If you're reading this chapter, you probably hated gym class and didn't play sports when you were in school. But does that mean you're doomed to be fitness-challenged during your pregnancy or for the rest of your life? No way! This chapter gives you the ins and outs of working out, explaining what to wear, how to stay injury free, and how to approach your first workout. You also find out how to set up a fitness routine that fits your interests, lifestyle, and goals.

Finding Fun Ways to Work Out

Your options for working out are nearly endless: You can exercise indoors or out, by yourself or with others, doing activities that range from walking and aerobics to swimming and cycling. This section helps you choose an activity that suits your personality and gives you a great workout. If you aren't sure what terms like *resistance bands* or *stair-stepping* mean, see Chapter 3 for a detailed explanation of what these activities are actually like.

You don't have to choose only one activity. By *cross-training,* you alternate activities every other day or combine two or more activities on any given day. So, you may decide that you like walking and cycling and alternate those every other day. Or, you may like the way weightlifting sculpts your muscles but want to include an activity that elevates your heart rate, so you use a stair-stepper and then lift weights directly after. Chapter 17 gives you tips and tricks for cross-training.

Honing in on your favorite activities

In order to stick to a workout routine, you have to like the activity you're doing. If you dislike walking, don't even think about taking it up. If you've never liked water, don't bother starting to swim. Instead, choose an activity that appeals to you — one that you'll look forward to doing!

The following list asks you a few questions and helps you narrow your list of potential workout activities.

- **Do you like being outdoors?** Walking is your best bet. After you deliver your baby, you can also try running, outdoor cycling, hiking, cross-country skiing, *snowshoeing* (walking or running in the snow with special shoes on), and any other outdoor activity.

  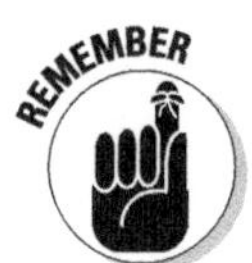

  Take care during summer months that you exercise only early in the morning or late at night, when the temperature is cooler. You need to avoid exercising outdoors during days when heat and humidity increase the possibility of heat exhaustion or heat stroke.

- **Do you dislike being outside in extreme weather?** Swimming, aerobics, yoga, indoor cycling, and any number of indoor exercises keep you out of the cold.

  One of the easiest ways to sculpt muscles is with an exercise ball, resistance band, or a weight bar. Chapter 11 describes how to use these low-cost, simple exercise methods, which are great complements to walking or other heart-pumping activities. Another simple (but not as cheap) way to work out is to buy a treadmill, stair-stepper, cross-country ski machine, elliptical trainer, or other piece of equipment (see Chapter 16). If you can afford this equipment and have the room, you'll develop a convenient workout routine, because you'll never have an excuse for not working out. If you don't have room for or can't afford this equipment, consider joining a pool or gym close to your home that offers indoor equipment. Also, you can purchase an exercise videotape (see Chapter 14) that lets you work out inexpensively in your own home.

- **Did you like riding a bike as a kid?** Chances are, you'll still like cycling now. Choose low-traffic areas that don't make you breathe exhaust, which can be bad for you and your baby. Also, if you're not yet adept at cycling, avoid riding outside until you deliver to minimize your changes of falling, and choose indoor cycling on a stationary bike instead.

- **Did you like swimming as a child?** People who love water tend to always love it, so take up swimming or water aerobics. Considered one of the safest activities in which you can participate, water exercises only require a swimsuit and a community pool for you to start working out. And, of course, you want to bring a towel — unless you enjoy dripping dry on the car ride home.

- **Do you want to work out with others?** Consider joining a gym or enrolling in a prenatal yoga, low-impact aerobics, or water aerobics class. See the "Finding a prenatal fitness class" sidebar for tips on finding a class that's right for you.
- **Do you prefer to work out alone?** You can do nearly any activity (using an exercise ball, walking, cycling, stair-stepping, weightlifting, and so on) alone, but staying motivated may be difficult. If you like being alone but need motivation now and then, consider joining an exercise group that meets once or twice a week (see Chapter 19). Also, when working out alone, keep a phone nearby at all times.
- **Are you looking for an activity that will calm you?** Yoga, swimming, and walking are activities that give you quiet time to meditate.
- **Do you need an inexpensive activity?** Swimming is among the least expensive activities you can find. Your swimsuit (usually around $80) and a membership to a pool (often $1 or $2 per visit) are your biggest expenses. Using exercise balls, resistance bands, or weight bars is also pretty inexpensive, because you don't need any special clothing or shoes (see Chapter 7). Walking is another inexpensive workout. If your community or employer offers a free or low-cost gym, nearly any indoor activity will be inexpensive, because they don't require much special clothing or other gear.
- **Are you easily bored?** Avoid indoor exercise equipment, unless you can set up a TV or other distraction in front of you. Choosing an outdoor activity or joining an aerobics or yoga class with a high-energy instructor are among your better bets.

Exercise is only horrible when you're doing something you don't want to be doing. The problem is, if you've never exercised, you may not know what activities you do and don't enjoy, so give them all a try until you find one you like. You can check out videos at the library, get a short-term (one- to two-week) membership at a gym or pool, or walk around your town. Don't invest in expensive clothing or equipment until you're sure, but remember that the proper gear does keep you from getting injured, so don't take too long to decide!

Choosing an activity that's truly a workout

A *workout* during pregnancy is any activity that takes your Rating of Perceived Exertion (RPE) to 12 to 14. (RPE is just like it sounds — how hard you think or perceive your workout to be — and 12 to 14 is considered "moderate" to "somewhat hard." See Chapter 3 for the lowdown.) This activity should be a *cardiovascular* (also called *cardio*) *workout,* meaning that it strengthens your muscles, heart, and lungs; burns a significant number of calories; and lasts for at least 15 minutes. With that definition in mind, here's a rundown of some activities and whether or not they constitute a workout:

- **Fitness walking:** Absolutely. If you're trying to begin fitness walking and aren't yet ready to walk briskly for 15 minutes, try a combination fitness walk/leisurely walk, in which you walk powerfully until you feel fatigued, and then begin walking slowly until you're ready to speed up again. Chapter 12 has more info.
- **Swimming:** Another great workout. The biggest advantage of swimming is that the water cushions your body, so you have little risk of injury. Swimming is also a whole-body workout that tones your arms and legs. See Chapter 13.
- **Cycling, stair-stepping, elliptical training, or cross-country skiing on indoor fitness machines:** Yes, ma'am — these are all great workouts. Be sure you're doing your stair-stepping on a step machine (such as StairMaster), and not in a high-intensity step-aerobics class, which may be too intense during pregnancy if you've never exercised before. See Chapter 15 for info on cycling and Chapter 16 for more on indoor machines.
- **Low-impact aerobics or water aerobics:** Doing aerobics is a terrific way to work out. Steer clear, though, of aerobic routines that offer breaks every five or ten minutes, because you'll miss out on the benefits of keeping your heart rate elevated for a sustained period of time and won't burn nearly as many calories as you do if you work out continuously. Chapters 13 and 14 give you the lowdown.
- **Yoga and Pilates:** Yes and no. Yoga and Pilates are excellent ways to move and breathe slowly and gently while still strengthening muscles, so they're recommended during pregnancy. Some yoga and Pilates routines, however, don't elevate your heart rate enough to strengthen the heart muscle, improve your breathing, and burn calories. Consider alternating yoga or Pilates (covered in Chapter 14) one day with another activity the next.
- **Exercise balls, resistance bands, and weightlifting:** Yes and no. Using resistance training is a tremendous way to strengthen and sculpt your muscles, but it doesn't elevate your heart rate and it doesn't burn many calories. Combining weightlifting with an activity that does elevate your heart rate makes for an ideal workout (see Chapter 17 for more on cross-training). Chapters 11 and 16 offer basic introductions to balls, bands, bars, and weightlifting machines; if you still have any doubts about how to weight train after reading those chapters, you may want to work out with a personal trainer or an instructor at a fitness club for your first few sessions.
- **Tennis:** Generally not a great workout for beginners, although if you and your partner are able to keep up long volleys and serve immediately after every missed shot, you can get a good workout. Most pregnant women, however, struggle with the quick stops and starts and have trouble balancing during their last trimester.
- **Golf:** Depends. If you walk for 9 holes (approximately 3 miles) or 18 (approximately 6 miles), you're getting an excellent workout. If you ride

in a cart, get out and swing your club, and get back in the cart, you're not working out. Keep in mind, too, that golf courses use a tremendous amount of chemicals to keep the fairways and greens free of weeds. To keep you and your baby away from these chemicals, you probably want to steer clear of golfing while you're pregnant.

- **Bowling:** Sorry, but no. Your heart rate isn't elevated for a continuous amount of time, you're not strengthening any muscles, and you're barely burning any calories. Bowling is fun, but it's not a workout. If you do bowl for fun, get a lane that isn't near smokers to avoid exposing you and your baby to secondhand smoke. Also be sure that your back isn't being stressed and that you're able to keep your balance as you play.
- **Strolling:** Probably not. In order to get the benefits of walking, you need to walk pretty fast — enough to elevate your heart rate and make conversing fairly difficult. Strolls tend to be more about sightseeing, window-shopping, and conversing, which is great, but they aren't workouts.

Are you getting the idea? Basically, you want to keep moving at a brisk pace for a minimum of 15 minutes, which means that activities that don't elevate your heart rate, that allow for plenty of rest, and that offer options to ride or sit instead of walk aren't going to get you very fit.

Finding a prenatal fitness class

If you want to work out with the support of other pregnant women and like the thought of having your exercise monitored by a professional, consider taking a prenatal fitness class. Before signing up, though, make sure the class offers the following:

- The instructor has a fitness or health-related degree and training in prenatal fitness.
- A health history and healthcare provider's consent are required before you can join the class. Even though your healthcare provider may have signed off on exercise, the trainer running the class should ask for this before you're allowed in.
- The facility is appropriate for prenatal exercise, offering a supportive floor, mats, restrooms, and a cool temperature.
- The class includes a warm-up, a cardio (heart-pumping) portion, strength and flexibility exercises, and a cool-down period. The exercises should also address pregnancy needs.
- The instructor is able to answer fitness and pregnancy-related questions. He or she talks about (or has posters hanging in the room about) the warning signs and symptoms to be aware of during prenatal workouts.
- You're given frequent exertion level checks and water breaks.
- Your progress is monitored and recorded.

If you're in a class that doesn't follow some of or all the preceding guidelines, look for another class or bring your concerns to the instructor.

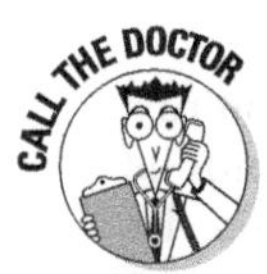

You've heard it before: Check with your doctor or midwife before beginning any exercise activity. Also check out Chapter 4 for more safety precautions.

Establishing Reasonable Expectations for Yourself

The key to starting and successfully maintaining a workout routine is to be reasonable with yourself. Your workout expectations while you're pregnant aren't about massive weight loss or a world-record pace. Instead, keep your expectations simple:

- **Proper weight gain:** Your healthcare provider will help you set a weight goal for each week, month, or trimester, and you can use your workout routine to stay within that weight range. You have to gain weight during pregnancy, of course, but if you can keep from gaining too much, you'll have an easier time getting back to your pre-pregnancy weight after you deliver. See Chapter 10 for additional information.
- **Overall health:** Focus on being healthy. Although you may hope to someday have a stronger, more muscular, lean body, now isn't the time to pursue that goal. Instead, focus on your overall health, taking care with what you eat, how much you sleep, and, of course, how briskly you exercise.
- **Small fitness improvements:** Have you ever watched participants in an Olympic event or a marathon and thought, "How can they get their bodies to do that?" The answer is simple: They did it over time. Elite athletes work for *years* to get their bodies to accomplish incredible feats. So goes your lifelong workout routine.

  The first day you work out, spend about 15 minutes on your activity. From there, gradually increase the time you spend exercising until you reach a level that fits your schedule and makes you feel fit. (See the "Creating a workout plan" section later in this chapter for details.) Over the course of many months, you may accomplish your goal of, say, exercising for 30 or 40 minutes per day, which isn't enough to win an Olympic event, but does make you a pregnancy workout champion.
- **A change in your lifestyle:** Ultimately, you want to exercise for the rest of your life, and your pregnancy is a great time to establish good habits and patterns. Heck, if you can work out during these nine months — when you need help getting out of bed and can't see your feet well enough to tie your shoes — you're tough enough to work out for the rest of your life.

The Basics: Warming Up, Cooling Down, Stretching, and Hydrating

Every workout routine — no matter what activity you decide to pursue — must include four important elements: warming up, cooling down, stretching, and *hydrating* yourself (drinking fluids). This section gives you a brief overview of these exercise basics.

Easing into each workout

Every time you work out, you want to start off gradually, giving your body time to warm up. This means that you ease into your workout, starting out more slowly than you intend to go during the bulk of your workout. The amount of time you warm up depends on how fast your body adjusts to physical activity, but for most people five or ten minutes is plenty.

If you're walking, start out by strolling for five minutes or so, and then begin to swing your arms and pick up your pace a bit, as discussed in Chapter 12. If you're cycling, cycle at a slow pace you know you can keep up for hours before increasing to a faster speed. If you're taking a class or watching a video, be sure the instructor eases you into the workout before doing anything difficult. And if you're doing any resistance training (balls, bars, bands, hand weights, or machine weightlifting), also do a bit of cardiovascular workout (for example, five minutes of walking), before beginning your resistance training routine.

Many people like to stretch *before* exercising, but this is an easy way to get injured. Stretching (discussed in the "Stretching afterward" section and in Chapter 8) can be as challenging to your body as the rest of your workout routine, so if you stretch *cold* muscles (muscles that have been resting), you're essentially working out without a warm-up. Instead of trying to warm up with a stretch, do your stretches after you finish your workout. Or, if you really feel the need to stretch before your workout, do a five- or ten-minute warm-up by walking or doing some other cardiovascular activity, stretch, work out, and stretch again. After you begin to stretch regularly after each workout, you'll no longer feel tight when starting a workout the following day.

Cooling down as you finish

As you near the end of your workout routine, gradually downshift to your warm-up pace again. This helps ease your body from the intensity of your workout and avoids stopping suddenly, which can cause muscles to tear.

Never end your workout with a big, ferocious finish and then stop — your muscles just can't downshift quickly enough, and a quick stop can also make you feel lightheaded or dizzy. Instead, spend about five minutes stair-stepping, walking, cycling, or doing any other activity at an increasingly slower pace than the one you held for the majority of your routine. This cool-down period helps you transition from a workout back to your ordinary pace.

If you work out for 15 minutes, the majority of your workout is spent warming up and cooling down. As you increase the length of each workout, keep your warm-up and cool-down periods the same, thus increasing the amount of time that you maintain your workout pace.

Stretching afterward

Right after you finish your workout — and before you sit down, take a shower, or relax in any other way — you need to stretch. Sure, you meet die-hard athletes who tell you they've never stretched a day in their lives, but the truth is, they've experienced far more soreness than they had to. Stretching today keeps you from getting sore tomorrow.

Over time, stretching also allows you to go a little farther and a little faster than you otherwise would be able to, because stretching makes your muscles better able to relax to their full length. Elastic muscles can move more fluidly than nonelastic ones, so when you stretch regularly, you're able to walk, cycle, and swim faster and more easily than if you don't.

Drinking plenty of fluids

After you work out and cool down, take time to hydrate your body. We're not talking about a sip of water — you need *a lot* of fluid! Drink at least 16 ounces (2 cups) up to 32 ounces (4 cups) of fluids within 30 minutes of completing your workout, and drink a total of 64 ounces (8 cups) throughout the day. See Chapter 9 for the lowdown on hydrating yourself.

Debunking "No Pain, No Gain"

Did you ever walk past the football players' weight room when you were in high school and see a large sign that read, "No pain, no gain"? This slogan was meant to convince teenage boys that in order to be at their fittest, they had to work themselves up to or beyond the point of pain. Granted, football is a difficult sport that does involve a lot of pain: After getting bruised from bumping into the corner of a coffee table, you can only imagine what it feels like to get tackled by a 200-pound guy who's running as fast as he can!

Even off the football field, the idea that you can't make fitness gains without feeling pain is still popular, but, in a word, it's a bunch of malarkey. In order to be at your fittest, you need to exercise regularly and with effort, but you shouldn't feel pain with any regularity. In fact, working out until you're exhausted and in pain just makes you not want to work out ever again.

Preparing to feel some soreness

During the first week to ten days that you work out — and anytime you start exercising again after taking time off — you will feel soreness. Soreness is different from pain, but because you've never exercised before, you may not immediately recognize the difference.

Pain comes from overdoing your activity; that is, exercising for too long or with too much vigor before you're ready to do so. *Soreness,* on the other hand, comes from working muscles you haven't worked before (or haven't worked for a long time), so chances are good (like, 100 percent) that you'll experience soreness. These underused muscles actually tear in miniscule amounts, and that causes soreness. When the tearing heals, the muscles are stronger (which is why you get more toned when you exercise) and more resistant to further tearing in the future (provided you continue to exercise regularly).

Soreness makes every muscle you use during exercise feel like a giant bruise, and it feels awful for the first day or two after you begin exercising. In fact, at that point, you'll probably be ready to burn your workout clothes and never try this again. But the main difference between soreness and pain is that soreness begins to fade after four to seven days (although it may not disappear completely for a few weeks), and as long as you continue exercising regularly, it won't come back. So, the price you pay for a fit pregnancy is feeling some pretty serious discomfort for a few days and some additional — but not nearly as intense — soreness for the next few weeks.

In those first few days of working out, you may wonder how muscles that you didn't even know existed can hurt so much. Although we want to help you avoid soreness altogether, it's a function of moving and using muscles that you haven't used for a long time, so you have to experience it. You can, however, reduce the degree of your soreness by starting slowly in your exercise program and avoiding large, sudden increases in intensity and duration (see Chapter 3). And always follow your workout with stretching, as discussed in Chapter 8.

One way to ease your soreness a bit is to continue to stretch and drink plenty of water. A warm (never hot) bath may make you feel a little better, as can a cold pack applied to sore areas. Stick with your workout routine in spite of your soreness. The only way to never experience this soreness again is to never get out of shape again. The soreness won't fade any faster by stopping your workouts; in fact, because you're moving your muscles, your soreness will likely disappear *faster* if you continue to work out.

Avoiding injuries

You've probably heard of athletes getting injured from their workouts and wonder how something so good for you can go so wrong. In general, injuries are caused by the following situations, so avoid them in your own training:

- **Doing too much, too soon:** The number-one reason why people get injured is because they try to train harder or longer than their bodies are ready for. Getting fit takes time, and you need to build up the length and intensity of your workouts very, very gradually. From week to week, never increase the average duration of your workouts more than 5 minutes: The first week, your average may be 15 minutes per workout; the second week, the average should be no more than 20 minutes; the third week, 25 minutes; and so on. And increasing even less than that is perfectly acceptable. See Chapter 3 for more information on controlling the intensity of your workouts.
- **Not stretching after a workout:** Many athletes spend time working out and then don't spend ten extra minutes stretching afterward. (See Chapter 8 for the lowdown on stretching.) What happens, instead, is that they finish a walk, complete a weight workout, finish the aerobics portion of a videotape, or do a workout on an elliptical machine, walk into the living room, and sit down to relax. Although this may seem like a sensible postworkout routine, without stretching, your muscles, ligaments, and tendons tighten up, becoming more prone to tears and sprains.
- **Wearing worn-out shoes:** Think about how much you spend on your car to ensure that you get safely from place to place. Thousands of dollars? Tens of thousands? Now think about what you need to safely get from place to place during your daily walk: a $70 pair of shoes. Yet, when that pair wears out, you may be tempted to wear it for a few more weeks, just to avoid parting with those 70 bucks. This is like not filling a flat tire or not fixing a dragging muffler, all to save some money: In the end, you'll just pay more. If the costs associated with having a baby are overwhelming your finances right now, try to find shoes on sale at larger sporting goods stores and at quality discount stores like Target or TJ Maxx.

  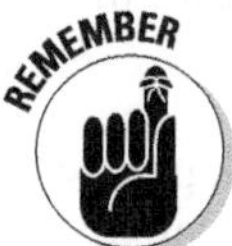

  The biggest challenge with workout shoes is that when they're worn out, they can actually still look pretty good on the outside, especially if you wear them only for working out and not for bopping around town. See Chapter 7 for details on knowing how often to replace your shoes.
- **Working out on hard surfaces:** This is where the analogy between a car and your body stops, because if you drive a car on dirt roads, it wears out faster than if you drive it on concrete. Not so for your body. The fact

is that concrete is the hardest surface on which you can exercise, and all that pounding can add up to an injury. Instead, work out on asphalt (blacktop) roads or bike trails (asphalt is far softer than concrete), dirt roads or trails, exercise mats or pads placed over a hard surface, or even a rug or carpet in your living room. You'll save yourself the wear and tear on your back, joints, and muscles.

Be wary if the shoulders of roads or trails are in bad condition or have lots of tree roots. Uneven surfaces can cause you to fall, and though falling doesn't necessarily put your baby at risk (your baby is like an egg wrapped in layers and layers of goose down and foam, so she's well protected), you want to avoid the possibility of an especially bad fall.

- **Not getting enough sleep:** Equating fatigue with exercise may sound like a strange idea, but think about this: If you had to run a marathon (a nightmare of an idea, we know!), would you run better or worse if you hadn't slept for 24 hours? The truth is, your body needs eight hours of sleep to recover from the stress of being pregnant each day, plus a little more to account for exercise. If you're planning to sleep five or six hours per night, work a full day, exercise, and be an incubator for your baby, you may as well make an appointment with a sports medicine doctor right now — you'll need his or her services when you get injured.

These aren't the only reasons for athletic injuries, but they're common ones that you can avoid.

Knowing your limits

Being new to exercise, you may think your greatest challenge will be making the time and getting the energy to work out. Surprisingly, though, exercise has an almost addictive quality, and after just a few weeks of consistent workouts, many women wouldn't dream of cutting back or taking time off from exercise. And though this devotion to an activity that's so good for you is admirable, if you're working out at all costs — regardless of how you and your baby feel — you can injure yourself, and worse, harm your baby.

Make a deal with yourself now that you'll wait until after you deliver a healthy baby before you get crazy about exercise. For the duration of your pregnancy, work out consistently, but don't go overboard. Now more than ever, you need to watch and listen to your body and limit your exercise if your body isn't responding well.

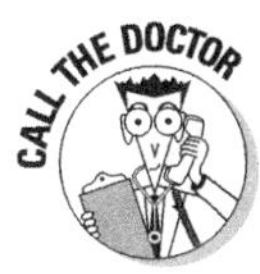

Contact your healthcare provider if you experience any of the important signs and symptoms discussed in Chapter 3.

Setting Up Your First Fitness Routine

Developing a fitness routine isn't easy, mainly because you've never had to include exercise in your day-to-day routine before. You can pick up a new habit, though, by doing an activity for just 21 days. This means that if you exercise today and stick to it for the next 21 days, in only 3 weeks, exercise will be a daily part of your life. Just think: You didn't always brush your teeth or floss every day, but you do now. (Don't you?)

To set up an effective fitness routine, you need to establish a convenient time to work out, set up a workout plan that includes some variation (so you don't get bored), keep track of your workouts, and stay motivated. The following sections get you started.

Carving time out of your day

To allow time to work out and stretch, you need to allot between 30 and 60 minutes each day that you exercise. Most women work out at one of three times throughout the day: morning (before work or other commitments), midday (lunchtime), and late afternoon or early evening (after work but more than three hours before bedtime so as not to interrupt sleep).

Starting the day with a workout

Many women find that working out first thing in the morning is the only way to ensure that they actually follow through with their exercise goals. Instead of coming home from work feeling hungry and exhausted, and still having to work out, you can exercise first thing in the morning and have the rest of the day to relax. You get to shower once (in the morning, after your cool-down and stretching), instead of feeling as though you have to shower in the morning before work and again later in the day. Besides the convenience, morning workouts are also beneficial because by getting your heart pumping early in the morning, you tend to feel energetic throughout the day.

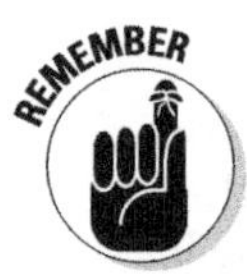

Unfortunately, morning workouts don't always work when you're pregnant. If you're feeling so nauseated that you can hardly get out of bed in the morning, chances are you're not going to feel like popping in your aerobics video or firing up the treadmill. In addition, morning workouts present two other drawbacks:

- **Working out in the dark:** In order to exercise before work, for at least part of the year you probably have to exercise when it's dark outside, which limits your outdoor activities. During these times of the year, you have to join a gym or pool or choose one of the indoor activities discussed in Part IV of this book.

- **Risking injury:** When you work out later in the day, your body has spent the day warming itself up. In the morning, however, your body is rather inflexible and not quite ready for prime-time activity. Be extra cautious about making sudden movements early in your morning workouts and warm up especially well. (See the "Easing into each workout" section earlier in this chapter.)

If you don't exercise in the morning, you have two other times to work out: lunch time and late afternoon or early evening. The following sections discuss the pros and cons of each of these options.

Taking time to exercise at lunch

Your lunch hour is a terrific time to exercise, especially if you get other people at work to join in. Using this time of day for exercise has the obvious drawback of not leaving you time to eat lunch, but if you still find time for a good meal after your workout, this may not be a problem. If your lunch time is an hour or less, however, you may not have enough time to work out, stretch, and shower or otherwise clean up before heading back to the second half of your workday. Ask your supervisor whether you can get to work a little early or leave a little later, freeing up more time at lunch.

Exercising outdoors in the middle of a hot, humid summer day may elevate your body temperature beyond what's healthy for your baby. To minimize your risk of overheating, talk to your healthcare provider if you're planning to work out at midday during the summer. You can exercise indoors in an air-conditioned facility. If you want to exercise outdoors in summer, switch to morning or early evening to avoid the hottest hours of the day. Because the sun rises earlier in the summer, you probably have enough daylight to exercise before work.

Working out later in the day

This option of working out in the early evening (before dinner) often presents a challenge if you plan to exercise at home, because by the time you run errands, drive home from work, and change your clothes, you may have also changed your mind about working out and decide instead to grab a bite to eat while you channel surf. However, if you can take a walk directly from your office, work out at a gym or pool that's on your way home, or meet with an aerobics or yoga class, you'll likely stick with your after-work routine. For many women, however, exercising in early evening presents an opportunity to destress before heading home.

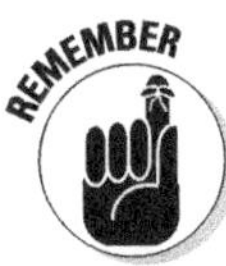

If you've been getting home right after work and eating dinner with your partner shortly thereafter, your new exercise routine may disrupt these well-established habits. Discuss your workout plans with your partner and see whether he wants to begin exercising, too (Chapter 19 has some ideas for getting your partner involved in your exercise routine). If not, perhaps he can find other activities that complement your exercise routine so that you both arrive home and eat later. If your partner expects you to be home to eat (or even make) dinner and resents your not being there, you'll probably abandon exercise before long.

A third option — exercising a few hours after dinner — isn't a good idea, because you're increasing your heart rate too close to your bedtime. Exercising less than two or three hours before your bedtime can interrupt your sleep and lead to increased fatigue the next day.

Creating a workout plan

Although a one-size-fits-all workout plan doesn't exist, Tables 5-1 through 5-3 give you an idea of what a beginner's exercise routine may look like. Modify these tables to match your own goals and the number of weeks you're into your pregnancy and always determine whether and how much you'll work out by how you feel and what your baby is telling you.

Tables 5-1 through 5-3 list the number of minutes to work out. If your form of exercise involves stopping and starting (such as with weightlifting or with exercise balls and resistance bands), don't count the minutes in between each type of exercise in your total minutes. And keep in mind that the minutes in these tables include time to warm up and cool down.

If you aren't sure whether you want to work out for four, five, or six days per week (Tables 5-1 through 5-3, respectively), think about your personality:

- Will you have an easier time developing a habit if you exercise every day, rain or shine, without having to remember whether this is a workout day or not?
- Are you more likely to quit exercising if you rarely get a break?
- How many days per week fit into your schedule?

You're far better off exercising four days per week than none at all, so simply follow a routine that works for you and don't feel as though you have to apologize for it.

We didn't include a seven-day-per-week table here because, when you're pregnant, exercising seven days per week is too challenging. During your pregnancy, exercise for no more than six days per week, although you can certainly do stretches every day. After you deliver your baby, feel free to add a seventh day of cross-training if doing so is appropriate for how you're feeling at that time.

The term *CT* in Tables 5-1 through 5-3 means "cross-train"; that is, switching from your normal activity to a very different one. See Chapter 17 for details.

Table 5-1 Four-Day-Per-Week Workout Plan

Week	*Monday*	*Tuesday*	*Wednesday*	*Thursday*	*Friday*	*Saturday*	*Sunday*
1 (60 min)	15	Off	15	Off	15	Off	15
2 (66 min)	15CT	Off	18	Off	18	Off	15
3 (70 min)	15CT	Off	20	Off	15	Off	20
4 (75 min)	15CT	Off	20	Off	20	Off	20CT
5 (80 min)	15	Off	25	Off	15CT	Off	25
6 (85 min)	20CT	Off	20	Off	25	Off	20

Table 5-2 Five-Day-Per-Week Workout Plan

Week	*Monday*	*Tuesday*	*Wednesday*	*Thursday*	*Friday*	*Saturday*	*Sunday*
1 (75 min)	15	Off	15	15CT	Off	15	15CT
2 (81 min)	15	Off	18	15CT	Off	18	15CT
3 (88 min)	20	Off	20	15CT	Off	18	15CT
4 (96 min)	20	Off	23	15CT	Off	18	20CT
5 (105 min)	25	Off	25	15CT	Off	20	20CT
6 (115 min)	25	Off	30	20CT	Off	20	20CT

Table 5-3 Six-Day-Per-Week Workout Plan

Week	*Monday*	*Tuesday*	*Wednesday*	*Thursday*	*Friday*	*Saturday*	*Sunday*
1 (90 min)	15	15CT	Off	15	15CT	15	15CT
2 (96 min)	18	15CT	Off	18	15CT	15	15CT
3 (103 min)	20	15CT	Off	20	15CT	18	15CT
4 (111 min)	20	18CT	Off	20	15CT	20	18CT
5 (120 min)	20	20CT	Off	25	15CT	20	20CT
6 (130 min)	25	20CT	Off	25	18CT	22	20CT

Wondering why each week increases? Because even though 15 to 20 minutes of activity is enough to raise your heart rate and expend calories, more is better, up to a point. Research varies, but for nonpregnant women, working out between 30 and 60 minutes per day, 4 to 7 days per week, is generally considered the ticket to excellent overall health and fitness. During your pregnancy, however, especially if you've never exercised before, 20 to 30 minutes per day, 4 to 6 days per week, is terrific.

Changing your routine

If you wore the same outfit each day, you'd get a little tired of it, wouldn't you? And maybe, after wearing the same thing day in and day out for weeks and weeks, you'd want to stuff the outfit in the trash and never see it again.

Vary your duration and intensity

Duration refers to the amount of time you work out in a given session; *intensity* refers to the effort you put into a workout.

Varying the duration means that you work out for a shorter duration one day (say, 25 minutes) and a longer duration the next day (for example, 40 minutes). By varying the duration, you don't get bored doing the same workout day in and day out.

If you're going to vary the duration, be sure you're ready for the longer duration. If you've never stair-stepped for more than 25 minutes, don't suddenly do a 40-minute workout just to avoid boredom. Keep in mind that you want to increase your workout times no more than 10 percent each week (for example, 150 minutes one week means no more than 165 minutes the next week).

Varying the intensity means that you work out harder for one workout session and easier the next, or you vary the intensity within a single workout. For example, you may do an intense workout, followed by two days of easier workouts, followed by another intense workout, and so on. Or, you can warm up for five minutes of a workout, go for a moderate pace for ten minutes, increase the intensity for five minutes, go back to moderate for ten minutes, and cool down for five minutes. Total workout: 35 minutes.

Mixing up your intensity can also brighten your mood and make you feel less fatigued. Seriously! A recent study at Auburn University discovered that people who mixed up high- and low-intensity work during a 20 to 40 minute workout were in even better moods and felt less fatigued at the end of their workouts than when they worked out at one intensity.

Varying the intensity of workouts during your pregnancy tends to be easier for experienced exercisers, not beginners, because in order to understand which efforts feel "hard," "moderate," and "easy," you need some experience with the sport or another activity. You also need to know how to listen to your body to ensure that you're not working out at too high an intensity for your level of fitness and stage of pregnancy. But with a little time and experience (and the details in Chapter 6), you, too, can start to fiddle with your intensity and duration.

Avoid increasing the intensity or duration of your workouts if you're experiencing any warning signs or symptoms. See Chapter 3 for a list of symptoms to watch for, especially on your days of longer duration or higher intensity.

In the same way, if you do the same workout — walk the same route, watch the same aerobics video, do the same exercise ball or resistance band steps in the same order — you'll get bored and may end up trashing your exercise routine altogether. Walk a different route every other day, buy two aerobics or yoga videos that you alternate, lift weights or use your exercise ball in a different order than you did the day before. Or go to a class two or three days per week and use a video on the other days. And if you're working out on a bicycle or other indoor equipment, see whether you can set up a small TV and VCR or DVD player and watch the news or your favorite movie as you work out.

A great, inexpensive way to spice up your routine is to cross-train. Chapter 17 gives you the details.

Keeping track of your workouts

You generally find two types of exercisers in this world:

- **Type-A exercisers:** Type-A exercisers plan their workouts days or even weeks in advance and write down details of every workout in an exercise log. They may also track how much they sleep, what they weigh, and what they eat each day. These are the overachievers that ruined the curve back in high school.

  Being a Type-A exerciser has its advantages. If you keep careful track of your exercise habits, you get a clear picture of what workouts tend to tire you or worsen morning sickness, for example. You also get to watch your improvement and decide whether to increase the amount you're exercising (see the following section). Of course, as with any planning and tracking, you may find yourself obsessing over exercise so that it becomes too important in your life. Remind yourself: Everything in moderation.

- **Type-B exercisers:** Type-B exercisers take each day as it comes, rarely planning a workout and never writing down the details of workouts after they're done. The idea is that exercise should be fun — not a planned activity — and as long as they're getting out and doing something, the details don't matter.

  Being a Type-B exerciser has its rewards, because your workouts correspond to how you feel, instead of fitting into a schedule that you set up weeks ago. The downside is that you may decide four or five days per week that your body is telling you not to work out. Although you really may feel awful and shouldn't be exercising, you may also be taking the easy road!

If you do decide to track your workouts, buy a calendar that has spaces for each day. Write down what workout you did and for how long. You may also want to note how you felt ("tired," "sore," "full of energy," and so on) and what may have contributed to that feeling ("got a great night of sleep," "bad morning sickness," and so on).

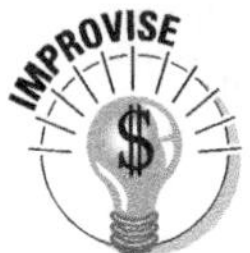

One simple, low-cost way to keep track of your workouts is to make a note in your daily planner. This way, you don't have to buy a separate journal or calendar, you're reminded to make exercise a priority, and whenever you feel a workout slump coming on, you can look back at your fitness progress for a strong dose of motivation.

Staying Motivated

Boredom, soreness, pregnancy-related pains, busyness, cold weather, rain, and countless other intruders may make you feel like straying from your workout routine. This section shares some tips for sticking to your workouts, even when the going gets tough.

Change from "have to" to "get to"

A sure way to have trouble getting motivated is to think of exercise as a "have-to" proposition: "I have to walk tonight" or "I have to go to aerobics class." When you find yourself falling into this trap, replace that thought with a positive one, and think about how fortunate you are to be able to exercise.

The next time you dread your workout and are saying with a sigh, "I have to go work out," try this: Think about your good fortune, smile, and say, "I *get* to go walking (or whatever other exercise you have in mind)!"

Keep inspiration close at hand

Each person is inspired in different ways, so find the inspiration that works for you and keep it handy. Here are some examples:

- A photo of a healthy baby (which yours will soon be)
- An inspirational movie or music that you watch or listen to during your workout

- A message to yourself that you write down or record when you're feeling great and read or play back when you're tired and grumpy
- The brochure of a walk, race, or bike trip that you intend to complete next year

Get a friend involved

One of the greatest motivators is someone who's waiting for you to show up for a workout. If you agree to meet a friend three mornings per week before work, you have to be there, or you leave her out in the cold. That doesn't leave you time to debate whether you're going to get up and work out or keep sleeping. (And remember that, in spite of the references to "her" and "she" that follow, your partner can also be a man.)

Be sure to take the following into account when choosing a training partner:

- Choose someone who's reliable (or you may be the one waiting out in the cold).
- Make a nonnegotiable pact that unless you're in labor or are experiencing one of the warning signs in Chapter 3, you'll both show up.
- Agree to be each other's motivators, which means neither of you can ever talk the other into going to the coffee shop instead of working out. But you can always *end* your workout with a visit to the coffee shop!
- Talk to her about some of the limitations you may experience throughout your pregnancy (see Chapter 3) and if she's not pregnant, make sure she understands those limitations.
- Make sure you live or work close enough that you can meet at a convenient place and time.
- Ensure that you both enjoy the activity (or activities) you choose.
- Take into account whether you're both at about the same fitness level. You don't want to be working out with someone who, for example, walks much faster or much slower than is comfortable for you. If the pace is faster than you're ready for, you can get injured. If it's slower than what you can handle, you won't get as fit during the time you spend walking as you would if you walked faster.

If you don't know of a friend who wants to work out, consider joining a class — it's like meeting a whole group of friends for a workout. Although skipping a class is a little easier than skipping out on a workout with one friend (see the preceding section), people are still expecting you to show up, and you're still accountable to those people if you aren't there.

If you can find a workout class meant specifically for pregnant women — aerobics, yoga, weightlifting, and so on — you'll get a double benefit: other pregnant women to share your workout and an instructor who's well versed in helping women get and stay fit during pregnancy.

Reward yourself

Nothing's wrong with a bit of self-bribery. Whether you reward yourself with a new pair of workout shorts, a relaxing bath, or a piece of furniture for your baby's room, the result is the same: You set a goal for yourself (such as, "Work out 20 days this month," or "Get in at least four 40-minute workouts this week), and when you reach it, you get the reward. Knowing that your reward is just around the corner makes getting out the door, turning on the aerobics tape, or driving to the gym that much easier.

Chapter 6

Exercise for Fitness Buffs and Competitive Athletes

In This Chapter

- Seeing how pregnancy changes your workouts
- Deciding whether to continue your current exercise routine
- Searching for exercises that complement your existing regimen
- Getting back to your current workouts after you deliver

If you've been an athlete — competitive or not — you may find yourself in a quandary: You're excited about being pregnant and want to do everything in your power to protect your growing baby, but you also kick yourself when you think about the fitness you may lose during your nine months of pregnancy.

Well, kick no more! Although your workouts need to change somewhat to keep you and your baby safe during your pregnancy, you can continue some of your routine, add to your routine with alternate activities, and maintain much of your fitness. And after you deliver a healthy baby, you can gradually ease back into your old routine and regain any lost fitness in just a few months.

This chapter helps you understand how a fit-pregnancy routine differs from your pre-pregnancy regimen. Be sure to also read Chapter 3, which discusses signs and symptoms your body may give you if you push yourself too hard while you're pregnant. And if you've never exercised before, skip this chapter and read Chapter 5.

If you're an elite athlete and hope to continue training at a high level during your pregnancy, consider being monitored by a physician or taking part in a supervised prenatal training program to minimize the risk of danger to you and your baby.

Understanding Physical Changes during Pregnancy

If you love to exercise or are a fierce competitor, you may think that nothing will change during the next 40 weeks: You'll just keep exercising the way you have been, deliver your baby, and not skip a beat.

It's a fine dream, but a dream nonetheless. *A lot* is going to change over the next nine months:

- Morning sickness (or any-time-of-day sickness) may interrupt your usual workout schedule.
- You'll be far more fatigued than you've ever been, so a seven-day-per-week workout schedule may no longer be possible.
- Your balance will be off, making you susceptible to falls and injuries and putting some forms of outdoor exercise off-limits.
- Your risk of injury is higher than it was before you got pregnant, because of a hormone called *relaxin* that loosens your ligaments and joints.
- Your weight gain (which is absolutely necessary to deliver a healthy baby) makes getting around more difficult than usual.
- The increasing size of your breasts and abdomen and the tenderness of your breasts may keep you from being physically capable of doing your pre-pregnancy exercises.
- You may experience a host of minor illnesses or other complaints that make you less able to start or finish a workout. These problems run the gamut, including (in alphabetical order) backaches, breathlessness, gassiness, headaches, heartburn, hemorrhoids, rashes, swelling and fluid retention, and urinary incontinence and increased urination. And that's just in the first trimester!
- Your body isn't going to recover nearly as fast as it has been able to, so you'll be able to do fewer hard workouts and will need more easy or rest days between harder efforts.

Modifying Your Workouts to Accommodate Your Pregnancy

Whether you need to modify your workouts depends on how you and your baby are faring during your pregnancy:

- Is the baby growing normally?
- Are you gaining weight normally?
- Do you feel good?

If you can answer "yes" to the preceding questions and your healthcare provider doesn't have any objections to you continuing your pre-pregnancy workouts, you don't need to modify your routine. If any of your answers to the three key preceding questions change, however, that's when you need to modify.

If all the physical stresses placed on your body during pregnancy sound terribly unfair given how fit your body was before you became pregnant, remember that, in just nine short months, you'll have a healthy baby as your reward. Until then, give yourself time to come to terms with the fact that your workouts will, indeed, change.

The following tells you how you may decide to modify your current routine:

- **Intensity:** *Intensity* refers to the effort you put forth as you exercise — hard, moderate, or easy efforts (see Chapter 3). In order to keep yourself healthy, you'll likely need to decrease the intensity of your workouts. If you can measure your workout intensity, expect your pace to slow down as you progress through your pregnancy. Don't fight this — simply do what you can while still feeling good the rest of the day. If you participate in a sport in which you can't measure intensity directly, pay careful attention to how your body feels during and after each workout. If you find yourself increasingly fatigued, are sore in muscles that have been long developed, or can't seem to work out as long as you used to, reduce the intensity of your workouts.
- **Duration:** *Duration* refers to the amount of time you spend exercising each day. If you want to continue the duration of each workout, and you feel great, do so. If you aren't feeling as good as you and your healthcare provider would like, consider reducing the duration. If, for example, you want to continue running 7-minute miles, you may find that you're comfortable running for 30 or 40 minutes per workout instead of 60. Or, if you don't want to reduce the duration, you can reduce the intensity: You may be able to run 60 minutes at 9-minute miles (reducing the intensity) and keep up the same duration (the 60 minutes of exercise). You can also alternate higher-intensity, lower-duration days with lower-intensity, higher-duration days.
- **Frequency:** *Frequency* refers to how often you work out — how many times per day and how many days per week. Even elite athletes tend to have trouble working out seven days per week while pregnant.

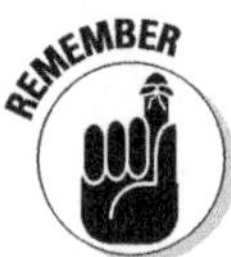

If staying in good shape isn't enough for you — that is, if you want to stay in the finely tuned, ready-for-competition shape that you were in before you became pregnant, you may need to rethink your ambitions. Trying to stay in top shape during the 40 weeks of pregnancy may mean making your workout routine a higher priority than your baby's health, a concept that may have tragic consequences. Your goal during pregnancy should be to not lose so much ground that you can't get yourself quickly back into shape after you deliver your healthy baby. But you're not going to run a marathon or play in a tournament a week after labor — you may, however, be able to perform at a high level four to six months after childbirth.

- **Competition:** The most notable change in exercise for a pregnant athlete is that your healthcare provider will likely advise you to stop competing by the second trimester (weeks 15 to 27). Although your healthcare provider may recommend that you stop competing earlier or later than the second trimester, the fact remains that pregnancy may set limits on your competition for at least a few months. Use common sense about this, thinking about what — if any — competitive gains you'll make by continuing your racing schedule and listening carefully to your healthcare provider's advice.

Many athletes have made successful returns to competition after delivering healthy babies, and some even find that time off from competition renews their interest in it and makes them more successful.

Finding Alternate Activities

If, after you reduce the intensity, duration, and/or frequency of your workouts, your body still isn't managing your exercise routine well and you're feeling fatigued or you and your baby aren't as healthy as you should be, talk to your healthcare provider about whether you can try a less-intense activity than the primary activity you've been doing. Table 6-1 gives you some ideas, but your healthcare provider may have others.

In order to quickly resume your training regimen after you deliver your baby, you want to work similar muscles with your alternate activity as you do with your primary activity. For example, cycling, speed-skating, and cross-country skiing all use similar muscle groups, but they use very different muscles than running, which is similar to walking and aerobics. So, if you're a speed-skater looking for an alternate activity, you want to choose cycling over walking.

For info on combining two or more activities into comprehensive workouts (that is, *cross-training*), see Chapter 17.

Table 6-1 Alternate Activities

If You Find That You Can No Longer...	*Try...*
Do step aerobics	Reducing the height of the step, switch to low-impact aerobics, or switch to a stair-stepping machine
Weight train with heavy weights, including squats, bench press, and incline bench press	Lifting lighter weights with more reps. Avoid deep-knee bends and pushing weights over your head when lying on your back or in an inclined position.
Mountain bike	Indoor cycling on a stationary bike
Perform gymnastics moves	Walking, low-impact aerobics, resistance bands, and/or weightlifting
Play soccer, basketball, or hockey	Weightlifting and either walking, using a stair-stepping machine, or using an elliptical trainer
Row	Weightlifting, swimming, and walking
Run or hike	Walking or low-impact aerobics
Ski (downhill or outdoor cross-country) or skate	Indoor cycling or a cross-country ski machine

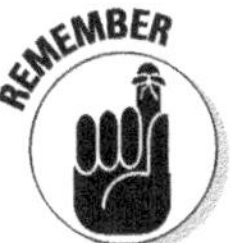

Even if you seem to be physically handling your workouts and don't want to reduce their intensity, duration, or frequency or change activities altogether, your healthcare provider may still ask you to change sports until after you deliver. This is especially true if you participate in very demanding activities like rowing and running, ball sports or contact sports that can result in blunt trauma to your baby (but may be considered okay), or activities that can result in a hard, serious fall that can hurt your baby. See Chapter 4 for additional information on sports that you may be asked to give up as your pregnancy progresses.

Easing Back into Your Routine after Delivery

As a fitness buff or competitive athlete, you may long for the day when you feel fit again, attack your workouts with vigor, and maybe even compete in your sport. Returning to your old routine will happen, but it takes time and patience. This section gives you a few tips, and Chapters 18 and 19 share even more ideas.

Take as much time as you need to get back to your old routine. Because you've likely reduced the intensity, duration, or frequency of your workouts, you'll need some time to build back up again. Most women need to take a minimum of two weeks off from exercise after the birth of their babies. This time allows you to recover from the stress of labor and delivery and allow your body to heal. In order to determine whether you're ready to get back into your exercise routine, ask yourself the following questions:

- Have you recovered from labor and delivery and do you feel ready to start exercising again?
- Is your baby feeding well, and is she on a feeding schedule that allows for a long enough break for you to exercise?
- Has your healthcare provider given you the go-ahead to start exercising?
- If you had a cesarean section or episiotomy, is your incision healed and are you able to move around comfortably and without pain?

If you feel ready to get started, start back slowly — and reduce or discontinue exercise if you experience any increase in vaginal bleeding or have pain or discomfort.

Although every woman and every pregnancy is unique, consider the following tips for a safe return to your old fitness routine:

- **Start your first postdelivery workouts as though you've never worked out before.** See Chapter 5 for some beginner's guides to working out, and follow whichever one allows you to work out without feeling any pain or significant discomfort. You may experience some muscle soreness and fatigue, but you shouldn't feel any sharp pains.
- **Increase your weekly minutes no more than 10 percent per week, no matter how antsy you feel about getting back into great shape.** This may mean that your return to your pre-pregnancy fitness level takes from four to six months.

  If you end up having a cesarean section, returning to your old exercise routine may take a couple of months longer than it will if you deliver vaginally. This timeline doesn't hold for all women, given that people heal at different rates, but is a general timeline to consider if you're trying to set goals for the year after you deliver.
- **Be cautious when stretching or doing any quick, stop-and-start movements for three to five months after delivery.** The hormone relaxin, discussed in the "Understanding Physical Changes during Pregnancy"

section earlier in this chapter, has made your ligaments and joints much less stable than they were before you were pregnant, making you more susceptible to sprains and torn ligaments.

- **Start with one high-intensity workout every one or two weeks and gradually increase to a maximum of two high-intensity days per week.** The demands of breast-feeding and new motherhood are hard enough on your body to consider doing more than two hard workouts per week at this stage.
- **Take one or two easy days (of lower intensity) after each hard workout.** Follow a hard-easy-medium-easy-hard-easy or hard-easy-easy-hard-easy-easy workout schedule.
- **If you're nursing, keep up your caloric intake so that you produce enough milk.** You may need as many as 500 more calories per day than you did before you became pregnant and started nursing. In fact, because of a nursing mother's high caloric needs, many healthcare providers recommend that you delay your full return to athletic activity if you're nursing, taking an additional four to eight weeks of low-key, gentle exercise after you deliver before turning up the intensity of your workouts. If you and your healthcare provider decide that a quicker return to your pre-pregnancy workout levels is appropriate for you, you need to ensure that you're getting enough calories and fluids (see Chapter 9). You may also require more sleep than you did before you became pregnant.
- **Don't try to lose weight too quickly, especially if you're breast-feeding.** By eating right (take a look at Chapters 9 and 10) and gradually increasing the intensity, duration, and frequency of your workouts, you'll naturally lose the weight in a relatively short time frame without dieting.

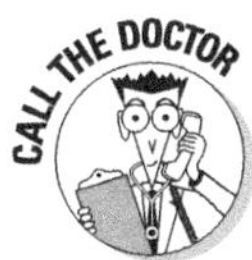

Continue to monitor your urine color, body weight, temperature, and overall physical well-being as your body returns to its pre-pregnancy state. Call your healthcare provider is your body isn't adjusting well to working out.

Chapter 7

Dressing for Success: Finding Workout Gear

In This Chapter

- Getting the right shoes
- Uncovering undergarments
- Dressing for summer and indoor activities
- Coming in from the cold with winter gear
- Finding a swimsuit that fits
- Brushing up on cycling gear

Designing, manufacturing, and selling fitness clothing is a competitive, highly profitable industry, because people — especially women — don't want to wear ratty, uncomfortable sweat pants when they work out; they want to look good and feel comfortable. Unfortunately, the industry hasn't kept up with a trend toward pregnant women working out, so the selection of pregnancy workout clothes probably isn't what you'd hoped for.

You can find a selection of clothing that's rather limited in terms of colors and styles available from companies that have made pregnancy fitness clothing a priority (see Chapter 23 for a listing). For some of your workout gear, you can (and should) buy clothing that's made specifically for pregnant women, but because it's pretty pricey and limited in its selection, you can use some non-pregnancy fitness clothes or nonfitness maternity clothes and get along just fine. This chapter helps you decide what clothing you need for the activities you have in mind.

Although this chapter covers some minor nonclothing gear, such as bike helmets and water aerobics flotation vests, this chapter isn't about larger equipment, such as bikes, weights, exercise balls, treadmills, and so on. Those items are covered in the Part IV chapters that discuss the particular activities requiring them.

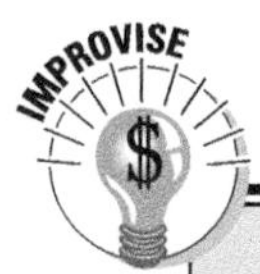

The bare necessities — a low-cost approach

The purpose of this chapter is to acquaint you with the types of clothing that people tend to buy and wear for a variety of activities. By perusing this chapter, you find out not only how to make yourself extremely comfortable while working out, but also how to carry on a fairly knowledgeable conversation with the salespeople trying to sell you this stuff.

However, you can spend a lot less money and sacrifice only a little in comfort by getting the following basic workout gear and doing away with the rest:

- **Good, sturdy shoes:** Although you'll get the best advice shopping at a specialty store for running, walking, aerobics, and so on, look for deals at nationwide sporting goods stores, such as Dunham's or MC Sporting Goods. And if you're willing to try on several pairs and go from store to store, don't rule out Target, TJ Maxx, and other discount stores.
- **Breast support:** Although a high-quality sports bra is ideal, some women find that by wearing two less-supportive bras (those found at Jockey stores and at many discount stores), they're just as comfortable and save money, too. If you're having a problem finding a comfortable bra, head to a department store that has a large lingerie department. The store may have someone on staff who is skilled in fitting bras and who may be able to help you find a bra that provides the best support.
- **Trim-fit shorts or tights:** These don't have to be intended for any particular activity or for workouts at all. Maternity shorts or tights probably fit best, but if you find something for your lower body that's comfortable during and after exercise and doesn't rub you raw with its seams, wear it. Look for *trim-fit* (close-fitting) shorts and tights in a larger size than the one you normally wear or check out the selection of men's clothing at your local discount store. Note that lightweight polyester materials tend to keep sweat away from your skin better than cotton does, so steer clear of cotton shorts.
- **A loose-fitting shirt:** This shirt can be lightweight or heavy; sleeveless, short-sleeved, or long-sleeved; with or without pockets or other decoration. As long as the seams don't rub, the shirt is the right weight for the temperature during your workout, and you're comfortable wearing the garment, a shirt doesn't have to be too technical. Many pregnant women like shopping in the men's section of discount stores to find comfortable shirts. Look for fabrics that *wick* sweat effectively, which means that they move sweat away from your body.
- **Socks:** You do need comfortable socks that soak up sweat, don't bunch up, and don't cause blisters, but you don't have to pay full price. Check out outlet stores specializing in socks, such as Socks Galore. Also check Target, Walmart, TJ Maxx, Shopko, Kmart, and other discount stores.

Sole Searching: Finding Shoes That Fit

Do you really need $100 Nike-Air-whatever shoes? Well, maybe yes, and maybe no. What you do need is the right shoe for the activity you're doing (a running shoe for running, a walking shoe for walking, an aerobic shoe for aerobics, a tennis shoe for tennis, and so on). You also need the shoe to fit your foot like a glove, which means that a shoe that's working great for your best friend or the salesclerk at the store may be all wrong for you. The perfect shoe should feel great the moment you put it on and shouldn't cause blisters, blacken your toenails, make your foot go numb, cause pain in your arch or heel, slip off your heel, or make your knee ache. (If these symptoms happen to you, you're probably wearing the wrong shoes or worn-out shoes. Take them back and ask to trade them in for a better pair.) So, if the right shoe for you costs $100, then yes, you need $100 shoes.

But if the right pair costs $45, you're getting a deal. When you go fitness shoe shopping, plan to reach that $100 mark so that you worry only about the comfort of the shoes (and not the price) as you shop. You can always celebrate later if your shoes cost substantially less.

Most major cities have at least one (if not more) running stores, which specialize in shoes, clothing, and gear for runners and — sometimes — walkers, too. That's where you want to go for running shoes and, with any luck, walking shoes. (To find a running specialty store, look in the Yellow Pages under "Running" or "Fitness" or search the Internet for running stores in your city or nearby towns.) For a good selection of aerobics shoes and tennis shoes, any sporting goods store should offer enough of a selection for you.

You need the assistance of a qualified salesperson to choose the right shoe for your activity and get the best fit, so never order your first pair or any model from a Web site or mail-order catalog. And if you're out shopping for an athletic shoe and you don't feel that the salesperson is listening to you or has enough experience to help you, make your exit. You're better off driving around a bit to find a great salesperson than getting stuck with a shoe that'll make you uncomfortable.

Throughout your first pregnancy, your shoe size will probably increase by a half size to a full size. And (we're sorry to have to be the ones to tell you this) that size will probably be your new shoe size for the rest of your life. If you're shopping for shoes early in your pregnancy, keep in mind that they probably won't fit by the second trimester, when you'll need a new pair. So, don't splurge on the first pair you buy, and assume it's going to last maybe three or four months. You can also buy a pair that's one-half to a full size larger than your normal size and wear very thick socks until your feet grow into them.

After your first trimester, buy the best pair for your feet and know that it'll last through the end of your pregnancy. Replace your athletic shoes about every six months — far more than those old loafers you've been wearing for five years — even if they don't look worn out. If you don't replace your shoes twice per year (or more often), you risk joint pain in your knees, ankles, and hips; shin pain; foot pain and/or bruises; and so on. It's like maintaining your car — do it before you need it, and you won't have any major repairs.

Making your shoes more comfortable

If your shoes used to be comfortable but aren't anymore, you're probably due for a new pair. If, however, a new pair of shoes seems almost perfect but is pinching a little or slipping off your heel, try this:

- If you feel numbness or tingling in your feet or if you're getting bruises or other soreness on the top of your feet, try relacing your shoes and skipping a few holes. Although the shoe manufacturer gives you a bunch of holes to lace through, you don't have to use them all. If your laces are too long after skipping a few holes, get yourself a shorter pair of laces and replace the ones that came with your shoes. If skipping holes doesn't relieve numbness or soreness, consider trying a wider (not longer) shoe. New Balance makes shoes of varying widths, as do some other manufacturers. Some pregnant women find that using a small *toggle* (that is, you thread the laces through it and pull to tighten instead of having to tie shoelaces) helps avoid the struggle of trying to lean over and tie your shoes late in pregnancy. Inquire at shoe stores to find a pair.
- If your shoe slips slightly off your heel with each step, try lacing through every hole as you normally would. When you're at the hole just before the top one, instead of going across the tongue to the top hole (the one closest to your ankle), loop the lace into the top hole *on the same side*. Repeat this on the other side. Now thread the ends of each lace through the tiny loop that you created on each side and tighten the laces. This may seem gimmicky and rather ridiculous, but it actually works! If this lacing trick doesn't end your heel slippage, consider trying a narrower (not shorter) shoe that some brands manufacture.
- If your shoes are pinching and the liner that comes with your shoe is replaceable (to find out, look inside your shoe, pull on the lining, and see whether it comes out), pull it out and replace it with a Spenco or other quality, cushy liner. The extra cushioning in the better liner can help alleviate the added wear and tear that pregnancy puts on your joints.

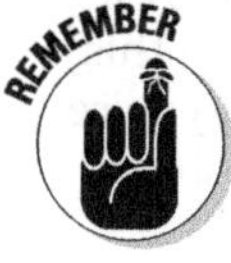

Pay special attention to the size of the *toe box* — that is, the area of a shoe that surrounds your toes — which varies greatly from shoe manufacturer to shoe manufacturer and from model to model. You want a toe box that's wide enough so that your feet don't feel pinched or go numb, but narrow enough so that your feet don't slide around and get blisters.

Getting Underneath it All: Undergarments

Although *undergarments* (the items that people don't see, such as a sports bra, underwear, and socks) aren't visible, they're extremely important for your overall comfort. If you're wearing an uncomfortable sports bra, the most comfortable T-shirt or shorts in the world isn't going to overcome the discomfort you feel because of that bra. So make the first layer you put on your most important.

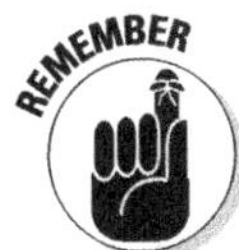

The principal element to look for in your undergarments is comfort, not fashion. After all, no one's going to see these articles of clothing except you. Also keep the following in mind as you shop:

- **Size:** Don't buy anything that feels too tight or too short. You're always better off with slightly loose clothing than gear that's too tight. If you're unsure about the fit of undergarments or haven't been able to find a comfortable sports bra or pair of maternity underwear, call your local department store to see whether they sell fitness and maternity undergarments and can size you at no extra charge. Yes, it's a little embarrassing to be poked and measured by someone you don't know, but these people know their stuff and can get you a perfect fit. Call first, though, because many department stores don't carry fitness gear, especially for pregnant women.

  Don't put a sports bra (or any bra) in the dryer — it may shrink or melt, and the elastic will wear out more quickly than normal. This goes for running shorts and cycling jerseys, too. Instead, use a clothesline or get a wooden drying rack to air-dry your delicate workout clothes.
- **Chafing points:** While standing in front of the dressing room mirror, move around to see where underwear or a sports bra may rub *(chafe)* your skin. You don't want your skin to be raw after you work out.
- **Fabric:** Everyone stopped buying polyester clothes in the late '70s, right? Well, maybe not. The truth is, the most comfortable fitness clothes have at least a percentage of polyester, sometimes under brand names like CoolMax (see the "CoolMax, DriFit, and more!" sidebar for details). The rest is usually cotton or *Lycra,* a fabric that makes clothing stretch and give a little.

CoolMax, DriFit, and more!

Is your head spinning from all the techno-names on the labels of fitness clothing? Just about every fitness clothing company has its own name for what's essentially the latest trend in workout gear: polyester clothes that breathe enough to allow air to flow through the fabric to your body and that *wick* moisture (carry moisture away from your skin) to keep you from getting clammy and cold.

CoolMax, a product from DuPont, is probably the most well known. To list every other name would take half a page, but some others include DriFit, Dryline, TransSPOR, and so on.

Keep in mind that one natural fabric — silk — is also a natural moisture-wicking product that breathes. Although it's expensive, silk will likely last longer than your CoolMax (and other brand-name) clothes, which tend to snag easily.

Sports bras

A *sports bra* (that is, a bra designed to support you during exercise) is essential for you. Not only will you gain weight in your breasts as you progress in your pregnancy, but your breasts may also be quite sore, such that any excessive motion is uncomfortable. So, to minimize the movement of your breasts as you work out, you need a well-fitted sports bra. Even if you're a small-busted woman who hasn't had to think much about bras in the past, you will now that you're pregnant.

Most sports bras are made of polyester and spandex, with a nylon/spandex lining, which really is comfortable. Look for wide, comfortable straps and buy the biggest size you can find that still gives you support, because a tight sports bra interferes with your breathing and blood circulation. Don't buy a running bra that makes you gasp for breath when you try it on, but do make sure that you feel supported. If necessary, take a brisk walk around the store with your sports bra on to see whether you feel supported. You may find yourself gasping at the price, though: Most cost between $25 and $40 at department stores, fitness stores, and running shops. Although you may be able to find comfortable, sturdy sports bras at a reduced price at some discount stores (such as TJ Maxx), the bras at discounters Walmart and Target generally don't offer the support you need while pregnant.

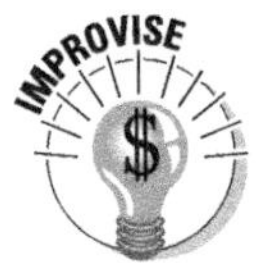

Instead of buying one very-expensive sports bra made of high-tech fabrics, some women wear two lower-cost cotton/nylon bras on top of each other to get great support without tight straps. Be sure to try on both bras together before you buy them, just to make sure they're not too tight.

Don't buy too many bras at one time — stick with one or two, because your breast size will change throughout each trimester. Plan now to go bra shopping at the beginning of each trimester or at any time that your sports bra feels too tight or unsupportive. You may, after you deliver, be able to go back to your pre-pregnancy or first-trimester bras, but many women find that some increase in breast size is permanent, so chances are that your second-trimester bras will fit best after you deliver your baby.

Some sports bras are also *nursing bras* (bras that easily fold down for nursing), which is really convenient if you're planning to nurse your baby. If you choose this option for your third-trimester bras, you may not need to buy additional nursing bras after your baby is born. Be sure the nursing sports bra really is a sports bra, though: Nursing bras are sometimes less supportive than sports bras, so be careful that one bra adequately does both jobs well.

Briefs

Briefs — a more polite way to say underwear or panties — aren't usually mentioned in polite society, but they can make a big difference in how you feel during your fit pregnancy. For the first trimester, you'll probably be able to wear the briefs you've been wearing, keeping in mind that cotton underwear is usually more comfortable than silky, polyester briefs; pure silk briefs are far and away the most comfortable. Although cotton briefs are fine for most sports, you don't want to wear them when cycling, because they quickly get soaked with sweat. Instead, most cyclists don't wear briefs at all or wear a very thin liner underneath cycling shorts (see the "Cycling shorts" section later in this chapter for details).

For your second and third trimesters, look for special maternity briefs, which accommodate your expanding abdomen with extra fabric (like a pouch for your belly) and a wide, comfortable waistband that fits either above or below your belly. Maternity briefs are available anywhere you find maternity clothing, even if the store or catalog doesn't sell pregnancy workout gear. Maternity briefs run from $5 to $20, depending on the quality of the material you choose.

Socks

As your body weight increases, the pressure on your feet increases, too, and all that's between you and the hard floor or ground are your shoes and a pair of socks. If you're doing any activity that pounds your feet on the ground (walking, running, weightlifting, stair-stepping, or aerobics, for example), take your socks seriously. For other activities that don't have that kind of pounding (cycling, swimming, and so on), just buy a six-pack of socks at your local discount store and call it a day.

Really good workout socks that you find in a specialty fitness store cost a bundle — sometimes $5 or $6 *each pair!* — but we recommend getting five or six pair, if you can. If not, ask the salesperson whether a multipack of socks is available that can cut down on the cost or whether he or she can recommend a cheaper substitute. Specifically, you're looking for the following features:

- **Weight:** You want the bottom portion of your socks to be cushioned and meaty. The extra thickness helps absorb some of the shock to your feet and legs.
- **Fabric:** You want at least some of the fabric to be made of CoolMax, a product from DuPont that wicks moisture away from your body and keeps your feet cool and dry (see the "CoolMax, DriFit, and more!" sidebar earlier in this chapter). The remainder of the fabric should be a blend of cotton (which absorbs moisture) and stretchy nylon or Lycra (which help socks retain their shape). Some people also like wool in their workout socks, although a substantial wool component can make socks a little hot in summertime.
- **Style:** For the most part, you want to wear ankle socks or footies that come pretty high on the ankle. If you work out outside and you're ever even slightly cold, make sure that whatever style you buy covers each

foot's *Achilles tendon* (the back of your foot between your ankle and your heel), because your Achilles can become injured if it gets too cold before or during a workout. Calf socks or knee socks aren't a good idea, because they can worsen varicose veins, a problem some pregnant women experience.

- **Size:** Buy socks according to your shoe size (a chart on the sock label usually tells you how the sock size relates to shoe size), looking at the label to make sure it's labeled "women's." (Men's and women's sock sizes are on two different scales.) Most women buy socks that are labeled with a "9–11" sock size.

Timing Yourself with a Sports Watch

If you work out on a machine or near a large clock (as is often the case in a pool), you don't need a sports watch. But if you walk or run outdoors (treadmills have timers built in) or do any other sort of activity that you want to time, stop by a sporting goods store or department store and get a name-brand watch (Timex, Casio, and so on) that suits your needs. You don't have to spend a lot, but don't buy a $10 watch that has an irreplaceable battery, because you'll just end up throwing the thing away in six months. If you watch the sales, you can probably find a simple name-brand watch for under $25 with a battery that will last about two years and can be replaced for $5 or less.

If you're considering buying a sports watch, you really don't need much: Look for one that has both a clock and a stopwatch and has a large, easy-to-read display so that a quick glance at it while you're exercising tells you how much time has passed. Some watches also have interval or lap timers and alarm clocks, but you probably won't use these features much.

Playing It Cool: Finding Summer and Indoor Gear

If you've shopped for summer and indoor pregnancy workout gear, you may be surprised at how little variety is out there. You can find comfortable clothing by contacting the companies listed in Chapter 23, but you'll be choosing from among one or two colors for each style. And because of the relative lack of competition in this industry, prices are still pretty high, although quality and comfort are quite good.

On the other hand, just about every major discount and department store carries well-priced maternity wear, some of which you can wear for working out.

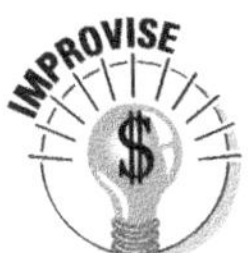

Instead of buying lots of workout clothes, consider buying a few high-quality items and airing them out or giving them a quick washout every day or two. You'll have to do a little more work than if you bought lots of different gear and threw it in the laundry basket every day, but you'll also spend a lot less.

As you consider the gear you need, look for items made of cotton, Lycra, and a pinch of polyester — that usually makes for the most comfortable clothing. Also steer clear of wild colors, which may not look great on you right now. Basic blues and blacks give an appealing, slimming look.

Running and walking shorts

Running shorts (which are also used for walking) are made of thin, lightweight material that doesn't cling to your legs as you sweat — see Figure 7-1. They range from short-shorts, which you probably have no interest in, to baggier, longer shorts that hit an inch or two above the knee, plus several lengths in between.

If you're going to be running or walking, get a couple pairs of maternity running shorts from one of the fitness pregnancy companies listed in Chapter 23. (You can also wear your partner's running shorts, but they look a little goofy, and the narrow elastic band may be uncomfortable on your waist.) Look for the thinnest material you can find, because they'll drape best on your legs as you walk or run. Plan to spend (gulp!) from $25 to $40 per pair.

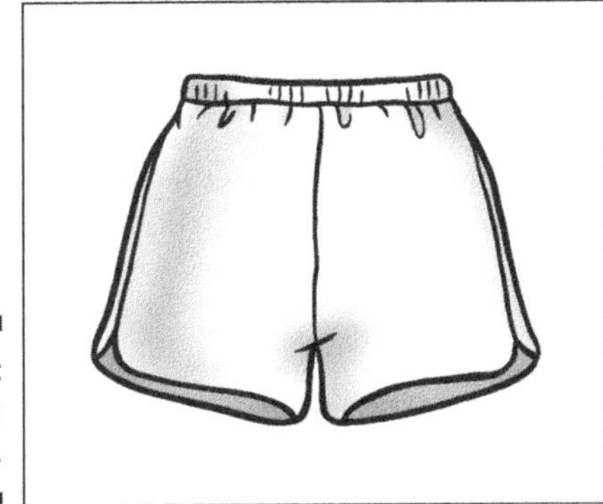

Figure 7-1: Running shorts.

Fitness shorts

Fitness shorts actually look a lot like cycling shorts (see the "Cycling shorts" section, later in this chapter), but they're made of a lighter-weight material than cycling shorts and are less padded. Fitness shorts are long, tight-fitting shorts that hit just at or above the knee (see Figure 7-2). You can wear fitness shorts alone or under traditional running shorts (so that less of your legs show when walking or running). These shorts work well for aerobics, yoga, and any of the exercise machines discussed in Chapter 16, and some people like them for running or walking, although they're usually less comfortable than running shorts because they can get heavy with sweat.

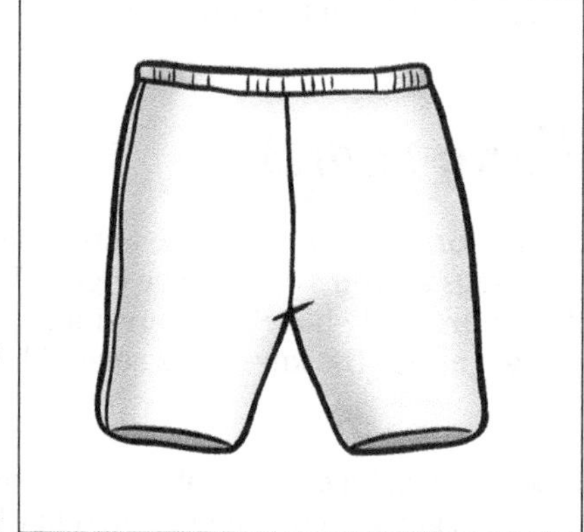

Figure 7-2: Fitness shorts.

Look for fitness shorts made from cotton and Lycra/spandex/Tactel (one or all those names may appear on the label). Don't bother with these shorts unless the ones you buy are specifically made for pregnant women — the nonpregnancy kind will ride up as your abdomen expands. The ones you buy should have an extra fabric pouch for your belly, along with a nice, wide waistband that doesn't pinch or bunch up. Most pregnant women prefer dark colors — navy blue or black — because they give a leaner line.

If you're thinking of getting a pair of fitness shorts, first try a unitard (see the following section), which has a similar fit as fitness shorts, but eliminates the need for a waistband of any kind.

Unitards: Onesies for women

A *unitard* is a one-piece item that combines shorts and a top into one (see Figure 7-3). The top portion is generally shaped like a tank top; the bottom portion can be long (down to the ankles) or short (hitting just above the knee). Many pregnant women buy one of each (long and short) and use them extensively throughout their pregnancies.

Gym bags that work

If you're working out at a gym or taking a fitness class after work, you need a bag that's large enough for your gear and a few other odds and ends. Consider the following when choosing your bag, which can run from $15 to $90:

- **Stay on your own side.** Look for a bag with a separate compartment for wet gear: a swimsuit, sweaty workout wear, or a wet towel. If bags with this feature are too expensive for you, tuck a couple of large resealable bags in your gym bag and stick your wet workout clothes in them before heading home.
- **Keep shoes down below.** Look for a bag with a separate area for shoes — often an extra compartment under the bottom of the bag that zips open and closed. In lieu of this feature, put your shoes in a plastic grocery bag to keep dirt and other gunk out of the rest of your bag.
- **Open wide.** Gym bags with a wide mouth (think of a carpenter's bag or doctor's house-call bag) are very convenient, because you can see everything in your bag — your balled up socks can't hide in the corner. Wide-mouth bags tend to be the most expensive gym bags on the market, so before spending money on this style, stop by your local hardware or Sears store and look at their wide-mouth tool bags. They often go on sale for $10 to $20, and many have enough amenities to make good gym bags.
- **Get a slim fit.** If you're locking up your valuables at the gym, make sure the bag you choose fits into the gym's lockers. This may mean that, if you're choosing from among several sizes of bags, you choose the smallest.
- **Strap on a mat.** If you're taking yoga and carry your mat with you, look for a bag that has outside straps for a mat. Check your local yoga specialty store or search online for yoga bags, and you'll find several bags that offer such options.
- **Let your back do the work.** If you're walking a long distance, consider getting a backpack instead of a gym bag. It doesn't have to be designed specifically as a gym bag, because even generic backpacks have at least two compartments (useful for separating shoes and wet clothes from dryer, cleaner items), and some have several smaller compartments that can hold everything from a wallet to keys to toiletries.
- **Make your shower efficient.** If you shower before heading home or to work, pick up a small toiletry bag for your shampoo, skin care, and cosmetics. In a pinch, you can put these items into a resealable bag, but you'll lose time fumbling around trying to find the item you need. Some gym bags also have built-in sections for your toiletries.

Unitards are incredibly popular for pregnant women because, by combining the top and bottom into one unit, you eliminate the need for a waistband, which is the feature of clothing that's often the most uncomfortable during pregnancy. They also create a long, slimming line, and the long ones never cut into your thighs. And if you don't like the idea of wearing a tank top, you can always wear a T-shirt over your unitard.

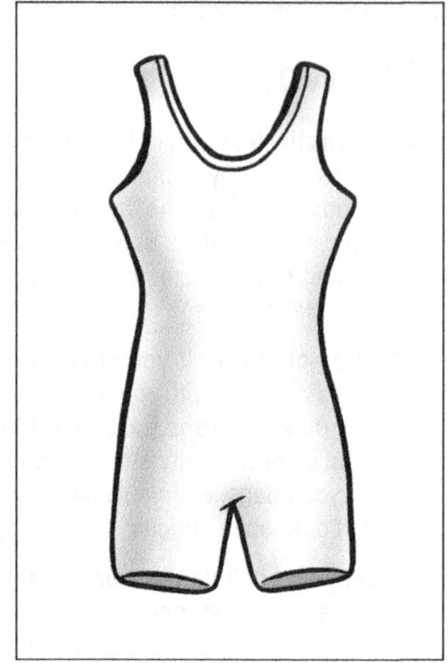

Figure 7-3: Unitard.

One downside to unitards is that they can be a pain to use when you have to go to the bathroom, and if you're like most pregnant women, you may feel the need to urinate pretty often, especially late in pregnancy. In order to take a simple bathroom break, you have to peel off the entire unitard.

If you're shopping at a fitness pregnancy company or store (see Chapter 23), your options in unitards will be limited to one or two styles, probably in black. When ordering from a catalog or the Internet, you may want to order more than one size and return those that don't fit you as well. Sizing is generally based on your pre-pregnancy size (so if you're a size 10 before pregnancy, you order a size 10 maternity unitard), although some come listed only as small, medium, large, and extra large. If that's the case, ask for assistance at the store or call the 800 number associated with the catalog or Web site.

T-shirts and tank tops

T-shirts and tank tops make up the bulk of your fitness wardrobe, and you probably want as many as the number of days per week you work out. Whereas sports bras, running shorts, and unitards can be worn for several days in a row without getting smelly or can be rinsed out and worn again the next day, you'll probably be most comfortable getting out a new T-shirt or tank top for each day's workout and washing them all at the end of the week.

Look for T-shirts and tank tops made of lightweight cotton or cotton with a touch of polyester. Heavy cotton T-shirts and tank tops are usually too warm for summer and indoor workouts.

Sun-protective clothing, like those made by Solumbra (`www.sunprecautions.com`), Coolibar (`www.coolibar.com`), and Solar Eclipse (`www.solareclipse.com`) offer excellent sun protection. Products range from hats and shirts to swimsuits and pants, and they block skin's exposure to the sun's harmful effects as well as or better than sunscreen does (especially given that sunscreen wears off as you sweat). Keep in mind, however, that only the parts of your body that the special clothing covers are protected from the sun.

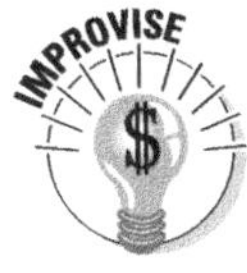

Some women wear their partner's shirts while pregnant, and this is an easy way to save money. Be careful, though, of tank tops that droop so low in the chest and armholes that you feel as though you're wearing nothing at all! You may also be able to get away with wearing maternity T-shirts that aren't necessarily meant for working out, especially if the material is a lightweight cotton that feels comfortable when you try it on. These can be a bargain at discount stores. Cut off any trim that can get caught on an exercise machine, however.

Most sports bras are designed to be worn alone, without a shirt over them, so if you're comfortable wearing just a sports bra, dispense with the T-shirt completely. If you're exercising outside, be sure to wear sunscreen, and put on a T-shirt after your workout if you start to get chilled by wind or indoor air conditioning.

Playing Outside: Rain and Winter Gear

If you're walking or doing any other safe outdoor activity during winter, be sure to use layers of clothing instead of, say, a heavy parka. If the weather is exceedingly cold, your first layer may be a turtleneck, followed by a long-sleeve T-shirt or thin sweat shirt, topped by a lightweight jacket. You may also want to wear two pairs of socks to keep your toes cozy. In slightly warmer weather, you may not need the second layer and may be able to wear a vest instead of a jacket. Using layers in this way allows air to move around your body so you don't overheat as you sweat.

Long-sleeved T-shirts and turtlenecks

If you're going to work out in breezy or even cold weather, purchase a few long-sleeved maternity T-shirts and turtlenecks wherever you buy maternity clothes. Look for lightweight cotton shirts that give you some room in your belly.

Tuck the layer of clothing that rests against your skin into your running pants or tights (see the "Tights and pants" section). This way, wind can't get up under your shirt and give you a bad chill. And when you get back home or to your office, immediately remove the layer closest to your body — especially if it's made of cotton — to get your skin warm and dry.

Many people believe that cotton is a no-no during winter, preferring CoolMax or silk long-sleeved Ts and turtlenecks under a jacket, because they pull moisture from your skin as you sweat. In extreme winter conditions (temperatures in the teens, single digits, and below zero), cotton does tend to quickly fill with sweat, making you damp and cold. In those conditions, silk clothing and polyester fitness products, discussed in the "CoolMax, DriFit, and more!" sidebar, keep you most comfortable. You'll probably feel as though you have too little on when you start your workout, but within a few minutes, you'll warm up. When temperatures are in the 20s, 30s, and above, cotton tends to work well for a lot of people. It still gets a little damp, but the thicker material makes you more comfortable when you're starting out, and you won't get a chill from the slightly damp clothes, because the temperature is relatively warm. Most experts recommend that you wear a moisture-wicking fabric, but you can decide what works best for you.

Jackets and vests

If you're going to be exercising on moderately cold days with occasional rain, a nylon jacket or vest may be all you need. (A *vest* is simply a sleeveless version of a jacket.) Buy an unhooded, lightweight jacket — preferably one meant for maternity or a size larger than your normal size — and wear it over a long-sleeved T-shirt, not a short-sleeved T. (Wearing nylon over a short-sleeved T-shirt — or on any bare skin — can be uncomfortably sweaty.)

If you live in an excessively rainy or very cold area, however, consider investing in a GoreTex jacket or both a GoreTex jacket and pants. GoreTex is a waterproof, windproof, and extremely breathable fabric that makes all but the most severe weather comfortable for exercising outdoors. GoreTex is the best-known brand of waterproof, breathable fabrics, but it's not the only one — ask whether a store or Web site sells other brands.

GoreTex is really expensive. Although you can find sales in February or March, regular prices start at about $150 and go up to about $250; GoreTex competitors may cost a little less. Because they're so expensive and can last for a decade or more, you want to avoid buying a maternity GoreTex jacket. If possible, get one that fits your partner, with the understanding that next winter, he'll wear that one, and you'll get a new one!

Tights and pants

Fitness tights are silky, lightweight, and made of tight-fitting Lycra/spandex. They're much thicker than the tights you wear under a skirt; they're more like thick leggings, but are made of materials that keep you dry and comfortable during a workout. Some fitness tights also have zippers on the lower backs of the legs that make putting them on and taking them off an easy task. Fitness tights fit snugly around your butt and legs, so most pregnant women wear them with a baggy shirt over the top. Maternity versions of tights are readily available — see Chapter 23 for details.

Before investing in maternity fitness tights, which cost from $25 to $60, consider getting a long unitard, which is like fitness tights and a tank top all in one. (See the "Unitards: Onesies for women" section.) Although unitards are more expensive than tights, most women find them more comfortable, because unitards don't have a waistband that rests on your belly.

Running pants (also called *fitness pants, exercise pants,* and plain-old *pants*) are like tights but are usually much thicker, so they're perfect for cold-weather walking. They're also baggier and don't have the sheen that tights often have, making them a little more attractive on pregnant women. Several of the companies in Chapter 23 offer excellent maternity versions; one even offers a during-and-after pant that fits (logically enough) during and after your pregnancy.

Another kind of pant is the kind that makes up the bottom half of a wind suit; the top half of the suit is a jacket. These are also called *wind pants* and are usually made of nylon, which you may want to avoid because of the swish-swish-swish sound they make with each step. (Wind pants also come in GoreTex, which is warmer and doesn't usually swish.) Wind pants range in price from $40 for nylon to $150 for GoreTex.

Hat, gloves, and a facemask

If you're planning to exercise outdoors during colder winter months and have gotten the go-ahead from your healthcare provider, invest in a pair of lightweight gloves or mittens and a lightweight hat. If you try to use the same wool hat and leather gloves that you use for nonathletic time spent outdoors, you may experience two problems:

- Your hat and gloves may smell sweaty when you want to wear them out to dinner.
- The heavy hat and gloves you need when you're cold and not working out are usually far too hot to wear during a workout, when you're raising your body temperature and sweating.

Even if you don't think you'll need a hat and gloves, take them with you in your pocket so you have them in case you do need them.

One of the best resources for lightweight hats and gloves is a specialty running store in your area; most stores carry several brands that you can try on. Expect to pay about $10 each for a basic fitness hat and well-fitting, lightweight gloves.

If you live in a severely cold area, consider getting fitness mittens, which are warmer than gloves because your fingers get to stay together and generate heat. Hind, a division of Saucony, sells a WindJammer Mitt that works almost miraculously to keep your hands warm. They look lightweight and flimsy, but they do an excellent job of keeping you warm. Plan to spend about $20.

If you live in a really cold area, you may also need a *face mask* or *balaclava* (like a ski mask, but made of much thinner material) to cover your entire face except your eyes (some even have holes for your nostrils and mouth) — see Figure 7-4. Look for one that's lightweight, not too tight, and that pulls down over your head so that you don't have to mess with fastening it every time. Don't think that you'll need a heavy one to protect from the wind and cold — you'll just end up ripping it off your face partway through the workout because it's so hot and stifling. Instead, look for one made of nylon, polyester, and spandex and plan to spend $15 to $25.

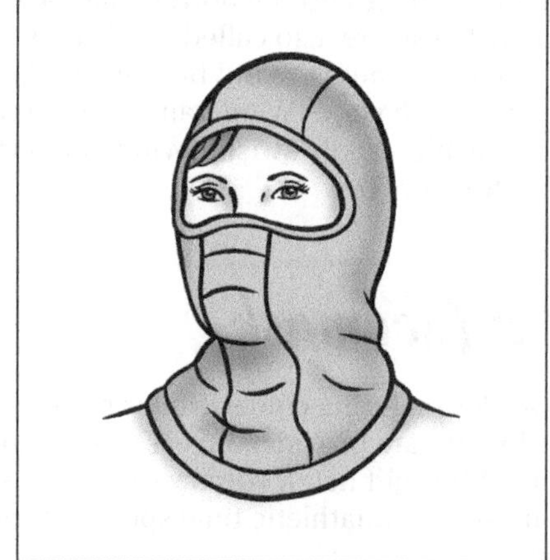

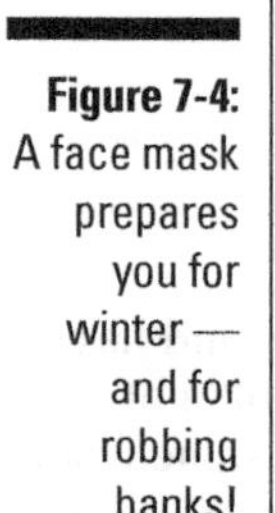

Figure 7-4: A face mask prepares you for winter — and for robbing banks!

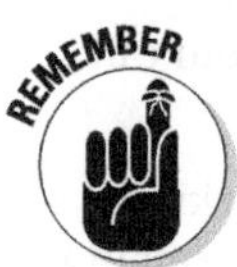

Always wear a hat in cold weather, even if you don't like the way your hair looks when you take your hat off. You lose about 50 percent of your body heat through the top of your head.

Water, Water Everywhere: Swimming and Water Aerobics Gear

If you've chosen swimming as your pregnancy fitness activity, you need only a well-fitting swimsuit and, if you want, goggles and a swim cap. For water aerobics, however, you may need additional products, ranging from a buoyancy belt (which helps you stay afloat and vertical) to hand weights. This section fills you in on the various water-related fitness equipment, shares some tips on buying each, and gives you some idea of what prices to expect.

Swimsuits

Swimming is an outstanding way to stay in shape while you're pregnant (see Chapter 13), but in order to take up or continue swimming, you need a maternity swimsuit as your pregnancy progresses. You may be able to wear your existing suit through your first trimester, although some women find that a nonmaternity suit gets a little uncomfortable as early as the beginning of the third month. You can find a pretty decent variety of suits for pregnant women, but many aren't for working out — they're for cavorting on the beach. Look for one that's specifically meant for working out, because it'll *chafe* (rub) less and be far more comfortable when you're swimming.

Look for a thick, quality fabric that will withstand frequent use and pool chemicals. The color isn't all that important, although many pregnant women feel most comfortable in navy blue and black. If you want to liven up your wardrobe, however, lots of prints in hot colors are available. Expect to spend between $25 (a bargain!) and $90 for a well-made, comfortable suit that you can use throughout your pregnancy.

Suits come in one piece or two:

- One-piece suits are shaped much like nonpregnancy suits, but with a pouch belly area for your expanding abdomen.
- Two-piece suits for working out usually consist of a bottom piece that looks like a traditional one-piece bottom (with a wide waistband that fits under or over the belly), paired with a top piece that fits all the way over your belly and overlaps a bit with the bottom piece.

The legs are cut with the same options as nonpregnancy suits — high (or French cut), medium, or low — and may include some ruffles or other trim, which can't hurt you, but won't wear well with repeated workouts and exposure to chlorine.

Look for a suit with a *shelf bra* (which is like a built-in sports bra), especially one that has a wide elastic band. If you don't think you're getting enough support for your breasts with the built-in bra, try a *racer-back* swimsuit style: two thick straps that crisscross on the upper back portion of your suit.

Look for a nylon/spandex swimsuit because it keeps its color well in chlorine. Be sure, however, to rinse out your suit with tap water after every use, hanging it up to dry. Every few rinsings, also wash with a gentle detergent. Forgetting to rinse your suit means that the chlorine will be trapped in the fibers of your suit, which quickly breaks down elastic.

Goggles and a swim cap

Goggles aren't a necessity, but they allow you to open your eyes underwater without discomfort. Goggles look a bit like glasses, but they strap on with elastic that wraps around your head, and the eyepieces are surrounded by plastic or rubber that keeps water out of your eyes. A good pair of goggles runs from about $7 to $20 and has the following features:

- **It keeps water out.** Silly as this sounds, some goggles allow water to seep under the rubber gasket that goes around the eyepieces. Before buying, ask whether the goggles are waterproof, and be sure you can return the goggles if they leak.
- **It's comfortable.** If you can't forget about your goggles while working out, you won't have a very intensive workout. Along with the eyepieces and head strap, make sure the nosepiece fits comfortably when you try each pair on in the store.
- **It doesn't fog up.** The purpose of goggles is to be able to see underwater; if they fog up, you can't see! Wear the goggles in the store for five or ten minutes to determine whether they fog up.

You can even get prescription goggles, which allow you to see in focus as you work out.

Whether to wear a swim cap is up to you (or may be a pool rule). If you have long hair, though, you may find that wearing a cap is more comfortable than not wearing one. Caps also protect your hair from chlorine, and most caps cover the ears, keeping them dry.

Made of latex, rubber, silicone, Lycra, or fabric (silicone being the most durable), swim caps also come with a chin-strap option, which helps hold the cap in place. Some also come with an inner seal that makes the cap extremely watertight. They cost from $8 to $25, depending on the material used to make them.

Water vest, weights, and shoes

If you're planning only to swim in water, you can do without any gear beyond a swimsuit and, if you choose, goggles and a swim cap. But to do water aerobics (see Chapter 13), your instructor may tell you that you need some of or all the following:

- **Buoyancy belt (also called water vest or flotation vest):** A buoyancy belt (see Figure 7-5) is made of a buoyant foam material that fits like a large belt around your back and belly. The belt keeps you afloat (with your head and shoulders above water) and in a vertical position as you work out. Buoyancy belts range in price from $25 to $60 and don't restrict your movements at all. Most pregnant women find that the AquaJogger Shape buoyancy belt, which is designed for women and has a four-inch longer wrap-around than other belts, is the most comfortable belt available. Ask for it by name at your local fitness store or shop online: It costs around $50.

  Some buoyancy belts are also shaped like a belt, but instead of being a consistent five- or six-inch thickness around your back and abdomen, these belts rise a little higher in the back (see Figure 7-5). These belts have better buoyancy and are meant for people with very little body fat who tend to sink in water.

  Some instructors prefer that you use a *flotation collar,* which wraps around your neck and keeps only your head above water. If you can, though, steer clear: Many people find that wrapping a flotation device around the neck feels a bit like being choked.

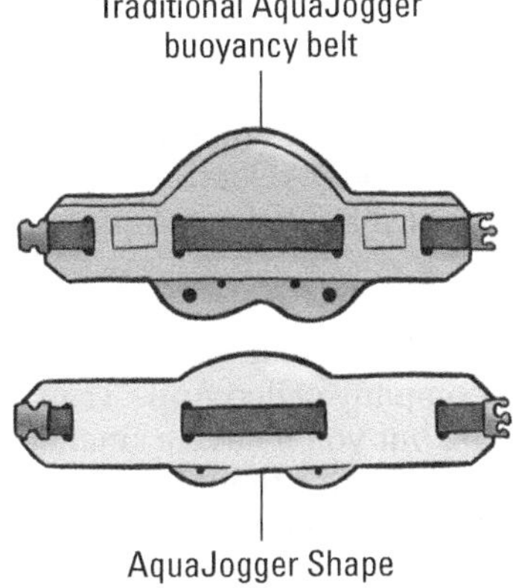

Figure 7-5: Buoyancy belts.

- **Webbed gloves:** Webbed gloves (also called water mitts), both those with full fingers and without, provide additional resistance as you move through the water, giving your arms, shoulders, chest, and back a better workout. Webbed gloves, shown in Figure 7-6, are quite thin and comfortable, so you have a full range of motion in your hands. They cost about $20 for a pair.
- **Water hand weights:** Water hand weights (also called dumbbells), which look a lot like standard hand weights (see Figure 7-6) but are buoyant and made of foam and other waterproof materials, range in weight and in how much resistance they provide. They cost from $20–$35 per pair and help sculpt your upper body.
- **Water or flotation shoes (also called aqua runners or aqua cuffs):** Water shoes (shown in Figure 7-6) do for your legs what gloves and weights do for your upper body: increase the resistance as you move through the water, thereby giving your lower body a better workout. The shoes slip on or attach with Velcro, depending on the style you choose. A pair costs $20–25.

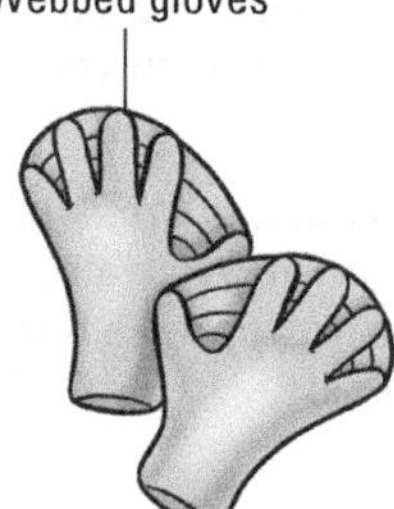

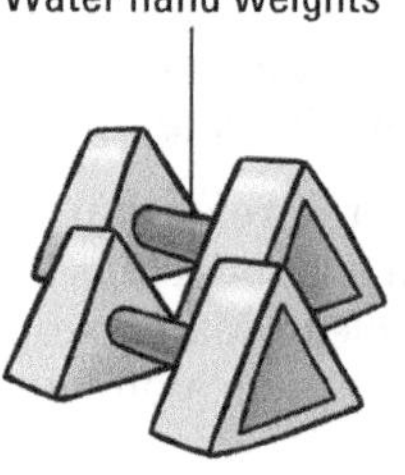

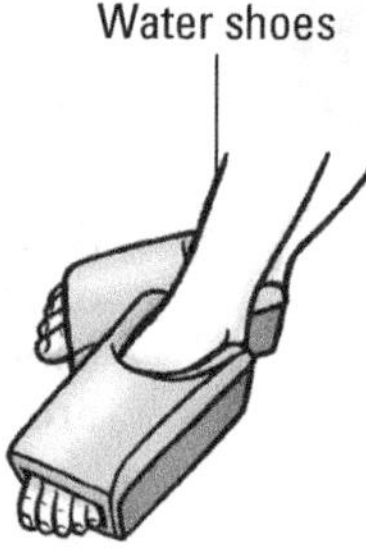

Figure 7-6: Water aerobics equipment: Gloves, weights, and shoes.

Most sporting goods and discount stores carry some water aerobics products, but don't be surprised if you find a poor selection. Consider ordering online from Kmart (`www.kmart.com`) or directly from AquaJogger (`www.fitdirect.com`).

Although AquaJogger is the undisputed leader in water products, don't overlook the flotation belt offered by a company called Aqua Trim. It's not quite as durable as AquaJogger's products, but you'll have a smaller upfront investment, because the company's prices are lower than AquaJogger's. Do a Web search for **Aqua Trim**, and you'll find numerous companies selling the company's products.

Your instructor may also ask you to invest in a *kickboard* (a buoyant board that keeps you afloat so that you can work out your legs), which you can get at any sporting goods store and which may be available to borrow at the pool you use.

Coming to Love Cycling Gear — Even Skin-Tight Shorts

Cycling has its own gear, all of which is designed to make you more comfortable, prevent chafing, and ease soreness. This section explains basic cycling clothing and other gear and tells you whether special maternity options are available.

You can buy all sorts of accessories for your bike, from water-bottle and tire-pump holders (plus the water bottles and tire pumps themselves) to a variety of sizes and styles of packs to carry stuff on your bike, such as locks, toolkits, and map holders. Given that your healthcare provider will probably ask you to train indoors on a stationary bike by the second trimester, this sort of gear is something to think about for the future, but not necessarily for now. In the meantime, start looking for an indoor bike — see Chapter 15.

Most fitness cyclists don't need *cycling shoes,* which are special, lightweight leather shoes that clip to your bike pedal and give you much more power with each push. (Note that these shoes are nearly impossible to walk around in after you get off your bike, although a few companies now make biking shoes that you don't have to hobble around in.) After you deliver your baby, you may want to consider getting cycling shoes if you're getting serious about cycling (that is, if you're training for long distances or are considering racing), but while you're pregnant and have your healthcare provider's okay to cycle outdoors, you're better off in regular shoes, because in a pinch you can easily get your foot off the pedal and onto the ground (instead of your foot being clipped to the pedal by the shoe). The same goes for *toe clips,* which are metal pieces on the front of pedals into which you can slip non-cycling shoes and get some of the same extra push that cycling shoes provide. In a pinch, though, your foot can get stuck in the toe clips, leaving you to fall over sideways.

Bike Nashbar (www.nashbar.com) has been an excellent source of cycling gear for decades, much of it at discount prices. The company doesn't sell any maternity clothing per se, but it offers such a wide range of sizes that you may be able to find clothing that works for you. Performance Bike (www.performancebike.com) is another great resource for cycling gear.

Cycling shorts

Cycling shorts, shown in Figure 7-7, are designed to pad your legs, crotch, and butt in the areas that tend to rub against the seat of the bike as you ride (the padding in the crotch of cycling shorts is often called the *chamois*). Cycling shorts also don't have seams where you tend to chafe. Made of moisture-wicking material, plus Lycra for stretchiness, everything about cycling shorts is tight, because cyclists want to keep wind out of the shorts and have the wind flow easily around the shorts, instead. In fact, most cyclists don't wear underwear when they cycle in order to keep their shorts as close to the body as possible and to prevent moisture from gathering in the underwear. Some, however, do wear a liner that is long and seamless, like the shorts themselves.

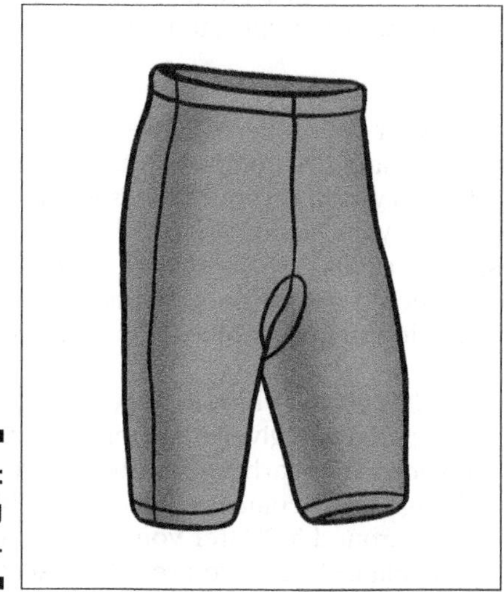

Figure 7-7: Cycling shorts.

Although you can find plenty of cycling shorts designed just for women, the problem with wearing regular biking shorts while pregnant is that they ride up as your belly expands. Chapter 23 shares the names of some companies that sell maternity versions of what they call cycling shorts (also called *biking shorts*), but they're often not well padded, making them identical to fitness shorts (see the "Fitness shorts" section earlier in this chapter). Although wearing fitness shorts as you ride is preferable to wearing anything shorter (such as running shorts) that can leave bare skin rubbing against the bike seat (and cause terrible chafing), true cycling shorts are even better because of the additional padding they provide for your inner thighs and butt. Expect to pay $25 to $50 for maternity or nonpregnancy cycling shorts.

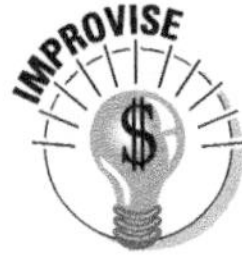

Baggy cycling shorts are becoming more and more popular for fitness cyclists, and if you can't find maternity cycling shorts, baggy cycling shorts may be comfortable for you. They're still padded in all the right places; they just aren't skin tight, so the waistband won't be as tight on your belly. If you're experiencing some chafing with baggy shorts, you have two options: Use a liner underneath the shorts (but this liner has a waistband that will be tight on your belly) and/or rub petroleum jelly on the spots where you're chafing before you set out on a ride.

You can also wear a unitard when you ride, but you may find that because your legs rub against the seat, your expensive unitard may soon wear in those areas. Also, cycling shorts come in long (down to the ankle) versions for cold-weather riding, but long cycle pants in maternity sizes is a rare find.

Cycling jerseys

Cycling jerseys, which are really just shirts designed for biking (see Figure 7-8), aren't the most attractive articles of clothing on the planet. Usually made of a polyester material that wicks moisture away from your skin, cycling jerseys are always longer in the back than in the front (because, as you lean over on your bike, a standard shirt pulls up in the back and exposes a line of skin), nearly always have a zipper in the front that runs from the top at your throat all the way below your sports bra (you can unzip this as you ride if you get too hot), often sport wild prints, and sometimes have one or two pockets in the lower back portion (for storing snacks). Most cyclists wear them skintight to reduce *drag* (the effect of wind slowing them down), although you can sometimes find varieties that look more like T-shirts that you can wear in a store without looking too out of place. Plan to spend from $25 to $50 for each jersey.

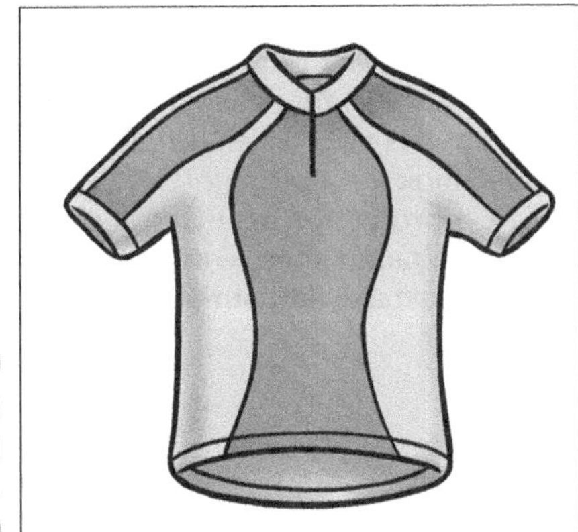

Figure 7-8: Cycling jersey.

If your healthcare provider has asked you to cycle indoors, you probably don't need one of these lovely jerseys, but if you're cycling outdoors, your ride will be far more comfortable if you invest in one or two. Look for synthetic fabrics (natural fabrics will retain moisture and become heavy with sweat), a comfortable fit, and enough length to cover your tush when you lean forward on your bike.

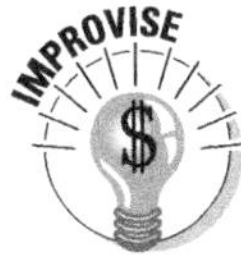

If you can't find cycling jerseys for pregnant women, consider buying one for fuller-figured women. You'll get the roominess you need.

Cycling jerseys also come in long-sleeved versions for colder days (they're too hot for summer training), and the cost starts at around $30. You can also buy a cycling *shell* — a windbreaker that's cut longer in the back — starting at $30 and going up to $200 for a completely water-repellent, yet breathable one. Many are super-compactable, so they fit easily into a bag attached to your bike.

Helmets

A bike helmet (see Figure 7-9) can save your life if you're thrown from your bike or involved in any sort of accident, making it the single most important piece of cycling equipment you can own. A helmet not only can save your life, but it also can reduce the risk of head injury by as much as 85 percent. Given what you've already invested in your bike, a helmet is an additional expense that isn't easy to swallow ($50 for last year's model, on sale, up to $150 for a fancy-schmancy racing type), but think of your investment in your helmet as life and accident insurance.

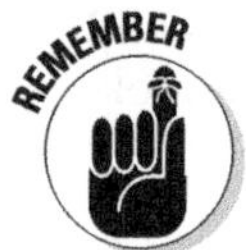

If your healthcare provider has asked you to ride indoors throughout your pregnancy, you don't need a helmet. After all, a helmet is meant to protect you if you fall, and the purpose of riding indoors is so that you don't fall!

When trying on helmets, keep in mind that the fit is everything — helmets don't protect the way they should if they don't fit properly. Pass on any helmet that doesn't fit snugly against your head, even if it does look totally cool. Most people prefer a helmet that has vent holes drilled throughout it — this keeps you cool as you ride. Also look for a rating of *Snell B95 Label of Certification,* which gives you the best protection against injury. If you're at a cycle shop, have someone on the store's staff show you how to properly fit your helmet and instruct you on how to make adjustments.

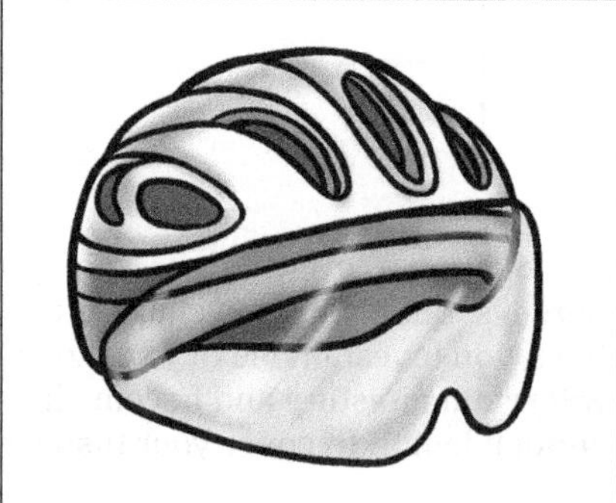

Figure 7-9: This cycling helmet has a shield to protect against sunlight and bugs.

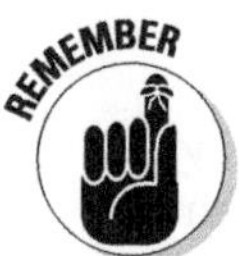

Your helmet won't last forever, because its cushioning ability is based on a foam core that breaks down over time. Think about getting a new one every four years or so; more often if yours is exposed to heat for long periods of time. Also replace yours if you take a fall and your helmet is hit hard or cracked.

If you're riding outdoors, you may also want to invest in a *windscreen* or *sports shield* (shown attached to the front of the helmet in Figure 7-9). This attachment not only reduces the glare of the sun but also keeps wind, dust, and debris from getting into your eyes as you ride. Sunglasses can have the same effect, as long as they provide some coverage around the sides of your eyes and not just on the fronts. You can also get a rearview mirror that attaches to the side of your helmet and lets you see who's coming up behind you.

Gloves

Like a helmet, padded cycling gloves are for riding outdoors, and most cyclists consider them a necessity. Gloves (see Figure 7-10) keep your hands from developing calluses and blisters that often result from gripping the handlebars and also absorb shock that would otherwise go to your arms, wrists, and shoulders.

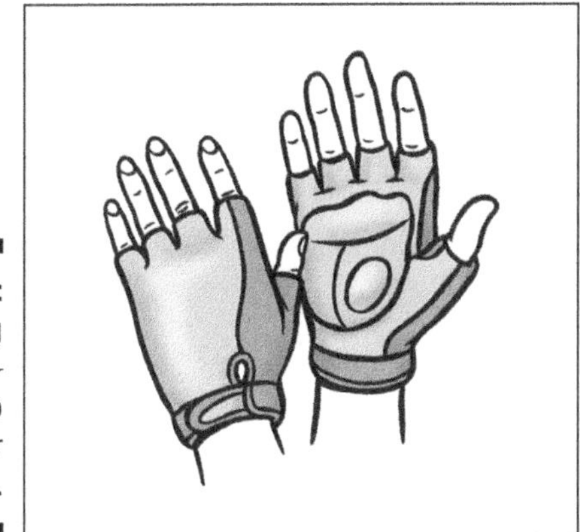

Figure 7-10: Cycling gloves — you can also use them for weightlifting.

Gloves come in full-finger or half-finger varieties and cost from $15 to $40. You can get gloves that are sized for a woman's hand, making them more comfortable. You want gloves that are well padded (with foam or gel) on the palm and water repellent on the rest of the glove. Most cyclists also prefer mesh on the back of the glove so that their hands don't overheat. Look for the lightest-weight, well-padded glove you can afford; heavy gloves will get too hot during your rides.

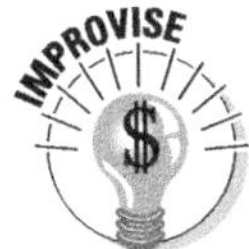

If you're cross-training with cycling and weightlifting (see Chapter 17), you can use cycling gloves as weightlifting gloves. Cycling gloves are a little lighter weight than weightlifting gloves, but they do the same thing: keep your hands soft in spite of grasping iron bars, which tends to cause calluses.

Chapter 8

Stretching the Truth: An Honest Look at Stretching

In This Chapter

- Considering the benefits of stretching
- Relaxing your upper body
- Stretching your lower back and hips
- Loosening your lower body

If you think that stretching is just a bother because it takes up your valuable time and doesn't add anything to your life, boy, are we glad you're reading this chapter. You may be surprised to discover that stretching can make the difference between developing an injury and staying healthy, can minimize low-back pain, and can be the most relaxing, enjoyable part of any workout.

Recognizing What Stretching Can Do for You

Many people don't view stretching as an important part of their workouts. They often take the approach of working out first, and then stretching only if they have the time. Rather than take this approach yourself, think of stretching as the second portion of your workout, not separating the two in your mind or in your workout. When you finish working out, stretch immediately, stopping only to drink fluids and, if you're really sweaty or cold, change your clothes. Don't, however, eat a meal, take a shower, or sit down with the remote before stretching, because you need to stretch your muscles while they're still warm. Plus, chances are, the stretching just won't happen, and you'll miss out on its valuable benefits. What are those valuable benefits? Read on and find out.

Warming up and stretching both make your body more flexible and ready to work out, but they do so in different ways. When you *warm up,* you ease into your workout by walking, swimming, cycling (or whatever) slowly and gently, gradually speeding up as your body becomes sweatier and warmer. In this way, your body is primed for more difficult exercise. *Stretching,* on the other hand, is a series of specifically designed exercises that you do after exercise and that help you become more flexible.

Stretch *after* your workout, not before. If you stretch before you work out, you may damage your cold (that is, un-warmed-up) muscles. If you decide to stretch on days that you don't work out, stretch extra gently and slowly so that you don't injure muscles.

Less soreness and lower risk of injury

Although some soreness is inevitable when you first start a workout routine, stretching can greatly minimize the discomfort you feel. If you were to put two people with similar genetics and experiences (say, twins) through the exact same workout routine, and one stretched and the other didn't, the non-stretcher would wake up the next morning feeling much less comfortable. And tight, sore muscles can become a chronic problem, increasing your muscle fatigue and putting you at a higher risk of injury.

When you stretch regularly, you experience much less stiffness when getting out of bed in the morning and when beginning your workout routine. Instead, your body feels limber and ready for action.

Jack-be-nimble joints

Stretching increases blood flow and aids in the supply of oxygen and nutrients to muscles and joints. It also increases your joints' range of motion, enabling them to move more comfortably and safely. Stretching helps decrease muscle tightness and allows for more normal movement throughout the range of motion. This ease of muscle movement can decrease the stress on your joints and decrease wear and tear, too. So, the bottom line is that your joints are going to move more easily and feel much better after a few days or weeks of consistent stretching.

Decreased low-back pain

If you don't stretch, tight *hamstrings* (the large muscles on the backs of your legs, between your butt and knees) are the result of many activities: walking, running, cycling, aerobics, and so on. In fact, many people who don't exercise at all have tight hamstrings just from standing, sitting, and driving a car. Eventually, your hamstrings can become so tight that your pelvic area begins to tilt, creating an S-curve in your back — this frequently happens during pregnancy. As you begin to stand and work out in this position, you may develop serious back pain. Stretching those hamstrings, however, can put the kibosh on back pain.

An added benefit to stretching is that you may also improve your posture. As your flexibility improves in your legs, your pelvis can return to its natural position, meaning better posture for you. Stretching all your back muscles allows your spine's natural curves to work effectively, absorbing the shock of weight-bearing activities.

Serious stress reduction

Stretching gently and slowly, without any bouncing or forceful movements, can feel almost like a minimassage. Add rhythmic breathing — exhaling as you move into the stretch and then breathing normally while holding the stretch — and stretching can feel almost meditative. All the tension you're feeling in so many areas of your body can melt away, leaving your body feeling refreshed and ready for your next workout — or, heck, ready for a nap.

Getting Loose: Basic Stretches

Although we don't have the space in this book to show you every stretch that has ever been invented, in this section, we give you some basic stretches that are targeted to fit your needs during pregnancy so that you can get started today. You may discover additional stretches — through additional reading, by watching a video, or by talking to your exercise class instructor — that are equally effective for you. You can also use the fitness ball exercises in Chapter 11 to stretch as you strengthen.

A few pointers before you begin

Keep the following pointers in mind as you perform these stretches and consider trying others:

- **Try to avoid lying on your back after your fourth month.** Although not every woman struggles with this problem, some women become lightheaded as a result of the baby's weight (during the second two trimesters) putting pressure on their blood vessels when they lie in this position.

Short bouts of a minute or two on your back shouldn't cause any problems, but if you do become lightheaded in this position, avoid any exercises that require you to lie on your back. If you become lightheaded while on your back, roll over onto your left side, a position that allows for better blood flow.

- **Avoid pointing your toes during a stretch, or you may find yourself dealing with a painful foot cramp.** Just keep your feet loose and unpointed throughout each stretch.

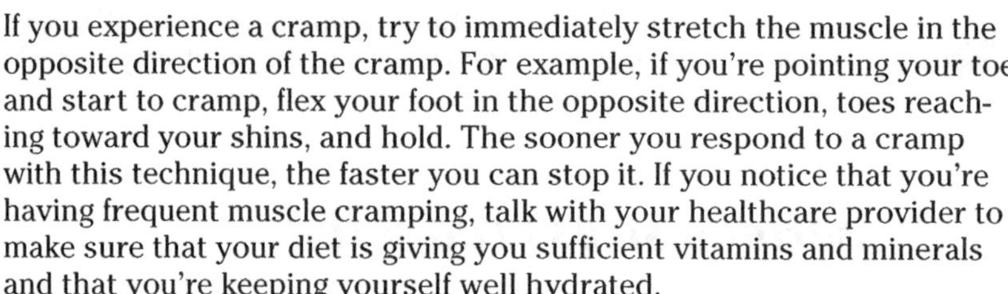

If you experience a cramp, try to immediately stretch the muscle in the opposite direction of the cramp. For example, if you're pointing your toe and start to cramp, flex your foot in the opposite direction, toes reaching toward your shins, and hold. The sooner you respond to a cramp with this technique, the faster you can stop it. If you notice that you're having frequent muscle cramping, talk with your healthcare provider to make sure that your diet is giving you sufficient vitamins and minerals and that you're keeping yourself well hydrated.

- **Breathe slowly, rhythmically, and naturally with each stretch.** Exhale as you stretch; inhale as you relax. Although you're holding the stretch, don't hold your breath.
- **Make each stretch last 10 to 20 seconds.** Stretch until you feel slight tension in the muscle, and then hold. As you feel the muscle start to stretch a bit more, take a deep breath, exhale, and stretch even farther until you feel slight tension again. Hold again. Continue to increase the stretch until you reach the 10- to 20-second mark. Do one or two repetitions.

If a stretch feels too tight, back off until the tightness eases, and then try again, stopping just short of where it felt too tight.

- **Don't bounce.** That just causes your muscles to tighten up in an attempt to protect itself.
- **Try not to stretch too far.** As a result of your pregnancy, your ligaments may be far more limber than they were in the past, but overdoing your stretches can lead to an injury.
- **Stay conscious of the area you're trying to stretch.** If you aren't feeling the correct muscle stretching, check your position to make sure you're doing the stretch correctly. Sometimes, a slight change in angle or position can improve the quality of a stretch.
- **If any stretch feels painful or uncomfortable in any way, stop that stretch and move on to another one.**

Stretching your upper body

Try the exercises in this section to stretch out your arms, shoulders, and chest.

Overhead wall stretch

This is one of the best stretches for releasing upper-body muscle tightness. It also helps improve posture.

1. **Stand with your back against a wall; arms out to your sides and against the wall with palms facing forward; and your feet, butt, shoulders, and head also touching the wall, as shown in Figure 8-1a.**

   Be sure to maintain a neutral spine, without flattening or curving your back.

2. **Take a deep breath and as you exhale, slowly raise your arms, keeping your hands against the wall.**
3. **Raise your arms all the way up or until you feel resistance, as shown in Figure 8-1b, and hold for 10 to 20 seconds.**

   If you can't keep your hands against the wall, ease up on the stretch by dropping your hands down until you're able to keep your hands against the wall. Hold this position until your muscles relax enough to try and stretch up a bit more. Don't force the stretch — give your muscles time to relax and move comfortably through the stretch.

4. **Return slowly to the start position and repeat several times throughout the day.**

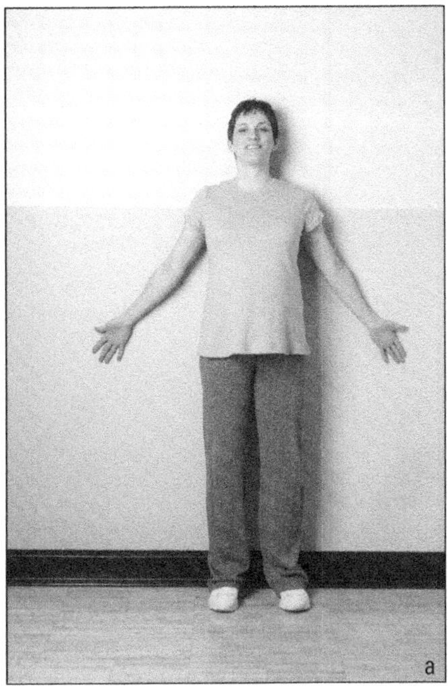

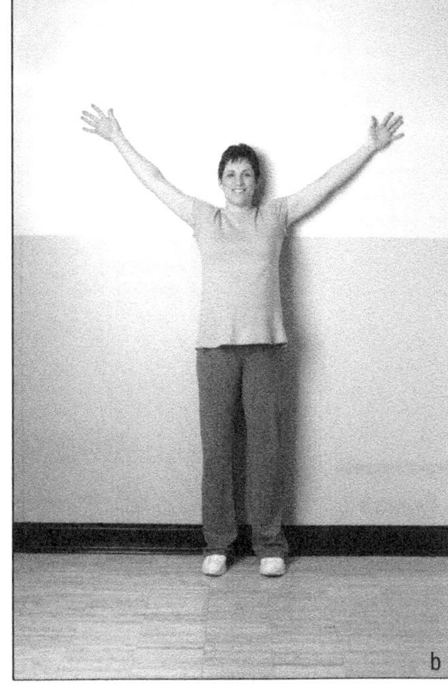

Figure 8-1: Overhead wall stretch.

Chest stretch against a corner

This exercise helps stretch both your upper chest and your calves.

1. **In a corner of a room, place one hand on each adjoining wall.**

   You can also do this stretch in a doorway by placing your hands on either side of the doorframe and leaning forward.

2. **Slowly lean forward with your elbows facing out until you feel a stretch in your chest and calves, as Figure 8-2 shows.**
3. **Hold the stretch for several seconds.**
4. **Repeat 2 to 3 times, several times per day.**

Loosening your back, hips, and groin muscles

Your low-back and hip area can be tough to stretch out. Use the two stretches in this section to ease through stiffness in this area.

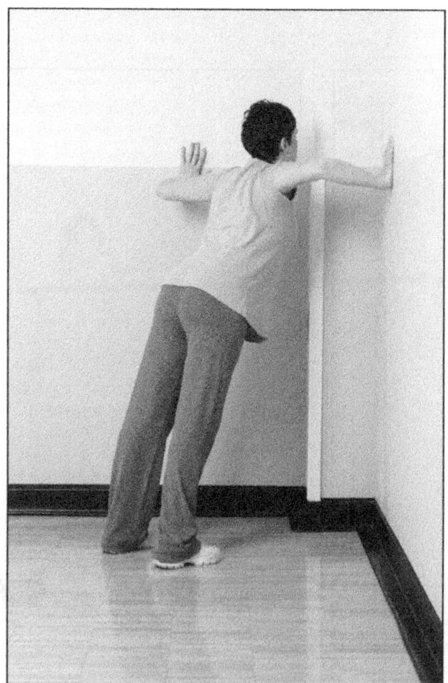

Figure 8-2: Stretching against a corner.

Chair stretch

The chair stretch is a great way to stretch out tight back, hip, and shoulder muscles, especially if you sit in a chair for long periods each day.

1. **Sit on a stable chair with your butt on the edge and your feet resting on the floor.**
2. **Slowly lean forward, allowing your arms to reach down toward the floor, as shown in Figure 8-3a.**
3. **Continue dropping forward from your hips until you feel a stretch in your back and hips.**

   If your belly doesn't allow you to bend forward very far, move closer to the edge of the chair and widen your knees until you can comfortably bend forward. Be careful, though, not to move so close to the edge of the chair that you slip off when you bend forward.
4. **Place your hands on your knees and slowly press yourself back up, as Figure 8-3b shows.**

   Don't rise back up without using your arms or you may put too much stress on your low back.
5. **Repeat this exercise throughout the day or whenever your back feels tight.**

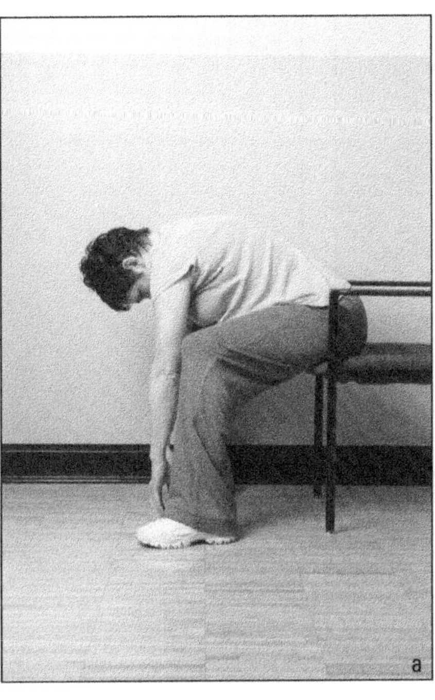

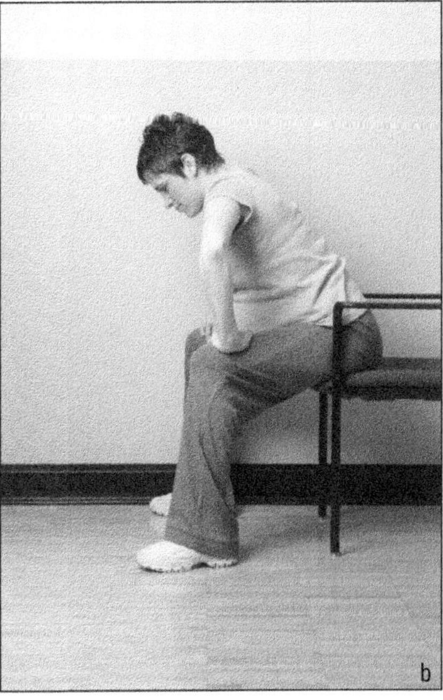

Figure 8-3: Chair stretch.

Standing back stretch

The standing back stretch is a quick, easy way to ease up low-back and neck discomfort.

1. **In a standing position, place your hands on your hips, as Figure 8-4a shows.**
2. **Lean your head back and gently bend back from your hips. Look up, bringing your shoulders back and pressing your chest out, as shown in Figure 8-4b. Hold for several seconds.**

   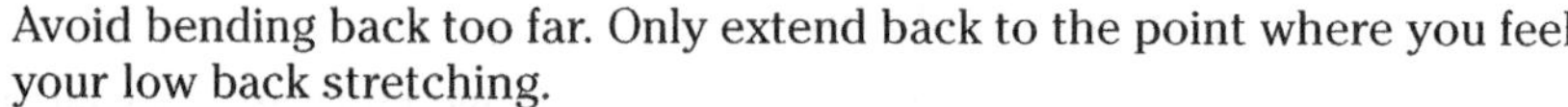

   REMEMBER

   Avoid bending back too far. Only extend back to the point where you feel your low back stretching.
3. **Relax and then repeat 2 to 3 times.**

Groin stretch

The groin stretch helps reduce inner thigh and hip tightness.

1. **Sit on the floor and place the soles of your feet together, as shown in Figure 8-5.**

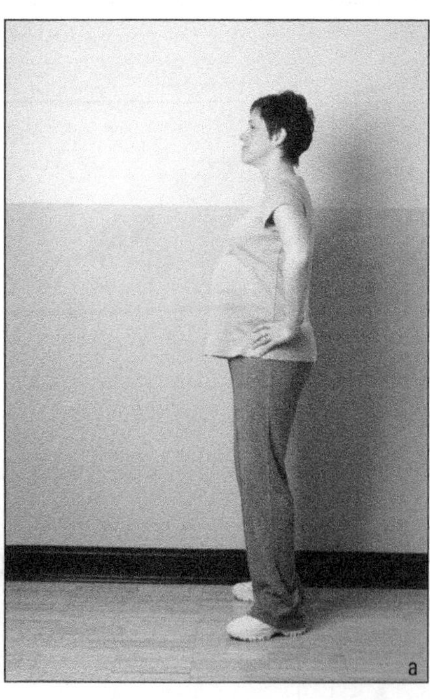

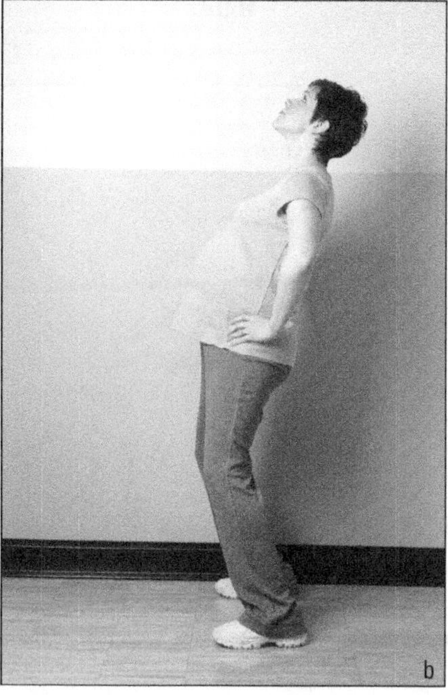

Figure 8-4: Standing back stretch.

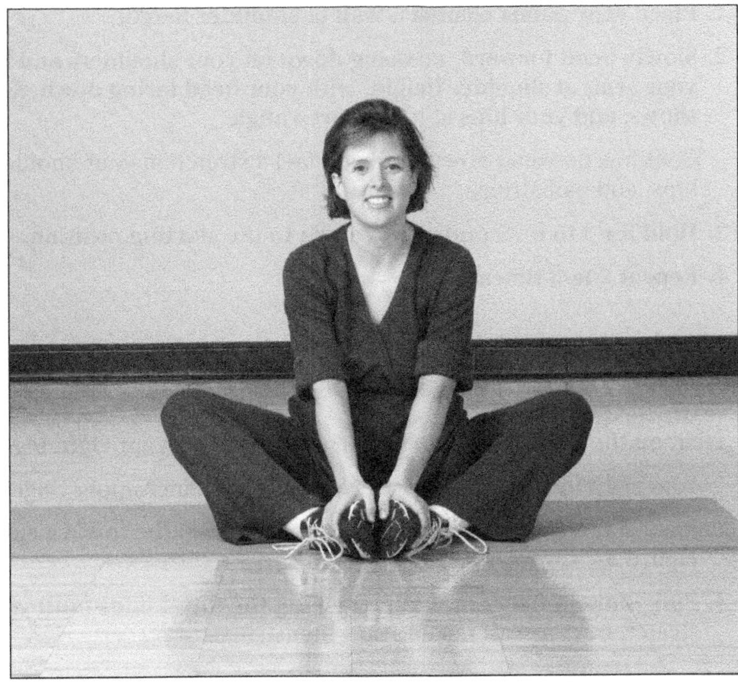

Figure 8-5: When stretching your groin, your legs look like a butterfly.

2. **Take a breath and as you exhale, press forward, bending from your hips without rounding your back, until you feel a stretch in your inner thighs.**
3. **Hold the stretch until you feel your groin muscles relax; keep pressing forward gently until you feel tension and hold.**
4. **Repeat 2 to 3 times.**

Loosening your legs

For many exercises, your legs bear the brunt of the workout — but even walking, standing, and sitting for long periods stress these limbs, so they need the gentle relaxation of a good stretch. Try the stretches that we describe in the following sections.

Ninety-degree wall stretch

Here's a stretch that helps several areas at one time: your upper arms, shoulders, back, and hamstrings.

1. **Place your palms against a wall at shoulder height.**
2. **Slowly bend forward, pressing down on your shoulders and keeping your arms at shoulder height, with your head facing down, as Figure 8-6 shows, and your hips at a 90-degree angle.**

   Continue pressing down until you feel a stretch in your shoulders, back, hips, and hamstrings.
3. **Hold for 3 to 6 seconds and return to the starting position.**
4. **Repeat 2 to 3 times.**

Hamstring stretch with a towel

The following stretch targets your hamstrings (the upper backs of your legs).

1. **Sit on the floor with your left leg straight and your right leg bent.**

   Your right foot should rest on your left leg's inner upper thigh.
2. **Place a towel around your left foot and grasp the towel's ends, as Figure 8-7 shows.**
3. **Pull yourself forward while grasping the towel ends until you feel a stretch in your calf muscle and hamstrings.**

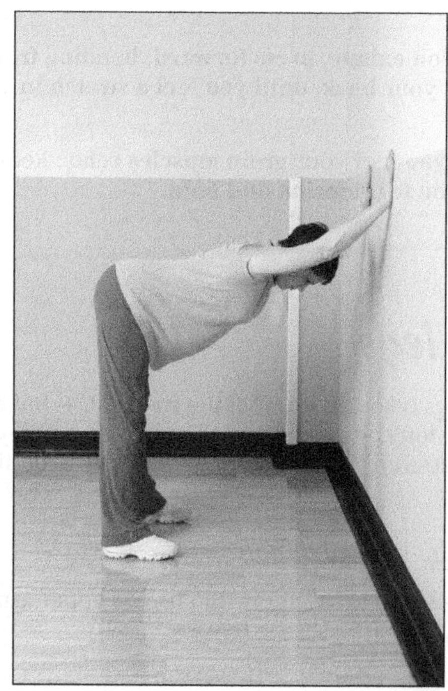

Figure 8-6: Bending at a 90-degree angle to the wall gives a good well-rounded stretch.

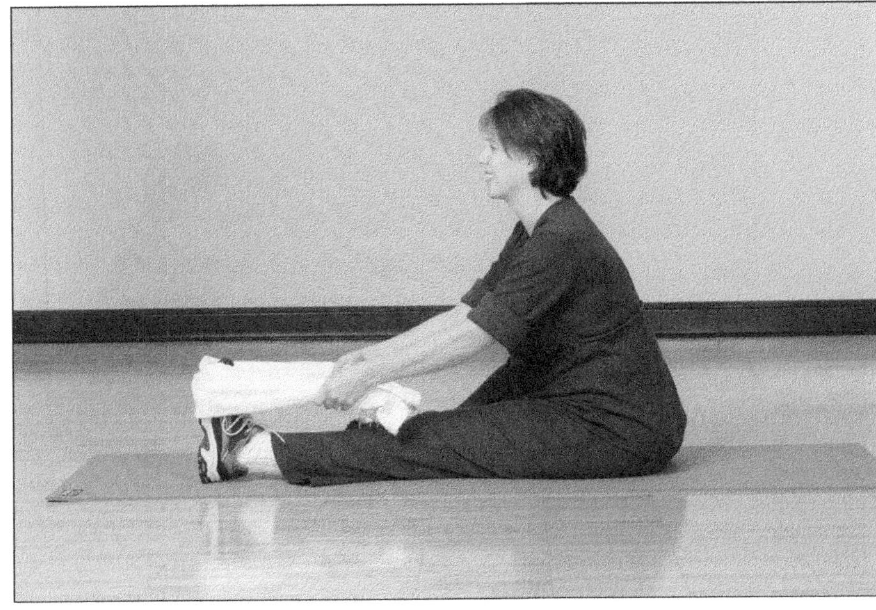

Figure 8-7: You can cop a squat while stretching the backs of your legs.

4. **Continue bending forward from your hips, keeping your back fairly straight.**
5. **Relax and repeat with your right leg, stretching each leg 2 to 3 times.**

Squat with a chair

Squats stretch the muscles of the hips, pelvis, and thighs. Doing this stretch is also a great way to practice the squat position for birth.

1. **Standing about arms' length away from a sturdy, heavy chair, grasp the chair's arms.**
2. **Lower your body into a squat position, keeping your feet flat, as shown in Figure 8-8.**

   Don't squat so low that you feel discomfort or pain. If you have difficulty keeping your feet flat as you squat, place your feet farther apart and rest your arms between your knees so that your weight is balanced.
3. **Hold this position only as long as it feels comfortable.**
4. **Rise back up to a standing position and repeat 2 to 3 times. Do this stretch throughout the day.**

   When you rise up, use your arms to help lift your body instead of putting all your weight on your knees.

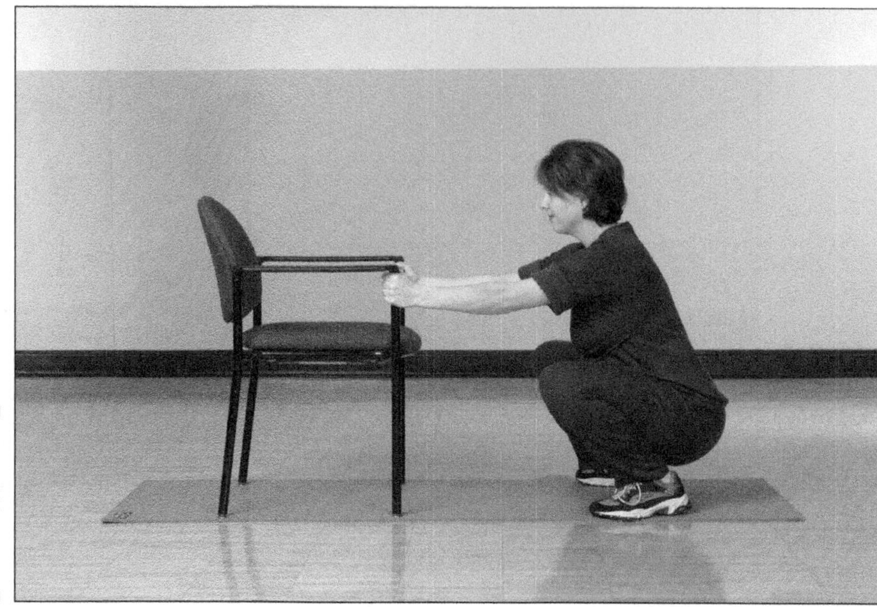

Figure 8-8: Performing the correct squatting technique.

Considering yoga

Some low-impact yoga classes and videos are essentially one long, intensive stretching session that leaves you feeling wonderfully refreshed. We've watched prenatal yoga videos (and we discuss them in Chapter 14) that make you feel good just listening to the soothing music and to the instructor's soothing voice. If you're looking for some serious stress reduction and want to focus on flexibility, consider incorporating a day or two of prenatal yoga into your workout routine. Alternating a prenatal yoga class or video one day with a more vigorous workout (for example, walking, swimming, aerobics, or cycling) the next day is an excellent way to gain flexibility while also increasing strength and improving your heart and lung function.

Keep in mind, however, that high-impact yoga (often called *power yoga*) is a different breed altogether. Although power yoga draws on the principles of yoga, it's a much more intensive experience that gives you an excellent workout, but hardly qualifies as soothing or relaxing. Unless you've been doing power yoga and have gotten the okay from your healthcare provider, we recommend steering clear.

Part III

Eating Well for Nine Months — and for Life

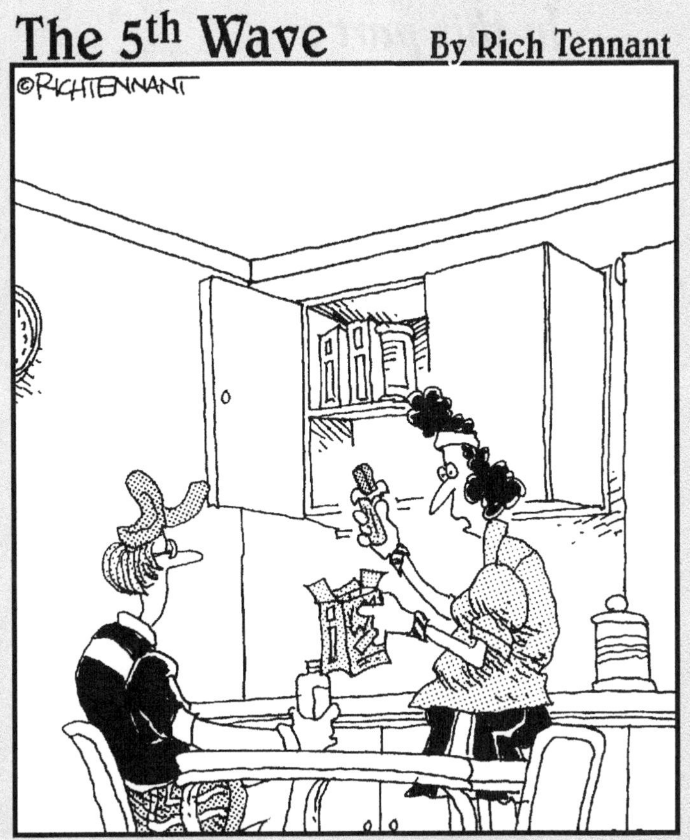

"They're energy bars for pregnant women. What flavor do you want, Ketchup and Pickles, Chocolate Potato Chip, or Sardine Blast?"

In this part . . .

We dish the dirt on nutrition and the weight that you need to gain in order to deliver a healthy baby. Eating and pregnancy just seem to go hand-in-hand, don't they? People talk about eating for two and nod wisely when a pregnant woman craves ice cream and pickles. So, in this part, you find out how to curb those cravings so that you take in only the number of calories you and your baby actually need. And you find out which foods, vitamins, and minerals are best for fueling your fit, pregnant body.

Chapter 9

Fueling Your Body with the Right Foods

In This Chapter

- Making the switch to nourishing foods
- Getting a basic understanding of carbs and fats
- Knowing which vitamins and minerals are critical during pregnancy
- Drinking enough fluids for your athletic body
- Avoiding certain foods that can harm your baby

If you've already had your first prenatal checkup, chances are, your healthcare provider has briefly discussed the importance of good nutrition, from selecting healthy foods to eating several small meals throughout the day to getting enough calcium and iron.

However, your healthcare provider may not have the time or training to give you specifics. So, this chapter gives you the lowdown on the food that fuels your body for prenatal exercise *and* that's best for your baby.

High blood sugar can trigger growth hormones that cause your baby to grow very large, which isn't healthy for you or your baby. If you've been diagnosed with prediabetes, had diabetes before you became pregnant, or developed gestational diabetes after becoming pregnant, talk to your healthcare provider about your special nutritional needs.

Developing Good Eating Habits

What you eat is largely a matter of habit, not a matter of searching for what your body really needs. If you detest vegetables or think the only way to eat meat is to deep-fry it, you're both ignoring the signals your body is sending you about the foods that truly nourish you and allowing lifelong habits to dictate what you eat. Most people make poor food choices because of three main habits:

- The foods you found comforting as a child (grandma's pie, mashed potatoes, ice cream, fried chicken) have a strong hold over you as an adult. When you eat those foods, you're getting a connection to what may have been happy times as a child.
- Commercials on TV, on the radio, and in magazine ads make you feel strongly as though certain foods are exactly what you're craving right now, even if you never would've thought of eating those foods without seeing or hearing the ad. And if you're out running errands and need a meal, your choices of healthy foods is severely limited, making eating poorly seem like the only option.
- The food served in restaurants, snacks and foods offered at parties and weddings, and the meals prepared by friends and family are meant to please and impress, not improve your health and longevity. You may believe that in order to be social and kind to your friends and family, you have to eat nonnutritious foods.

Because of these three factors, you can easily begin to believe that eating well is a pipe dream: The foods that bring you comfort, the foods advertised all around you, and the foods served at every social gathering you attend are all foods that you know to be unhealthy and nonnourishing, making healthy eating impossible, not to mention boring and un-fun.

But we're going to let you in on a little secret: If you want to feel great, radiate good health, wake up refreshed and energetic and stay that way all day long (well, most days, anyway), avoid major health problems, and provide all the nutrients your baby needs, you must regularly eat well. Here's how:

- **Fill up on the good stuff.** When you need a snack, grab an apple or banana, not a cookie or box of crackers. Eat before heading out for errands and bring healthy snacks with you in your purse. When you've had a bad day and think that the pint of Haagen-Dazs (or whatever your favorite comfort food or memory food) is the only way to solve your problems, first make a big stir-fry with lean chicken (or pick up a pint of this at your local Chinese takeout restaurant), drink a large bottle of water, and then — if you're still hungry and stressed — put a scoop or two of ice cream in a small dish and see how that feels.
- **Don't completely deny yourself anything tasty.** A doughnut once a week doesn't compromise your health, but a doughnut every day, combined with other unhealthy eating habits, quickly has negative effects on your health.

- **Turn off or otherwise ignore all food-related advertisements.** The companies advertising food don't care about you — they care about profits. Whether you struggle with illness or general feelings of blah is completely irrelevant to them, as long as you keep buying those foods. Take charge of your eating by eliminating the influence of commercials on your healthy lifestyle. This goes double for the many unhealthy recipes found in the food section of your local newspaper, many home and garden magazines, and gourmet food publications. Look for publications that cater to healthy eating, especially those that provide recipes that are low in fat and include fresh vegetables.
- **Immediately look for the one or two healthy choices upon entering any restaurant, party, or other social gathering.** If you're not doing the serving or bringing a dish with you (as is the case at a restaurant or wedding), search for the veggie plate, a big salad, a lean meat option *without* any sauces, or a legume or whole-grain food.
- **Serve or bring healthy foods and limit the number and size of treats.** If you're serving the meal, offer an enticing array of brightly colored vegetables, legumes, whole grains, and lean meat, and then offer small slices of a delicious fruit pie with a spoonful of low-fat frozen yogurt. Your guests will be amazed at how colorful and delicious a nutritious meal can be and will be clamoring for recipes. If you're at a potluck gathering, such as an office party or baby shower, bring one or two healthy dishes that you know you'll eat, and quickly evaluate what other healthy foods are available at the gathering.

When you embrace a healthy way of eating, you do limit the unhealthy foods that you eat, but in a short while, you won't miss them. The key is to not think of healthy eating as temporary or something to be endured, but to come to love the foods that are healthy more than the ones that aren't. After relishing grilled chicken or turkey breast, a greasy sausage loses its appeal. If, in a straight-up taste test, you compared the natural goodness of a treat like grapes or strawberries to a high-fat cookie, you'd be amazed at how much more delicious natural fruit is to anything Mrs. Fields makes.

All that said, if you're unable to keep food down during any part of your pregnancy, find foods that you can tolerate and, until you're able to keep down other foods, don't worry about whether what you're eating is healthy. Sometimes, pregnancy causes you to reject even the healthiest foods, so make gaining weight normally your number-one priority, with healthy eating number two on that list. That doesn't mean for you to completely disregard everything this section just told you, but common sense tells you that you're better off eating something that isn't so great for you than *not* eating the good stuff. Chapter 10 offers more advice on managing morning sickness and nausea at other times of the day.

Sorting through the Hype about Carbs and Fats

Had it with the hype? Carbs are good; carbs are bad; protein is the answer; fat is good; fat is bad — everything you hear one day comes around and sounds like the opposite a year or two later. We don't blame you for being frustrated, but the reason for all the mixed messages is that food is far too complex to be labeled as "good" or "bad" all the time. Take some examples:

- Most carbs are great.
- A few types of carbs aren't good for you.
- Protein is good for you, but too much can be a burden on your body.
- For the most part, you want to eat low-fat foods, but a few high-fat foods are actually good for you.
- Most fats aren't good for you at all.

We don't kid ourselves into believing we can end all your frustration just by offering this small section, but in the two following sections, we try to simplify what's clearly a difficult subject.

Understanding why low-carb is no good

If you're one of the growing number of people latching onto a low-carb diet, keep in mind that avoiding or reducing carbohydrates and working out just don't mix. Carbohydrates act as a fuel for your exercising body; without a decent supply of carbs in your diet, you tire faster and recover from workouts more slowly than your carb-eating counterparts.

Low-carb eating has good intentions at its roots. Carbohydrates come in two forms: simple carbohydrates (also called simple sugars) and complex carbohydrates. Simple sugars are found in sugar (which is in many prepared products), honey, candy, some very sweet types of fruit, cookies, pastries, many processed snack foods, sugary cereals, sweet corn, and so on. Simple carbohydrates' main job is to quickly replenish *glucose* (readily absorbed fuel) that your muscles and other tissues need right after very strenuous exercise (like when training for a marathon). But most people don't work out hard enough to need those simple sugars directly after exercise. Yet, simple sugars make up the bulk of most people's diets, and the result of eating all these sugars that the body doesn't need and can't effectively process is a host of health problems, because those extra calories are stored as fat. Over time, this can lead to obesity and increase your risk of developing some diseases.

Analyzing energy bars

If you've been to any sporting goods store, specialty fitness store, or even health-food store lately, you've seen a tremendous array of *energy bars,* with brand names like PowerBar, Clif Bar, Balance Bar, and Carb-Boom. Energy bars were invented as a healthy equivalent to candy bars for hikers and cyclists, who needed something quick and easy to carry with them, but wanted something a little healthier than candy bars. Originally aimed at high-mileage athletes who have trouble eating enough food to maintain their body weight, energy bars are dense in calories, high in carbohydrates, and lower in fats than candy bars.

What has happened since their invention, however, is that people who aren't in any danger of wasting away from too much exercise and not enough food are eating them, too — sometimes eating several per day because, you know, they're "healthy." Yes, they may be made with whole-wheat flour instead of white flour, and they may have some oats or other good sources of carbohydrates, but energy bars are anything but healthy, and some have enough calories in them (300 to 400) that eating just four or five per day would supply all your caloric needs for an entire day! When compared with a banana, apple, a cup of oatmeal, half of a whole-grain bagel, or other foods, energy bars don't look so appealing. And they're really expensive, too, so you'll save money by eating other foods.

If you tend to grab an energy bar (or candy bar) while you're out and about because you get hungry and need a snack, plan ahead by bringing a snack of your own. Even a medium-size purse can hold an apple, small bag of gorp (good old raisins and peanuts), a bagel in a resealable bag, a can of low-sodium V-8, or whatever other healthy options appeal to you.

Limiting the simple sugars in your diet (with the exception of several half-cup servings of fruit or fruit juice each day) is a great idea; you'll feel better. However, the other type of carbohydrate — the complex carbs found in vegetables, whole grains (like dense whole-wheat breads, slow-cooked oatmeal, and whole-wheat pasta), and some less-sweet fruits (such as partly green bananas) — are an excellent source of energy and fuel for someone who's exercising and shouldn't only *not* be eliminated, but should make up from 50 to 70 percent of an exercising adult's diet.

Low-carb eating is a reaction against the typical high-sugar diet and asks its adherents to limit the sugars in their diets, which sounds like an excellent plan. However, whole-grain foods that are low in simple sugars but dense in complex carbs show up as no-nos on a low-carb eating plan, and instead, low-carb eaters are often encouraged to eat low-carb, high-fat foods such as cream, bacon, and other foods high in saturated fat. Although this does eliminate or at least reduce the simple sugars, it also eliminates the incredibly healthy complex carbs and encourages people to fill up on unhealthy high-saturated and high-trans-fat goods (see the "Avoiding saturated and trans-fats and discovering the good fats" section). And foods that are high in protein and fats aren't efficient forms of fuel, so when you exercise, your body has to work very hard to break down and use these types of foods.

Low-carb dieting would be an ideal way to eat with the following modifications:

- Eat an unlimited variety of brightly colored vegetables.
- Eat dense, whole grains.
- Eat four or five half-cup servings of unsweetened fruit each day.

  Keep in mind that the sweeter a fruit tastes, the more sugar it has in it. Although pineapples, strawberries, grapes, oranges, and other sweet fruits are an exellent treat, you don't want to eat a lot of those fruits at one sitting, nor do you want to eat them frequently throughout the day.
- Substantially reduce your intake of saturated fat and trans-fats.

Ideally, you want to substantially limit your simple sugars, get the majority of your calories from complex carbohydrates that are low in trans-fats, and supplement these complex carbs with low-saturated-fat proteins, such as chicken and turkey breast, seafood that's approved for pregnancy, lean cuts of beef and pork, and low-fat dairy products.

Table 9-1 Trading Less Nutritious Carbs for Nutritious and Fiber-Filled Sources of Carbs and Proteins

Simple Carbohydrates to Limit or Avoid	*Complex Carbohydrates to Eat Instead*
Cookies	Apples, bananas, and other unsweetened fruits
Highly processed snack foods, including crackers and chips	Air-popped popcorn or popcorn cooked in olive or canola oil (which are low in saturated fat), Rye-Krisps Broccoli, cauliflower, asparagus, squash and zucchini, beans, and all other green vegetables; salads, especially those made with a range of lettuce types; red and orange vegetables
Sugary, light-colored cereals; instant oatmeal	Whole-grain cereals with little or no added sugar; slow-cooked oatmeal
White rice	Brown rice
White tortillas, white bread, and white-flour bagels	Whole-wheat tortillas and any dense, heavy, whole-grain bread and bagels

	Low-Fat Proteins to Eat, Too
	Nonfat and low-fat milk, cheese, and yogurt
	Low-fat soy products (especially useful if you're lactose intolerant)
	Eggs, especially egg whites and products such as Egg Beaters
	Legumes (beans, split peas, lentils), especially when combined with brown rice at the same or nearby meal
	Poultry breast (legs and wings tend to be high in saturated fats, as are poultry sausages)
	Lean cuts of beef and pork cuts with the words "loin" or "round" in the name

Another reason not to eat a high-fat, low-carb diet is that it tends to contribute to morning sickness and to feelings of nausea at other times of the day. Chapter 10 has the lowdown.

Avoiding saturated and trans-fats and discovering the good fats

Are you confused about whether fat is bad for you or good for you? For years, you've heard conflicting information telling you that all fat is bad, some fat is bad, fat isn't the problem — carbs are, and so on. But, although this may be a bit of an oversimplification, some fats are good, and some are bad.

Bad fats come from the following food sources and should be limited:

- **Saturated fat from animals:** Animal fat, including hamburger, lamb, dark meat from chicken and turkey, fatter cuts of beef and pork, pork rinds, poultry legs and wings, jerky, high-fat dairy products, butter, and lard contain saturated fats that tend to clog arteries and can lead to increased body fat.

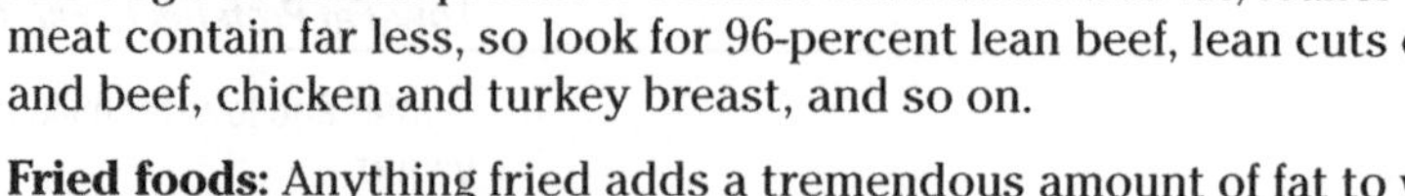

Although all animal products contain some saturated fat, leaner cuts of meat contain far less, so look for 96-percent lean beef, lean cuts of pork and beef, chicken and turkey breast, and so on.

- **Fried foods:** Anything fried adds a tremendous amount of fat to what could be good foods, such as lean meats and vegetables. Although you can fry in *unsaturated* oils, which don't have the heart-clogging properties that saturated fats have, you've still added fat to a product that probably tastes terrific without frying. If you must fry, however, your best bet is to fry in canola, flaxseed, or olive oils.

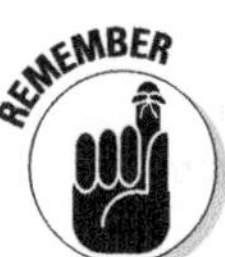

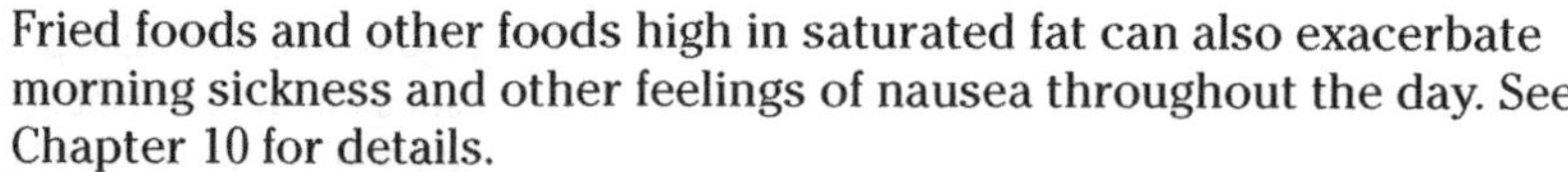

Fried foods and other foods high in saturated fat can also exacerbate morning sickness and other feelings of nausea throughout the day. See Chapter 10 for details.

- **Trans-fats and hydrogenated oils:** Trans-fats are in a lot of snack foods, and although the label may give you the name of a vegetable oil, trans-fats are altered in such a way that your body reacts to it just like lard! Chips, crackers, cookies (even low-fat cookies), granola bars, pastries, microwave popcorn, many types of bread, many cereals, and most peanut butters often contain trans-fats.

  By reading food labels carefully, however, you can avoid trans-fats. Look for the words "hydrogenated" or "partially hydrogenated" oils on labels and avoid those products that use hydrogenated oils, especially when near the top of the list. Keep reading labels and don't give up: For every ten cereals or microwave popcorn products that have trans-fat, you find one that doesn't.

Some foods contain what appears on the food label to be a lot of total fat, but the fats aren't saturated or trans-fats; they're unsaturated fats that protect your heart and other organs. These foods include:

- Avocados
- Canola and flaxseed oils
- Fatty fish, such as salmon and mackerel
- Nuts and seeds
- Peanuts (not technically a nut) and peanut butter made only from peanuts and salt
- Olives and olive oil

Fill up on low-fat foods and eat good fats in moderation. At the same time, limit your intake of bad fats, using Table 9-2 for some ways to cut back.

Table 9-2 Alternatives to Trans-Fat and Saturated Fat Foods

Potential Trans-Fat and Saturated Fat Source	*Healthy Alternative*
Breads (trans-fat)	Breads made without hydrogenated oils; you can also make your own in a bread maker with sesame, canola, or olive oil instead of lard, shortening, or butter
Butter and cream (saturated fat)	New olive- and canola-oil-based spreads that say "No trans-fat" on the label; fat-free half-and-half
Cereals, especially granola and other high-fat cereals (trans-fat)	Cereals made without hydrogenated oils; cereals with lower overall fat content
Chips and crackers (trans-fat)	Rice cakes, nuts, and seeds (watch the label, though, for trans-fats and hydrogenated oils!)
Cookies (trans-fat)	Homemade oatmeal cookies made with sesame or canola oil instead of shortening or butter
Dark poultry meat (saturated fat)	White poultry meat
Fried foods (saturated fat)	Nuts, seeds, rice cakes, and other healthy snacks; grilled or baked meats, poultry, and seafood; steamed vegetables
Granola bars (trans-fat)	Fruit
High-fat dairy products and meats (saturated fat)	Low-fat or fat-free dairy products; meats labeled as having lower fat content
Margarine and shortening (trans-fat)	New olive- and canola-oil-based spreads that say "No trans-fat" on the label
Microwave popcorn (trans-fat)	Air-popped popcorn or popcorn popped the old-fashioned way (a stir-popper) in olive or canola oils
Pastries (trans-fat)	Pumpkin dessert (pumpkin pie without the crust) or banana bread made with sesame or canola oil instead of shortening or butter
Peanut butter (trans-fat)	Natural peanut butter that's made only of ground peanuts and salt
Sausage (saturated fat)	96-percent lean ground beef

Complete protein = legumes + whole grains

A *complete protein* is one that contains all eight essential amino acids that your body needs for optimum health. Most meats, poultry, and seafood contain enough complete proteins to fuel your body, which is why Western culture puts such an emphasis on eating animal products. However, with some simple math, you can create a complete protein at a meatless meal by combining legumes with dairy or whole grains. Some examples include:

- Meatless chili served over brown rice
- Peanut butter served on whole-wheat toast
- Split-pea or lentil soup and a hunk of dense bread
- Hummus (made from chickpeas) served on whole-wheat pita bread

You can also eat legumes at one meal and whole grains at the next and get the same benefits.

If you're used to eating meat at most meals (or at least at dinner), you may wonder how to make a satisfying meal that still offers the nutrients that a meat-based meal does. Simply plan a meat-free meal that offers plenty of *legumes,* a vegetable family that includes black beans, split peas, lentils, chickpeas (also called garbanzo beans), peanuts, and so on. Legumes are mostly low-fat, nutrient-dense, filling foods that make you feel satisfied after you eat them. And though you can buy dried legumes and make them into soups and other hearty dishes, you can also buy canned varieties that you can whip into a meal in just 10 or 15 minutes. By combining legumes with whole grains (discussed in the following section), you can create a complete protein that's just as good as any meat product. See the "Complete protein = legumes + whole grains" sidebar for details.

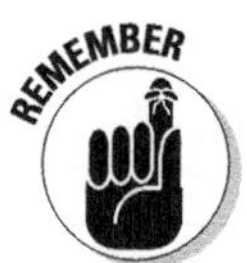

During your pregnancy, you need 8 to 10 grams of protein for every 15 pounds of body weight. (Read food labels to determine how much protein is in various food products.) You want these protein-rich foods to be as low fat as possible and to be complete proteins, whenever possible.

Getting Your Vitamins and Minerals

Although everyone needs certain vitamins and minerals to stay healthy, energetic, and injury free, pregnant women need more of certain vitamins and minerals than men and nonpregnant women do. If your healthcare provider hasn't already prescribed a prenatal daily vitamin, you'll probably get one soon. But you can also get the important vitamins and minerals from the foods you eat. This section dishes the dirt.

Discovering the wonderful benefits of folic acid

Folic acid, also called folate, is on the mouths and lips of every OB/GYN, because taking folic acid has been directly shown to reduce birth defects involving the brain and spinal cord, including spina bifida. Folic acid also may reduce the risk of certain congenital heart defects. Timing is critical, because the greatest benefit to your baby is when you take folic acid before you conceive and during the first trimester.

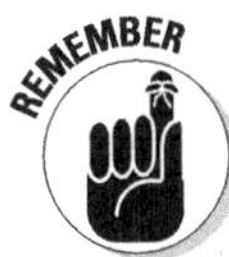

Depending on what your healthcare provider suggests, you need between 0.4 and 4 mg of folic acid every day. Many women get their folic acid from a prenatal vitamin, but you can also find this important nutrient in legumes, leafy green vegetables, orange and pineapple juice, sunflower seeds, orange vegetables, and nuts.

What if you're a vegetarian?

If you're a vegetarian, you need to be especially careful about your eating habits while you're pregnant, or you may not be able to get the nutrients you need to help your baby grow properly. Vegetarians tend to fall into one of two categories:

- **Lacto-ovo vegetarian:** This sort of vegetarian doesn't eat the flesh of animals, which means no meat, poultry, or fish, but does eat other animal products, such as milk, cheese and eggs, along with a host of grains, legumes, vegetables, fruits, and so on. If you're a lacto-ovo vegetarian, be sure you eat plenty of milk-based products. In addition, in order to mimic the complete proteins found in meat, combine whole grains (such as brown rice or whole-wheat pasta) with legumes (dried beans, split peas, lentils, and so on). Eat these together at the same or a nearby meal, and your body will get all it needs to make the protein complete.
- **Vegan:** A vegan doesn't eat any foods that originate with animals, which excludes the obvious ones like meat, poultry, and seafood, but also rules out dairy products and eggs. A vegan has to get all her nutrients from plant-based sources, such as legumes, grains, nuts, seeds, vegetables, and fruits. Vegans need to plan carefully to get all the required nutrients when *not* pregnant; being a pregnant or nursing vegan is even more challenging. Like a lacto-ovo vegetarian, if you're a vegan, you want to combine whole grains with legumes to create complete proteins. In addition, because plant foods don't contain vitamin B_{12}, you probably need a B_{12} supplement (ask your healthcare provider). Because you're not ingesting dairy products and other animal sources, you may also be lacking in calcium, vitamin D, iron, riboflavin, and zinc. As soon as you find out you're pregnant, tell your healthcare provider that you're a vegan and read up on ways to get all the nutrients you need for you and your baby to thrive.

Eating calcium-filled products

Developing babies need calcium, and yours will get what he needs, which then diminishes your calcium supply. For this reason, you need extra calcium — at least 1,200 milligrams per day. Obvious food sources include dairy products, but you may not realize that other foods contain calcium, too:

- Milk
- Cheese
- Yogurt
- Whole sesame seeds
- Broccoli
- Spinach and other dark green lettuce
- Canned salmon and sardines with bones (a rather disturbing thought, but a good source, if you can stomach it)
- Tums

If you have problems digesting dairy products (and a substantial percentage of the population does), you may have trouble with any one of the components of dairy: the sugar (lactose), the protein, or the fat. If you have trouble digesting the lactose or the fat, you're in luck, because you can buy lactose-free and fat-free dairy products, or you can take tablets that help you better digest lactose. However, if you're allergic to the protein in milk, no dairy product is going to work for you. Try getting your calcium from other sources, including calcium-fortified soy "milk" products and orange juice. If you're allergic to or intolerant of dairy products or don't eat them because you're a vegan (see the "What if you're a vegetarian?" sidebar for details), tell your healthcare provider early in your pregnancy so that he or she can prescribe a supplement with calcium and/or direct you to other food sources.

Becoming an iron kid

You and your baby are red-blood-cell-making machines! That's right, every day, you and your baby make new red blood cells, and in order to do this efficiently, you need to give your body more iron than you need when you're not pregnant. If you don't get enough iron, your body may stop making as many red blood cells, causing you or your baby to become anemic, a condition characterized by weakness. (And you can't do much working out when you're weak!) Prenatal vitamins contain iron, but you can also get iron from legumes, pumpkin and squash, red meats, seafood, chicken, pork, and nuts.

Discovering a few other essentials

In addition to folic acid, calcium, and iron, your pregnant body needs lots of other vitamins and minerals, and ideally, you get most of these by eating a well-balanced diet. Your healthcare provider may prescribe prenatal vitamins, but you can also get many of the vitamins and minerals you need from healthy food sources. Table 9-3 lists the vitamins and minerals considered most important for pregnant women (including folic acid, calcium, and iron), the amount most women need, and some common food sources for them.

Table 9-3 Vitamin and Mineral Sources

Vitamin/Mineral	*Amount*	*Food Sources*
Calcium	1,200–1,500 mg	Dairy products, seafood, almonds, soy, leafy green vegetables
Essential fatty acids	Not measured	Nuts, soybean and canola oils, soy milk, and other products. Avoid trans-fats (see the "Avoiding saturated and trans-fats and discovering the good fats" section)
Folic acid	0.4–4 mg	Legumes, leafy green vegetables, orange and pineapple juice, sunflower seeds, orange vegetables, nuts
Iron	13–30 mg (first trimester) 18–30 mg (second and third trimesters)	Legumes, pumpkin and squash, green leafy vegetables, red meats, seafood, chicken, pork, nuts
Magnesium	600–900 mg	Leafy green veggies, legumes, seafood, nuts and seeds
Potassium	435 mg per hour of exercise	Bananas, many dried fruits, avocados, potatoes, oranges
Selenium	200 mg	Legumes, mushrooms, garlic, Brazil nuts
Vitamin E	400–800 IU	Many nuts and seeds
Zinc	30–60 mg	Lean beef, fish, egg yolks, oysters, bran

Drinking Enough Fluids

Throughout every day — whether you've exercised that day or not — you need to drink plenty of fluids. Plan to drink a minimum of eight cups of fluids per day (and remember, that's a minimum!).

Water

Good old-fashioned water is far and away the best way to get your fluids. Water is critical for proper functioning of your organs, so you want to get the majority of your fluids by drinking water. Keep a water bottle with you at all times: on your desk, in your purse, and in your car.

If you don't like the taste of water, you may have substances in your water that create an off-taste. Note, however, that most bottled water is just a bottled version of whatever's in your tap, so the flavor isn't much better, and you waste a bundle of money. You can try filtering your water: Brita and other companies make low-cost filter systems that attach to your kitchen or bathroom faucet. If you're still not thrilled with the taste of water, try squeezing a slice of lemon into each glass.

Sports beverages

Sports beverages include Gatorade, Powerade, Accelerade, and so on, and if you've never tried them, they're actually quite palatable — most taste just like Kool-Aid. The advantage of a sports beverage over water is that it includes *electrolytes* like potassium, magnesium, calcium, and sodium that you lose as you sweat. Sports beverages can also keep you from getting a stomachache after exercising.

The disadvantage is that sports beverages are pretty high in calories, and although you need to add calories while you're pregnant and nursing, if you get in the habit of thinking of sports beverages like water, you can easily gain weight when you're no longer pregnant or nursing. If you really feel that you need a sports beverage after workouts, try to limit your daily intake of sports beverages to 12 ounces, just after you finish exercising.

Sports drinks are expensive if you buy them in individual bottles. To save money, buy the powdered version at your local grocery store. You simply mix the powder with water, and you pay less than one-tenth the price with the exact same flavor. And you can dilute sports beverages with extra water to reduce calories and sugar content.

Carbonated sodas and carbonated sports drinks

Most physicians and midwives want you to steer clear of carbonated beverages, especially sugary sodas, because they add calories to your diet without adding any vitamins or other nutrients and they don't contain the electrolytes that sports beverages offer. One alternative is the new variety of carbonated flavored water. However, all carbonated beverages, even carbonated water, also contain phosphates, which can interfere with calcium absorption and may lead to bone-density problems. A treat now and then isn't going to hurt you. But if you love those fizzy bubbles and don't want to drink anything else, ask your healthcare provider whether it's safe for your baby.

Juice

One-hundred-percent orange juice is rich in potassium, vitamin C, and other important vitamins. However, it's high in calories and doesn't really fill you up, so go easy on it. One small glass per day (six to eight ounces) is about all you need. You get a better bang for the buck by eating the whole fruit, so when you have a choice, eat the fruit — fruit is more filling than juice and provides additional nutrients.

Milk

Two or three 8- to 12-ounce glasses of low-fat or fat-free milk are an excellent source of calcium, but you may not be able to stomach a glass of milk right after working out. If not, try drinking a glass of skim milk just before bed (warm it up in the microwave, if you like). In addition to getting much-needed calcium, the protein in milk helps many women fall asleep quickly.

Coffee and tea

Coffee and tea are hot, tasty beverages, but a better choice is water. Caffeinated beverages can cause more frequent urination which, of course, can put a cramp in your workout! It can also keep you up all night. Healthcare providers don't have conclusive guidelines about how much caffeine is a problem during pregnancy. What we can tell you is that the 300 mg or so in two regular mugs of coffee or tea (or one very, very large mug) doesn't appear to pose a significant risk. More than that may be a problem for some women, especially during your first trimester, so talk to your healthcare provider if you're a hard-core coffee drinker.

However, coffee and tea are fluids that count in your daily total of eight cups, and if you look forward to your mug(s) of coffee or tea everyday, you don't need to stop drinking it completely. Check with your healthcare provider if you're concerned about the effects of caffeine on your pregnancy.

Recognizing Which Foods to Limit or Avoid Completely

In nearly any pregnancy-related book, you find a list of foods to avoid eating, because those foods have the potential to cause serious complications for you and your baby. Although this isn't a general pregnancy handbook — instead, everything in this book is geared toward the specific topic of working out during pregnancy — we include this section because the information is so important. Besides, if you or your baby aren't gaining weight properly and otherwise feeling well, you won't be able to work out, so avoiding these foods gives you more opportunities to work out!

Soft cheeses and unpasteurized milk

Pasteurization is a process that destroys bacteria (including salmonella, listeria, and *E. coli*) in foods that tend to sour easily by heating the foods to a specific temperature for a specific amount of time. Milk, cream, cream cheese, and yogurt almost always go through the pasteurization process, which is why you can keep them in your refrigerator for a couple of weeks or longer without making yourself sick.

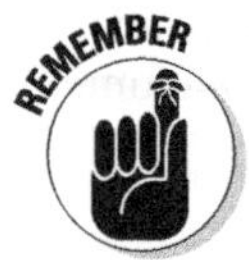

However, many gourmet cheeses (such as bleu, Feta, Brie, and Camembert) are made from *raw milk,* which is a fancy way to say unpasteurized milk. When these cheeses are aged less than 60 days, the bacteria can remain in the cheese, potentially causing infection, premature labor, or miscarriage. Pâté can also contain these bacteria.

Undercooked or raw meat, eggs, or seafood; pâté

If you like soft-cooked eggs, pâté, and rare (you know, bloody) meat and seafood, you may want to rethink your tastes, because these foods frequently contain bacteria that's killed when cooked at a high temperature but lives when not cooked hot enough. And bacteria has the potential to cause infection; while you're pregnant, it can also cause premature labor and even miscarriage. Always cook your eggs and seafood so that no part looks undercooked; cook meat until it's medium well to well done. Avoid pâté altogether when you're pregnant or nursing.

Certain seafood even when well cooked

Seafood is an excellent source of protein and many other nutrients and, if possible, is a food source that most people should eat every day. But not every type of seafood should be on your list of good foods to eat — at least, not while you're pregnant — and you want to limit your intake of all seafood to 12 ounces per week. Both from natural sources in the environment and from industrial pollutants, methyl mercury (a form of mercury) exists in the waters inhabited by and foods eaten by certain types of fish, and the mercury passes through their bodies and into yours, and from yours into the nervous system of your baby.

The fish with the highest levels of methyl mercury are shark, swordfish, king mackerel, tilefish (also called golden snapper), and tuna (steaks or in cans), so try to avoid these completely. Other varieties that are specific to your area may also be on the no-no list, so check with your local health department. In addition, marlin and sea bass sometimes contain high levels of methyl mercury (but sometimes don't), so you may want to avoid those while you're pregnant or nursing, too.

Alcohol

These days, avoiding alcohol seems like a no-brainer that we don't even need to mention in a book for pregnant women, but just in case you've been living in Upper Mongolia for the last ten years, here's the bottom line: Regularly consuming alcohol when you're pregnant puts your baby at risk of *fetal alcohol syndrome,* the leading cause of mental retardation and physical birth defects. Chances are, a sister, cousin, girlfriend, co-worker or someone else has shared advice from a healthcare giver saying that an occasional glass of wine during pregnancy isn't a problem, but this information usually comes from a physician who's trying to calm the fears of a newly pregnant woman who had a large glass of wine on Friday night and found out she was pregnant on Saturday afternoon!

If you do have an occasional alcoholic beverage during your pregnancy, don't beat yourself up over it: Many a healthy child has been born to women who drank some alcohol during their pregnancies, and studies don't verify that drinking small amounts of alcohol during pregnancy causes fetal alcohol syndrome. But the bottom line is that alcohol isn't good for your baby, so avoid it throughout your pregnancy if at all possible. In fact, the motto of the National Organization on Fetal Alcohol Syndrome is "No safe time. No safe amount. No safe alcohol. Period." That's a pretty strong statement.

Chapter 10

Healthy Weight Gain during Pregnancy

In This Chapter

- Knowing how much weight gain is ideal
- Finding ways to subside nausea
- Discovering the calorie content of common foods
- Giving into cravings but with healthier foods

Pregnancy isn't a time to lose weight, but rather to manage your weight. You *must* gain weight to deliver a healthy baby, and your healthcare provider can guide you as to how much is healthy for you.

For some pregnant women, managing their weight actually means they have to work hard to even gain enough weight to support a baby. In fact, for some women, nausea and vomiting are so severe that they simply can't gain enough weight. If this problem applies to you, this chapter gives you a few tips to help keep food down.

For other people, weight management means limiting pregnancy weight gain to only the amount your doctor tells you to gain so that you and your baby are healthy, but you're not faced with an overwhelming amount of weight to lose after your baby is born. You manage your weight during pregnancy by eating a variety of healthy foods (see Chapter 9), by selecting your foods carefully with the full knowledge of their calories and other nutritional content (which we discuss in this chapter), and by exercising.

Adding Up the Numbers: Normal Weight Gain

In order to have a successful pregnancy, you have to gain weight — and not just the six to eight pounds that your baby will weigh when he's born, but also extra fat stores, blood, and body fluids that your baby needs to survive.

Your healthcare provider can help you establish weight-gain goals for each week, month, and/or trimester of your pregnancy.

The average weight gain is 27–30 pounds, and it breaks down like this (see Figure 10-1):

- 7.5 for the baby
- 7 in fat stores that you need to sustain your pregnancy
- 4 in extra body fluids
- 3–4 in extra blood
- 2 in amniotic fluid
- 2 in the uterus
- 1–1.5 in the placenta
- 1–2 in the breasts

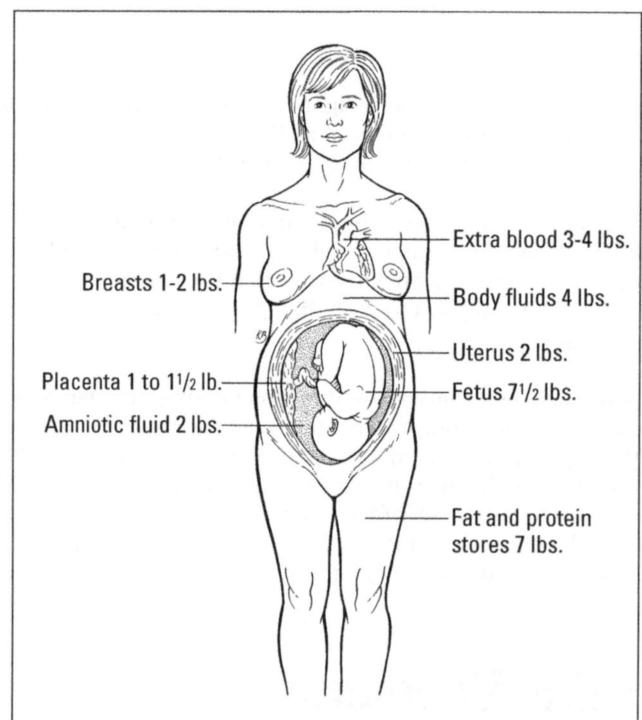

Figure 10-1: How pregnancy weight gain disperses throughout your body.

Keeping Food Down during the First Trimester

Some women are unable to gain the amount of weight they need because they vomit or feel nauseated whenever they eat. And if you're not gaining weight as you're supposed to, your healthcare provider may ask you to stop exercising until you begin to gain weight normally.

Although nausea and vomiting are usually limited to the first trimester and tend to occur only in the morning, note the two following not-so-usual characteristics of so-called morning sickness:

- Nausea and vomiting can occur at any time of the day. In fact, some women feel best in the morning and can't tolerate foods at other times of the day.
- For some women, this period of sickness extends beyond the first trimester.

If you're experiencing sickness in the morning or any time of day, try the following tips:

- Eat several small meals throughout the day and have a snack just before bed. If you get too hungry (for example, after going 12 hours between dinner and breakfast), your nausea will likely become unbearable.
- Keep crackers or another nonperishable, nonspicy snack on your nightstand and eat it before you get out of bed in the morning, especially if you tend to feel nauseated as soon as you get out of bed.
- Keep your meals small. Overeating exacerbates the nausea and can also create or worsen heartburn.
- Focus on eating low-fat, high-carb foods and low-fat dairy products. These foods are much easier to digest than fried foods and high-fat, low-carb foods.
- Limit or completely avoid sweet foods, which tend to increase nausea.
- Try eating ginger, which is an ancient remedy for nausea. You can buy it whole in the produce section of your grocery store; you simply peel it, cut it into cubes, and bake or boil it. You can also find it ground in the spice aisle; sprinkle it on pudding, yogurt, or ice cream or add it to a smoothie or milkshake. If you can find ginger ale (such as Vernor's or Canada Dry) in your area, try that or try ginger tea.

- Avoid overdoing fluids with meals. Drinking fluids with your meals can make you feel overly full.
- Take your vitamin on a full stomach, during or just after a meal.
- If you're unable to get much of anything down, experiment with different types of foods at different times of the day, forgetting everything you know about what healthy foods to eat and when to eat them. If you crave a certain type of food, try it — your body may be telling you what it wants. Even if the food you crave doesn't qualify as one of the healthy foods described in Chapter 9, don't worry too much about the quality of your food choices until your nausea and vomiting disappear — getting some calories in you is your most important priority at this point.
- Avoid tight-fitting clothing, especially during exercise. See Chapter 7 for advice on maternity exercise clothing that doesn't put pressure on your belly.

Keep drinking water, even if you can't keep anything else down. Vomiting quickly dehydrates you, but keeping up your water intake helps keep you from becoming dangerously dehydrated. Also try keeping a cup of ice chips handy and dissolving a few in your mouth every few minutes; this a good way to hydrate when you're feeling nauseous. The same goes for frozen juice: You just chop it up into pieces and eat it.

Eating Enough without Overeating

For a long time, people have thought of pregnancy as 40 weeks of weight gain, followed by 40 years of trying to take the weight off. Over the last few years, however, researchers have found that women who exercise while pregnant gain less fat than their nonexercising counterparts and, after they deliver, have an easier time losing what weight they do gain.

Before getting pregnant, many women are careful about their body weight. Although not everyone is going to have — or even want — a supermodel's body, as a pre-pregnant woman, you probably tried to keep any weight gain to a minimum by watching what you ate and, perhaps, incorporating exercise into your daily routine. For most of your adult life, you've likely had some idea of which foods are high or low in fat and calories. And you have a pretty clear picture of how much you can eat before you start to gain weight.

But now, like Renee Zellweger training for her role in *Bridget Jones's Diary,* you're actually supposed to gain weight. Weight gain during pregnancy is essential for your baby's health. But how much is too much? Will it come off right after the baby is born? Does the necessity of gaining weight mean you throw everything you know about weight control out the window? This section helps you solve the riddle of gaining weight — but not too much weight — during your pregnancy.

Dispelling the eating-for-two myth

The bottom line is that, without exercise, you need only about 300 extra calories per day to gain enough weight to feed and support your developing baby — not twice as many calories as you needed before you became pregnant. That's not a lot, considering that each of the following fast food choices have more than 300 calories, and you're not getting much bang for your 300-calorie buck:

- 1⁄10 of a large Godfather's pizza (305 calories)
- Large Coke at McDonald's (310 calories)
- Starbucks everything bagel (320 calories)
- Grande caramel Frappuccino at Starbucks (350 calories)
- Krispy Kreme glazed cream-filled doughnut (350 calories)
- Regular chocolate cone at Dairy Queen (360 calories)
- Medium fries at Burger King (370 calories)

What happens to many pregnant women is that they follow the "eating for two" advice and see pregnancy as a time to eat whatever they want in whatever quantity feels good — and pregnancy can make you feel very hungry! And they gain more than the weight of the baby, placenta, extra blood, and other essentials of pregnancy.

Finding alternatives

Given that the food choices listed in the preceding section aren't good ways to get your extra calories, what alternatives do you have? Consider the following tips:

- **Go crazy with vegetables.** To maintain a healthy weight, eat all the vegetables you want. Eat your vegetables raw or cook them by grilling or steaming (frying adds fat and calories; boiling washes away many of the vegetable's nutrients). Don't add sauces, and use just a sprinkle of salt, if other herbs aren't flavorful enough.

  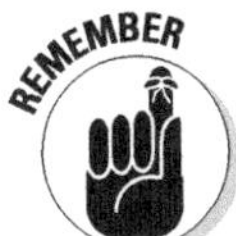

  Don't, however, overload on fruits. Pound for pound, fruits are much higher in calories than vegetables. And though most fruits are full of vitamins and low in fat, if you eat all the fruits you want until you're full, you'll probably exceed your required supply of calories for the day. Aim for four or five half-cup servings of fruit each day.

- **Eat complex carbs that are high in fiber.** Look for whole-grain, high-fiber foods like whole-grain pasta, whole-grain breads, whole-grain cereals, and oatmeal. Reduce your intake of foods that don't offer much nutritional benefit for their calories, such as white rice, potatoes, and white bread. See Chapter 9 for more information on your need for carbohydrates.

- **Drink plenty of water and skim milk.** Avoid sugary sodas, milkshakes, and other high-calorie drinks. Fruit juice offers many vitamins and minerals, but it's rather high in calories, so don't avoid fruit juice completely, but don't go overboard, either. Note that vegetable juices, such as low-sodium tomato juice or V-8 (excess sodium can cause swelling during pregnancy), are far lower in calories than fruit juices and are full of vitamins.

Also use Table 10-1 to help you determine the calorie count of some common, healthy food choices.

Table 10-1 Calorie Count of Healthy Foods

Food	*Calories*
Apple (med)	80
Asparagus (1 cup)	45
Banana	105
Blueberries (1 cup)	80
Broccoli (1 cup)	45
Brown rice (1 cup)	150
Cantaloupe (½)	95 (***Note:*** ½ of a honeydew melon has far more: 225 calories.)
Carrot (one)	30
Cauliflower (1 cup)	30
Celery (1 stalk)	5
Chicken breast, skinless and baked (¼ pound)	100
Chicken drumstick (baked, no skin)	75
Date (a good alternative to cookies, but limit the number you munch on)	23
Egg white	15 (the entire egg has 75 calories)
Kiwi	45
Lean ground beef (1 cup)	200
Mango	135
Unsweetened oatmeal (1 cup)	145
Peanuts (¼ cup)	165

Food	Calories
Plum (med)	25
Raisins (1 cup)	435 (limit to small handfuls)
Red pepper (one)	20
Salmon (3 ounces)	150
Tangerine	35
Tomato (one)	25
Zucchini (1 cup)	35

Tying in to the exercise-calorie connection

Staying fit during pregnancy makes you conscious of how your body feels, so you're far less likely to think of pregnancy as a time to throw caution to the wind and overindulge. When you like the way your strong arms feel or how firm your thighs are getting, you make better choices about the foods you eat.

In addition, you're burning more calories than if you don't exercise, so when you respond to your hunger and odd cravings and take in more calories than the extra 300 you need, you don't gain as much weight. Here's a sample of the approximate calories you burn for 30 minutes of various activities if you weigh 125 pounds (you burn slightly less if you start out weighing less; slightly more as you gain weight in your pregnancy):

- Swimming: 300
- Using an elliptical trainer: 270
- Cycling 12 to 14 miles per hour: 240
- Running 10 minutes per mile: 240
- Stair-stepping: 180
- Doing low-impact aerobics: 165
- Dancing: 165
- Gardening: 135
- Brisk housecleaning: 135
- Walking 17 minutes per mile: 120
- Yoga: 120

Compare these activities to sitting (34 calories for 30 minutes), and you see that exercise helps you burn far more calories than if you don't work out.

Pickles and Ice Cream: Feeding Your Cravings

Ah, yes: the old pickles-and-ice cream cliché. For generations, the cravings of pregnant women have been both held up as an undisputed fact and mocked as pure fiction. But whether cravings are in your mind or in your body, if you feel a craving, you feel it!

If you find yourself raiding the fridge late at night (or at any time) and, as a result, you're not eating very healthy foods, keep some of the following healthy snacks in your fridge or pantry:

- Peeled baby carrots, celery sticks, zucchini or yellow squash sticks, and pepper slices
- Small, portable fruit, like apples, bananas, tangerines, plums, peaches, and so on
- Fat-free, low-calorie gelatin, pudding, and yogurt in single-serve packages
- Low-salt, fat-free rice cakes
- Reduced-fat, low-salt crackers made without hydrogenated oils (check the label)
- Single-serve cans of low-sodium V-8 or other tomato juice
- Cubes of low-fat or fat-free cheese
- Sorbet, low-fat sherbet, low-fat frozen yogurt, or low-fat ice cream
- Frozen fruit juice bars

Alternatively, don't stock your pantry and fridge with any of the following. If your partner likes this stuff, too bad — he'll have to go without for these 40 weeks, because if a craving sets in and the high-fat, high-calorie object of your desire is within reach, chances are, you'll eat it.

- Cookies and candy
- Chips and other processed snack foods
- Sugary cereal
- White bread
- High-fat milk, cheeses, yogurt, and ice cream

The best news you've heard all day

Are you ready for some great nutritional news? A recent Finnish study linked eating chocolate during pregnancy with happy, confident babies. Seriously! At six months of age, babies born to women who regularly ate chocolate during pregnancy showed more happy traits (smiling, laughing) and demonstrated less fear of new situations than babies born to women who didn't eat chocolate while pregnant.

One caveat: All the women in the study, chocolate eaters and abstainers alike, felt stress during their pregnancy, so these effects may not exist for that one woman in 10,000 who somehow manages to be stress free during pregnancy. And researchers aren't yet ready to say without a doubt that other factors aren't contributing to this link between chocolate and happy babies. But given how happy eating chocolate can make you, why wouldn't babies feel just as good about it?

Also keep trigger foods out of the house. A *trigger food* is one that causes you to overeat every time you eat it. Each person has different trigger foods, from chocolate to crackers to cookies to pie. Now, if your trigger food is broccoli, no need to limit it at all, but for most people, trigger foods aren't exactly healthy or wholesome!

Part IV

Fun and Healthy Activities for Pregnancy and Beyond

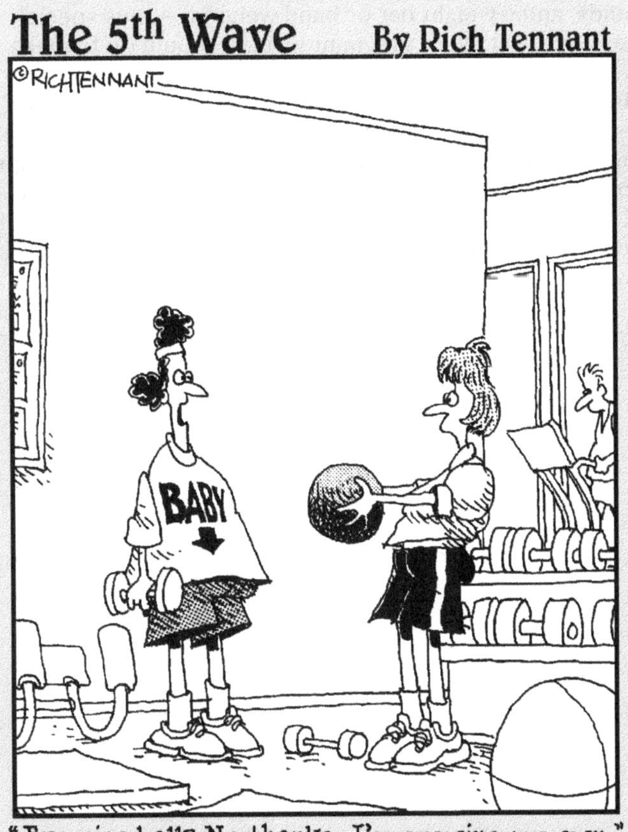

"Exercise ball? No thanks, I'm growing my own."

In this part . . .

We introduce you to a world of fun activities that, done regularly, get you into terrific shape. From the first chapter on how to use an exercise ball, resistance bands, and a weight bar or hand weights — plus special exercises that every pregnant woman should do to make delivery easier — to chapters on fitness walking and running, swimming and water aerobics, yoga and low-impact aerobics, cycling, and indoor machines, this part discusses the equipment you need, shows you techniques, and helps you design a workout plan for these activities. At the end of this part, you also find a chapter on cross-training, which helps you incorporate two or more activities into one workout plan.

Chapter 11

Balls, Bands, Bars, and Mats: Simple, Inexpensive Workouts

In This Chapter

- Discovering cheap workout equipment
- Building your core strength
- Using an exercise ball to build strength and flexibility
- Getting strong with exercise bands
- Toning with a weight bar or set of hand-held free weights

In this chapter, you discover the least-expensive workouts you can create: All you need is an exercise ball, a set of resistance bands, or a weight bar or set of free weights. (If you're not sure what these doohickeys are, check out the following section.) By using this type of equipment, you keep your financial investment low, you eliminate the need to buy special clothing, and you make getting started right away easy to do, because you can do the exercises right in your living room or dining room. And one of the best benefits of using balls, bands, or weights is that you can build your upper body strength. Having a strong upper body reduces your risk of back injury and helps prepare your body to lift and carry your baby.

For best results, combine the strength-building exercises in this chapter with other inexpensive forms of exercise that give a cardiovascular workout, such as walking (see Chapter 12) or using an aerobics video (see Chapter 14). And if you've never worked out before, see Chapter 5 for important information about how to monitor your workouts and make adjustments based on how you're feeling.

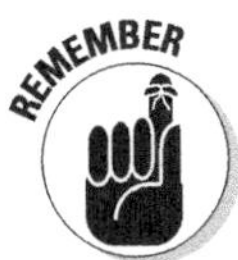

For any of the exercises in this chapter, wear comfortable clothing (see Chapter 7). You can go barefoot, wear socks, or wear aerobics shoes. If you're going barefoot, you may want to invest in an exercise mat that provides some traction. Look for these mats at any sporting goods store or through any store catalog that sells yoga equipment.

Introducing the Cheapest Exercise Equipment You Can Buy

By watching advertisements on TV or talking with friends, you may begin to think that you need to spend a lot of money on exercise equipment or on a gym or pool membership in order to get fit. Nothing is further from the truth. You can give yourself a great workout by using the following equipment:

- **A workout ball:** A *workout ball* (sometimes called an *exercise ball*) is a plastic, air-filled ball on which you can sit, bend, and stretch to get a great workout that doesn't hurt your back. Because you have to work hard to stay balanced while on the ball, your balance improves, along with your posture, strength, and flexibility. During pregnancy, the ball supports your additional weight and helps you work out in spite of your changing center of gravity. As you use the ball more, you become more proficient and comfortable on it. See the "Working with a Workout Ball" section for details on purchasing a workout ball and for some exercises to try.
- **Resistance bands:** *Resistance bands* are like giant rubber bands — they provide resistance both as you stretch a band apart and as you slowly allow it to return to its natural position. With a set of resistance bands, you can perform dozens of strengthening exercises in a small space and with very little financial investment. In fact, just about everything you can do with hand weights (see the following bullet), you can do with resistance bands, such as bicep curls, shoulder press, and so on. See "The Irresistible Lure of Resistance Bands," later in this chapter, for details on choosing the right bands for you and for some specific resistance-band exercises.
- **Hand weights or a weight bar:** *Hand weights* — small dumbbells that you hold in your hands — are inexpensive, easy to use, and a cinch to maintain. However, if you need to buy several sizes for different exercises (such as a set of one-pound weights, three-pound weights, five-pounders, and ten-pounders, for example), your costs can add up. For this reason, weight bars, like the one shown in Figure 11-1, are becoming increasingly popular. You can use just the bar or add small doughnut-shaped weights to each end. The disadvantage of weight bars is that they force you to use both arms at the same time, whereas free weights allow you to use one arm at a time. See the "No Holds Barred: Bars and Hand Weights" section for details and a listing of some common exercises. Also check out Chapter 16 for a discussion on using weight machines, which are far more expensive but use many of the same muscles.

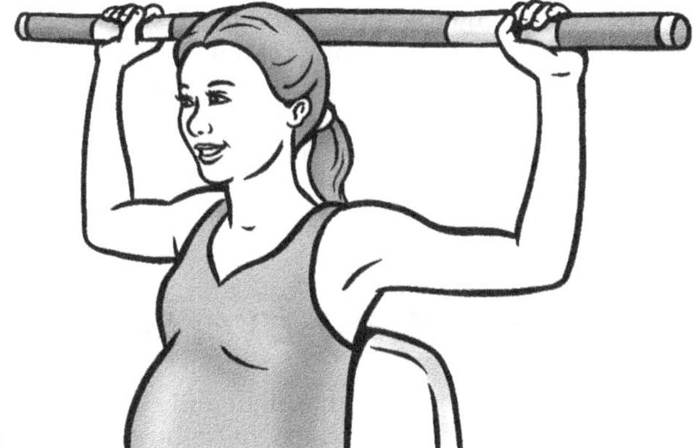

Figure 11-1: A weight bar.

Weider makes an all-in-one kit that includes an exercise ball and pump, resistance bands, wrist or ankle weights, and a jump rope. It retails for around $40 and is available at sporting goods stores and many discount stores that carry exercise equipment. Recently, this kit went on sale at Sears for $25, and with a $10 Sears coupon that came in the newspaper, we bought the whole kit and caboodle for just 15 bucks!

Don't forget to breathe!

Be sure to keep breathing normally and correctly (exhaling as you lift or stretch; inhaling as you relax) when you do any of the exercises in this chapter, rather than holding your breath, as you may be tempted to do. You may not think you need instructions on how to breathe, but the truth is many people don't breathe efficiently when they exercise their core muscles (or, for that matter, when they do any kind of exertion, like lifting a baby, as discussed in Chapter 18). If you tend to hold your breath when you're making an effort, try practicing a better way to breathe:

1. **Lying on your back or in a semireclined position, place your arms out to the side and bend your knees with your feet resting on the floor.**

   Keep a natural curve in your back — don't try to flatten your back against the floor.

2. **Breathe in, letting your belly fill and rise.**
3. **Breathe out, pulling in your abdomen.**

To double-check whether you're breathing correctly, place one hand on your belly as you breathe in and out, checking that your belly rises as it fills and collapses as it empties. Your tummy, not your shoulders, should rise and fall with each breath.

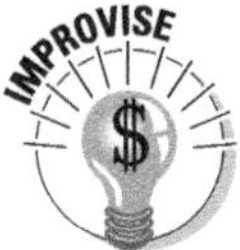

If $15 still sounds like too much money, how about free? Any item that's easy to hold and that weighs enough to build muscle functions as a hand weight. For a really inexpensive set of weights, take empty milk or juice containers and fill them to varying levels with sand or pebbles. Use your bathroom scale to see how much each one weighs. Cans of food — soups, veggies, fruits — and bottles of syrup or juice also work well.

Doing Core Strengthening Exercises

Your *core* muscles are those that keep you upright and stable as you walk and exercise — the muscles in your abdomen, hips, back, butt, and pelvic floor. Because these muscles are all layered and interconnected, you want to do exercises that reach several of the muscles at one time. (These exercises are usually called *core strengthening exercises,* but they're also sometimes referred to as *functional exercises* or *spinal stabilization.*) After exercising multiple core muscles, you'll find yourself standing up straighter and taller, and your coordination and strength will improve throughout your body.

You don't need special equipment to do core strengthening exercises, just a mat or towel to lie on and a pillow or rolled-up towel to put under your head.

Pelvic floor (Kegel) exercise

Your *pelvic floor muscles* play an important role — both during pregnancy and throughout your life — in maintaining function and support of your pelvic organs (bladder, reproductive organs, rectum). The pelvic floor muscles form a figure eight around your urethra, vagina, and anus, spanning from the front of your pelvis to your tailbone — see Figure 11-2. Doing pelvic floor exercises with control strengthens the pelvic floor muscles and, at the same time, gets you used to what it feels like to contract and relax your pelvic floor, which comes in handy at pushing time during delivery. Pelvic floor exercises (also called *Kegel exercises*) are simple to perform after you get the hang of which muscles to contract.

One way to locate your pelvic floor muscles is to notice the muscles that contract when you stop your flow of urine: Those muscles responsible for stopping the flow are the pelvic floor muscles. Use the urine stop-and-start test when sitting on a toilet to figure out how to locate and isolate the pelvic floor muscle group. After you've figured out how to contract your pelvic floor muscles, use the following exercise to strengthen them.

To do the pelvic floor exercise:

1. **Slowly contract your pelvic floor muscles throughout a count of 5.**
2. **Hold for 5 seconds and then release for a count of 5.**

   As you contract the muscles, think of drawing them up and, like an elevator, going up several floors. Figure 11-2 shows what the pelvic floor muscles look like when they're relaxed and what happens when you contract them.

As you do Kegel exercises, keep these suggestions in mind:

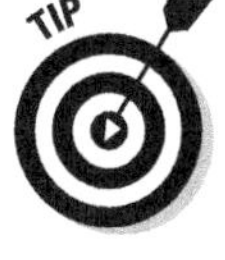

- Start with 10 to 20 slow repetitions (reps), twice a day, and build up to 25 or more reps, twice a day. If your pelvic floor muscles fatigue quickly, do fewer reps each time, but do the exercises more than twice a day.
- Remember that no one can tell you're doing these exercises, so you can do them anywhere. In fact, try to use certain activities (for example, driving to work, brushing your teeth, or taking a shower) as your cue to do your exercises.
- Contract your pelvic floor muscles each time you lift, laugh, sneeze, or cough to provide support.

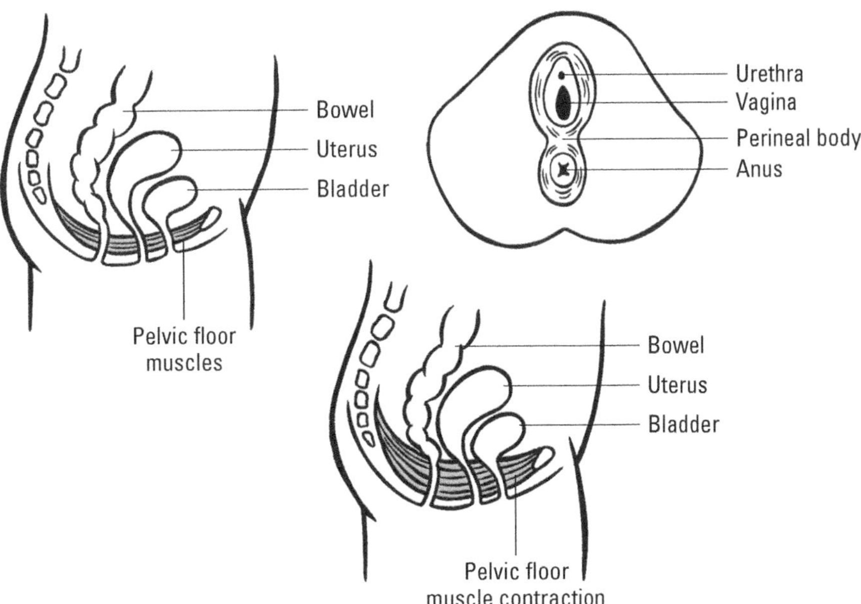

Figure 11-2: The pelvic floor muscles relaxed and contracted.

Don't fatigue your muscles to the point of being unable to perform any more pelvic floor contractions. If you're unable to hold for 5 seconds, alternate slow contractions and holds with the *quick-contraction technique:* Contract your pelvic floor muscles by quickly squeezing and releasing, repeating for up to 20 or more reps. Keep in mind, however, that the longer you hold each contraction, the more effectively you build pelvic floor strength, so your ultimate goal is to build your reps and contraction hold times from 5 seconds to 10 seconds or more.

Four-point abdominal exercise

Your abdominal muscles provide support for your back and your abdominal organs. During pregnancy, however, the expansion of your tummy can cause your abdominal muscles to lose some ability to support your spine, which also makes traditional sit-ups difficult and not very effective. Instead, focus on gently strengthening your abdominal muscles without putting stress on your low back, using the four-point abdominal exercise in this section.

The following four-point abdominal exercise strengthens the abdominal muscles.

1. **Get on your hands and knees on a soft surface, as shown in Figure 11-3.**

   If you have carpal tunnel pain, rest on your knuckles instead of your hands.

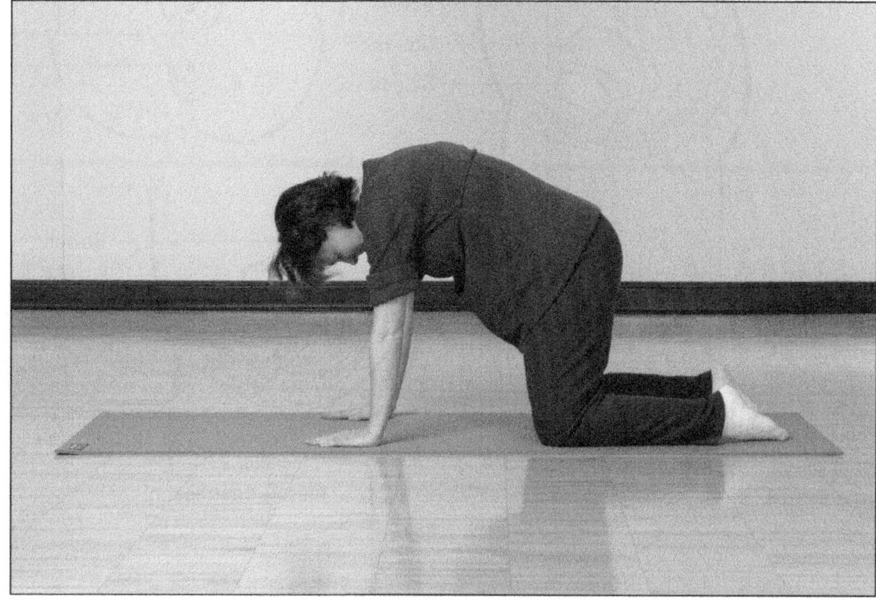

Figure 11-3: Maintain a neutral spine while doing the four-point abdominal exercise.

2. **Maintain a neutral spine, without overarching or swaying your back. Count to 5 while slowly contracting your abdomen.**

   Think of pulling your belly button up toward your spine as you contract.

3. **Hold for 5 to 10 seconds, breathing normally as you hold, and then relax slowly to a count of 5 and repeat 5 to 10 times.**

Four-point strengthening and balance exercise

The four-point strengthening and balance exercise targets your abdominal muscles and also improves your balance and overall strength. Start this exercise slowly, and don't raise your arm and leg higher than a height that feels balanced for you. If you feel as though you're going to lose your balance, lower your arm and leg to the point were you feel balanced again.

1. **Get on your hands and knees on a soft surface, as shown in Figure 11-4a.**

   If you have carpal tunnel pain, rest on your knuckles instead of your hands and use a padded mat.

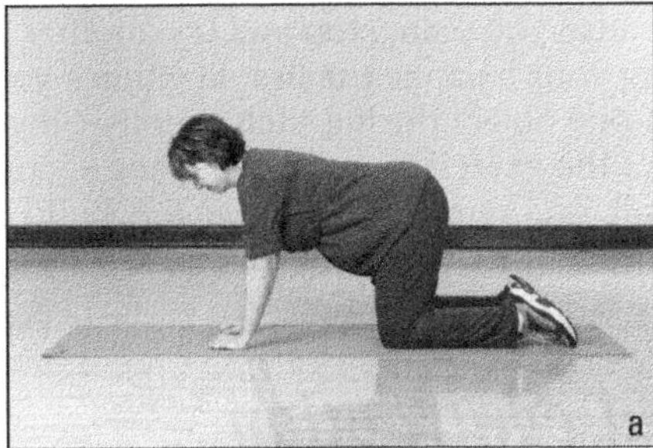

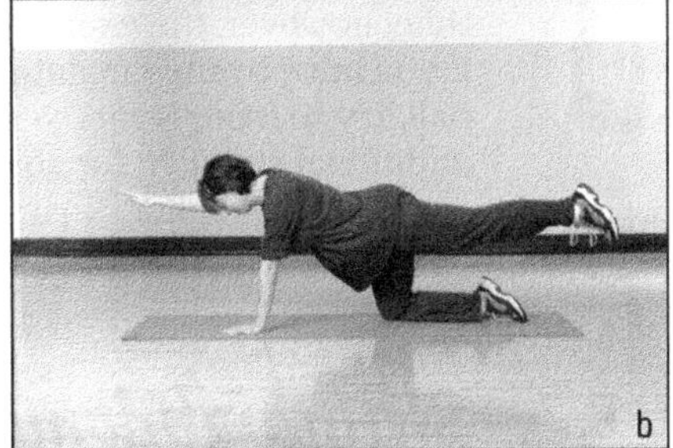

Figure 11-4: Doing the four-point strengthening and balance exercise.

2. **Slowly extend your right arm up until it's level with your right shoulder.**

3. **Slowly extend your left leg out until it's level with your left hip, as Figure 11-4b shows.**

   Try to keep your back in a neutral position, not overarched or swayed.

4. **Hold for 5 seconds and return to your starting position. Repeat with your left arm and right leg. Build up to 5 reps each side.**

Working with a Workout Ball

Workout balls come in different diameters. If you get a chance to try a ball before buying, sit on it and put your feet flat on the floor. If the ball fits you correctly, your thighs will be perfectly horizontal and parallel to the floor. If you aren't able to try the ball before you buy, use the following guidelines:

- If you're between 4'11" and 5'3", use a 55-centimeter ball.
- If you're between 5'4" and 5'10", use a 65-centimeter ball.
- If you're 5'11" or taller, use a 75-centimeter ball.

Keep in mind, however, that if your legs are particularly short or long, you may want to go one size down or up, respectively. If you're ever in doubt about which size to choose, or if your height is right between two sizes, always choose a larger ball, not a smaller one.

Because an exercise ball can lose its air fill, be sure to buy a ball that includes a pump or purchase a pump separately. Although you can work out on an underinflated ball (that is, you won't ruin the ball), the ball won't be as firm and stable as when it's properly inflated. The ball should feel firm and supportive but still respond to the weight of your body and provide some give.

After you purchase a ball and inflate it, try the following exercises. If at any time, however, the exercises cause you pain, stop and try another exercise. If you have trouble maintaining your balance the first few times you use the ball, try to focus your eyes on one object during each exercise. If you want additional stability, for some of the exercises in the following sections, you can place the ball against a wall. And remember to *gradually* build up to the number of repetitions (reps) noted for each exercise.

Sitting abdominal contraction

The sitting abdominal contraction strengthens the abdominal muscles like the core strengthening exercises do (see the "Doing Core Strengthening Exercises" section), but you perform the exercise while sitting on an exercise ball, which may be more comfortable during pregnancy than working out on the floor.

1. **Position yourself comfortably on the ball with your feet flat and your hands resting on your tummy, as shown in Figure 11-5.**

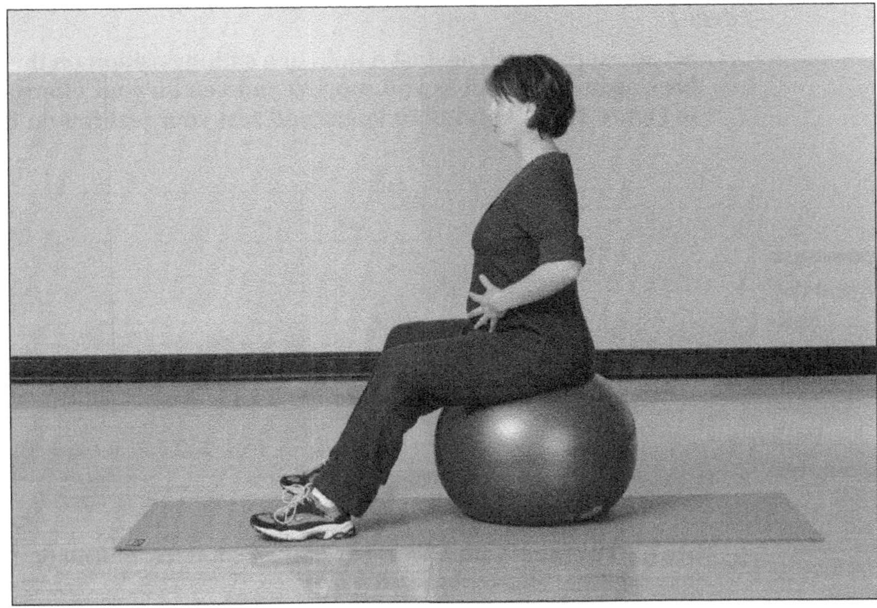

Figure 11-5: Sitting on a workout ball and contracting your abs.

See the "Working with a Workout Ball" section for information on selecting and using an exercise ball.

2. **Take a deep breath and, as you exhale, slowly contract your abdomen as tightly as you can.**

   As you contract, focus on pulling in the muscles below your belly button.

3. **Keep breathing normally as you hold for a count of 5.**

4. **Relax to a count of 5; repeat 5 to 10 times.**

Semireclined abdominal exercise

The following progressive, two-level exercise is adapted from what's known as the *Sahrmann abdominal exercises.* Sahrmann exercises (discussed further in Chapter 18) are a safe and effective way to strengthen the muscles below your belly button without hurting your back. You start with level 1, and when you're able to do 20 reps with each leg, move up to level 2. The exercise has been modified from a back-lying position to a semireclined position to make it more comfortable for pregnancy.

Level I

1. **Set an exercise ball against a wall. In a sitting position on the floor, lean back against the ball as you support yourself on your elbows, as shown in Figure 11-6a. Bend both knees and rest your feet flat on the floor.**

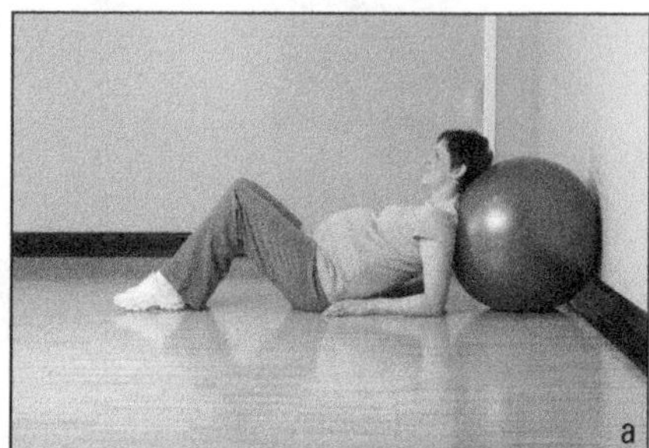
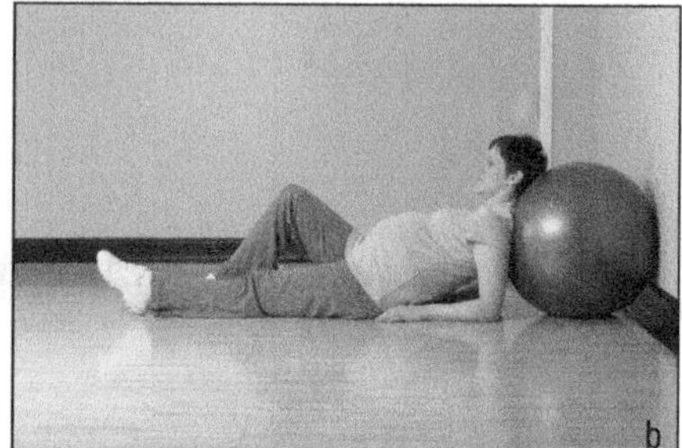

Figure 11-6: Semi-reclined abdominal exercise, Part I.

   See the "Working with a Workout Ball" section for information on selecting and using an exercise ball.

2. **Take a breath and, as you exhale, contract your lower abdominal muscles and hold as you slowly slide your left leg out along the floor to a count of 5, until it's straight, as Figure 11-6b shows.**

   Remember to keep breathing normally as you hold the contraction.

3. **Slowly bring your left leg back to its starting position, using a count of 5 and keeping your abdominal muscles contracted.**
4. **Relax your abdominal contraction and repeat with your right leg; build up to 20 reps on each leg.**

Level II

1. **Get into the same position as Part I of this exercise describes in the preceding section.**
2. **Take a breath, exhale, tighten your tummy, bend your left leg, and bring it up toward your chest, as shown in Figure 11-7a.**

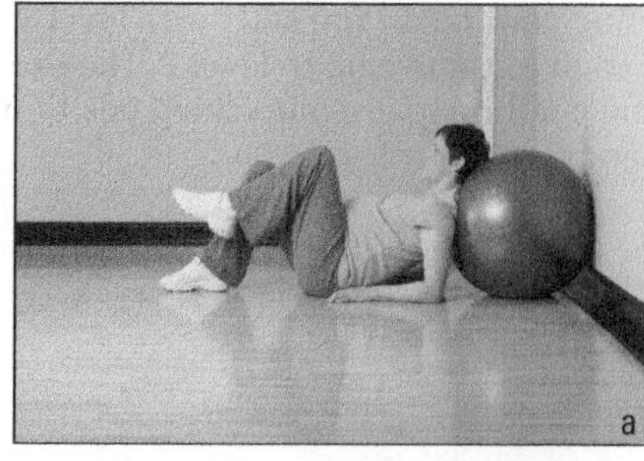
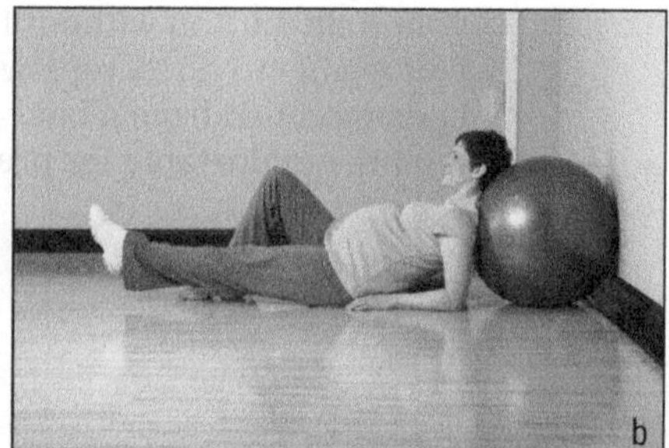

Figure 11-7: Semi-reclined abdominal exercise, Part II.

3. **Continue contracting your abdominal muscles and slowly extend your left leg out, using a count of 5, until it's parallel with floor, as shown in Figure 11-7b.**

   Keep your leg up an inch or two from the floor.

4. **Slowly bring your left leg back, using a count of 5, to its starting position.**
5. **Relax your abdominal contraction, and then repeat the sequence with your right leg, building up to 20 reps on each leg.**

Ball back extension

The ball back extension exercise feels wonderful on your back. It effectively stretches your entire spine and your chest. Use caution when doing this exercise, however, because you need to maintain balance. Avoid rising up too far onto the ball and make sure your feet are securely planted on the floor throughout.

1. **Sit on the floor with the ball behind you and your feet placed securely on the floor or on an exercise mat.**
2. **Extend your arms back onto the ball and slowly press your back into the ball. Raise your bottom up off the floor until you roll your body partially up onto the ball.**
3. **Relax your head and neck back onto the ball as you drop your arms to the sides, as shown in Figure 11-8.**

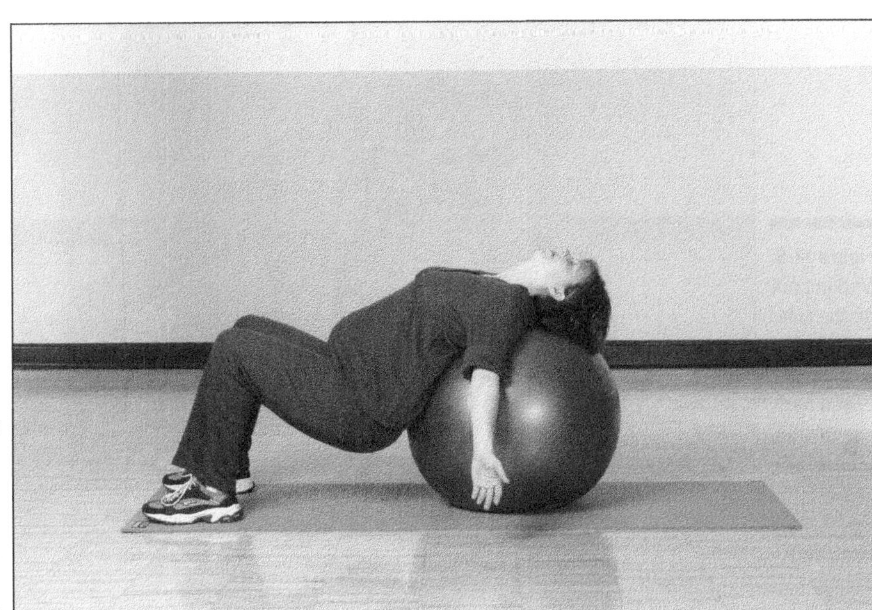

Figure 11-8: Leaning back in the ball back extension.

4. **Gently roll back and forth a few inches.**
5. **Slowly roll back down to your starting position. Repeat 2 to 3 times.**

Ball side shoulder and back extension

The following exercise works the sides of your body — the muscles in your shoulders and back — by having you bend sideways over the ball. For greater stability, brace the ball against a wall.

1. **Kneel on the floor and place the ball on your right side.**
2. **Straighten your left leg out to the side and point your left toe, keeping your foot on the floor. Remain kneeling on your right knee.**
3. **Slowly stretch your body sideways over the ball, as shown in Figure 11-9.**

   Lift your left arm overhead as you stretch and, if necessary, grasp the ball with your right arm to help provide stability. Avoid stretching beyond the point where you feel comfortable.
4. **Repeat on the other side.**

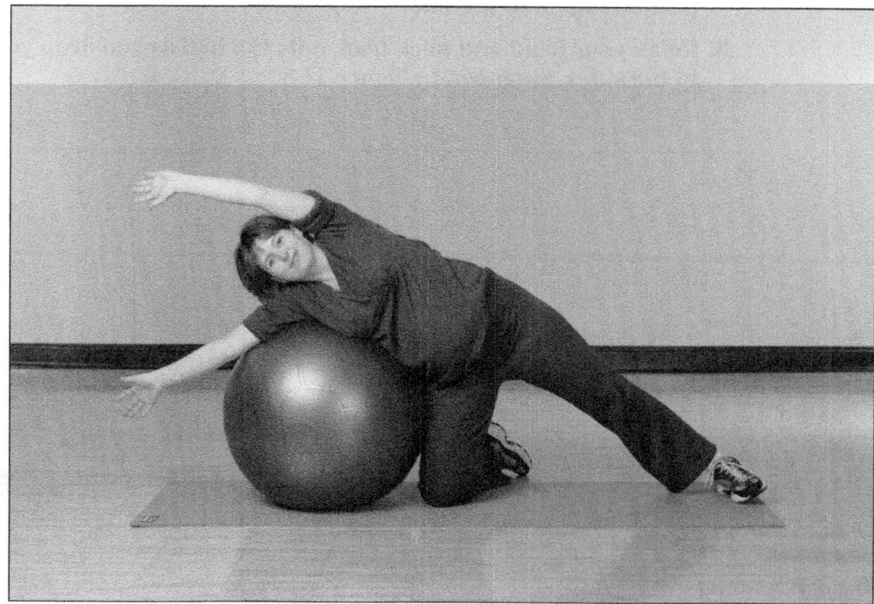

Figure 11-9: Working out on the side: The ball side shoulder and back extension.

Ball forward spine extension

The ball forward spine extension exercise stretches and strengthens your entire spine.

1. **Kneel on the floor with the ball in front of your body.**
2. **Place your hands on top of the ball and face your head down.**
3. **Slowly lean forward, rolling the ball away from your body until your arms are straight and you feel a stretch throughout your back and hips, as shown in Figure 11-10.**
4. **Hold the position for 5 seconds and roll back to your starting position.**
5. **Press forward again, this time angling your body to the left until you feel a stretch in your right arm and back. Hold for 5 seconds.**
6. **Roll back and repeat, angling your body to the right.**
7. **Repeat all three forms of this exercise 2 times.**

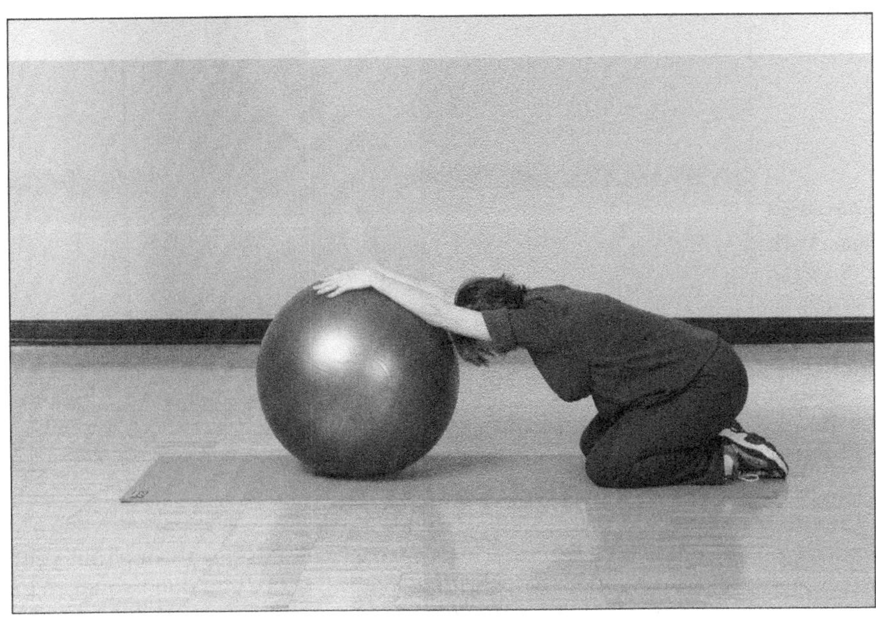

Figure 11-10: Leaning forward in the ball forward spine extension.

Ball pelvic tilt

The ball pelvic tilt stretches and increases your range of motion in the muscles surrounding your pelvis and hips. Take care that you don't push past the point of comfort; make this a gentle stretch.

1. **Sit securely on the ball with your feet on the floor and your hands on your hips, as Figure 11-11 shows.**
2. **Using slow, gentle motions, gently rock your pelvis forward and tilt backward, repeating 2 to 3 times.**

   You can also hold each position for several seconds to enhance the stretch.

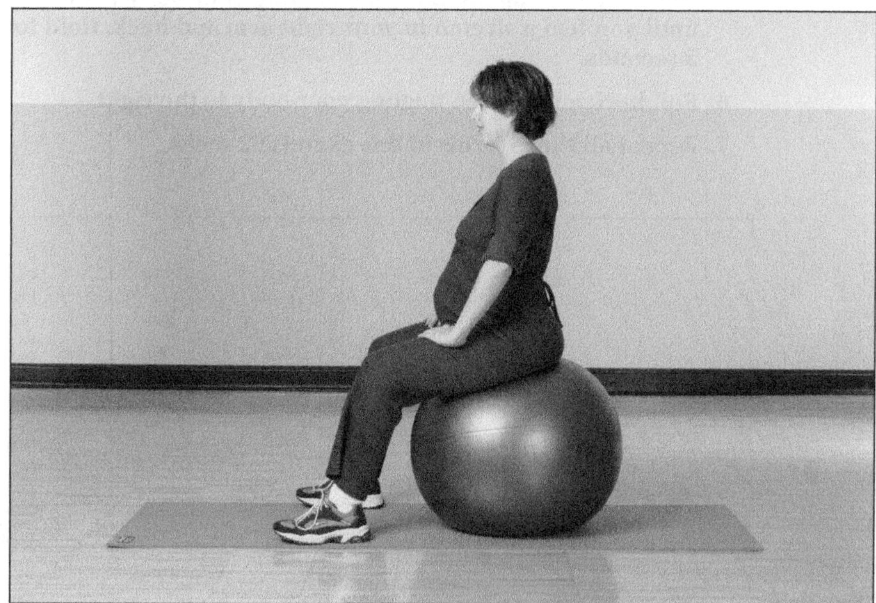

Figure 11-11: Sitting up straight for the ball pelvic tilt.

Ball lift and squat

The following exercise works a variety of muscles throughout your legs, back, and arms and also helps with balance. Be sure you don't squat so low that your knees hurt or that you have a hard time rising up out of the squat position.

1. **Squat down with your feet shoulder-width apart and grasp the ball with both hands so that you're holding it at shoulder height, as Figure 11-12a shows.**

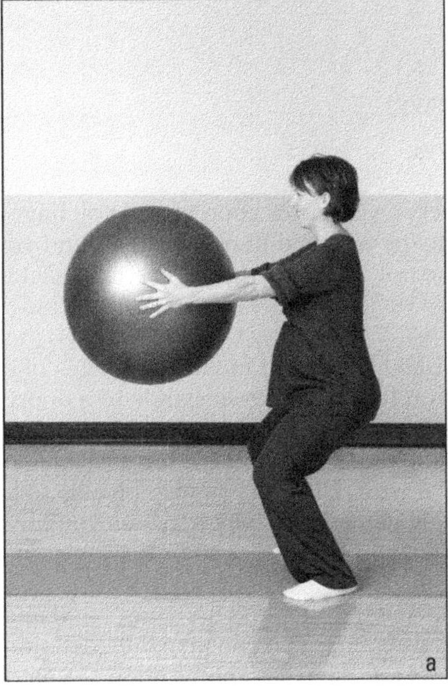

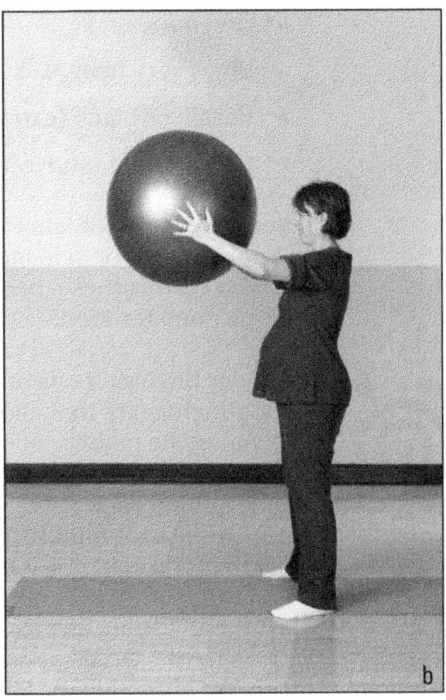

Figure 11-12: Squat and lift to tone your legs, back, and arms.

2. **Slowly rise to a standing position by straightening your legs, keeping the ball in front of you and lifting it to eye level, as shown in Figure 11-12b.**

   Make sure that your back remains straight.

3. **Return to your starting position and repeat.**

The Irresistible Lure of Resistance Bands

Resistance bands come in a variety of colors, each related to its thickness and the amount of resistance it offers. The thicker the band, the more resistance the band gives, which means the harder your workout will be and the fitter you'll get. You need to determine which band to use by finding the level that allows you to do 10 to 12 reps without straining. As you become stronger, move up to the next level. The colors are, from thinnest (least resistance) to thickest (most resistance):

- Tan (very thin)
- Yellow (thin — many people start with this color)
- Red (medium — many people start with this color, too)

- Green (heavy)
- Blue (very heavy)
- Purple or black (extra heavy)
- Gray or gold (super heavy)

If you're using a nonlatex variety (which is a good idea if you have an allergy to latex), the color scheme may be a little different. Call around your area to see who carries these, because not every store that carries resistance bands has the nonlatex kind.

Consider buying a resistance band kit, which includes all sizes of bands, plus door attachments that allow you to connect your bands to a doorframe, thus expanding the number of exercises you can do. Also look for resistance bands that have handles, which may be more comfortable for you than looping the tubing around each hand. And, if you're lucky, you may be able to locate some newer resistance bands that you can adjust, which means you buy only one band, but you can adjust it from light resistance to heavy resistance.

Start the following exercises with a thinner, less-resistant band and work your way up to thicker, more-resistant bands. You can also increase the band resistance by shortening the length of the band (wrapping a loop around your foot). Do each exercise slowly and deliberately. If you start with a thicker band or if you do your exercises too quickly and lose control, the snap from the band can really hurt. (Think of how much a small rubber band hurts as it snaps back at you, and then multiply that by about 100.) This snapback is also a reason to buy the highest quality resistance bands you can afford — after all, if a cheaper band breaks midexercise, the force of that snap against your skin can lead to a serious injury. In the same way, if you see a hole, tear, or worn spot in the tubing, replace that band so that it doesn't snap midexercise.

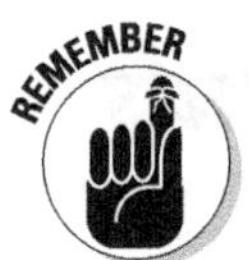

When using resistance bands or lifting weights (see the section "No Holds Barred: Bars and Hand Weights," later in this chapter), don't lock your knees or elbows; instead, keep them bent slightly. Use a slow, controlled motion when you lift the weight or band and when you return to your starting position. You may want to use a count of 1, 2, 3 as you lift and again as you return to your starting position. Build up to 1 or 2 sets of 10 to 12 reps of each exercise.

Band bicep exercise

The following exercise works your *biceps,* which are the muscles on the inside of your upper arms.

1. **Stand with the band under your feet, the ends in your hands, and your arms extended toward the floor, as shown in Figure 11-13a.**

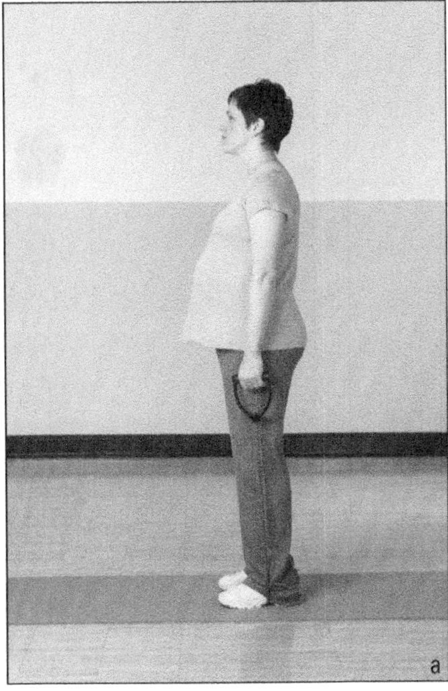
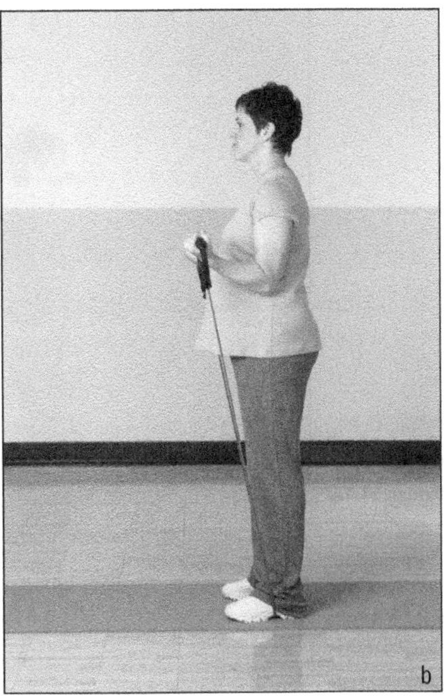

Figure 11-13: Tone your biceps by using a resistance band.

2. **With your palms facing up, slowly curl your hands up toward your chest by bending your elbows, as shown in Figure 11-13b.**

   The only movement in your body should be in your lower arms and elbows. Keep your upper arms, legs, and back perfectly still so that the exercise focuses on your bicep muscle. Most people find that holding the upper arms and elbows tight against your sides helps reduce movement.

3. **Return to your starting position at the same speed and repeat. Start with 10 to 12 reps and gradually build up to 2 sets of 10 to 12 reps.**

Band tricep exercise

The following exercise works the *triceps,* which are the muscles at the back of your upper arms. (These muscles are the ones that cause many sleeveless shirts to hide out in the backs of closets.)

1. **Stand with the end of the band under your left foot. Bring the other end up behind your back and grasp it with your left hand.**
2. **Bend your left elbow up to be level with your head and place your right hand under your left arm for support, as shown in Figure 11-14a.**

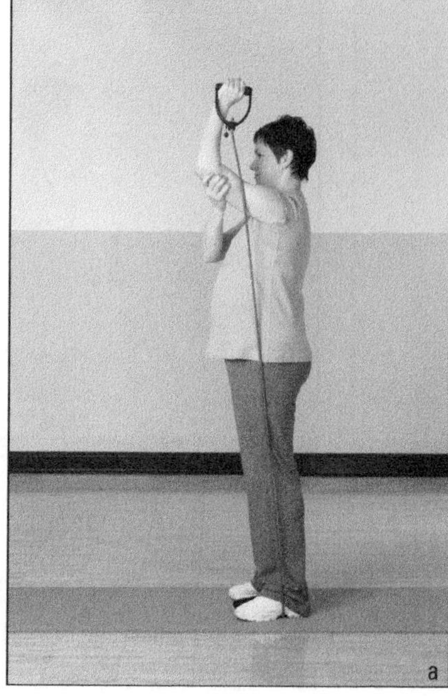

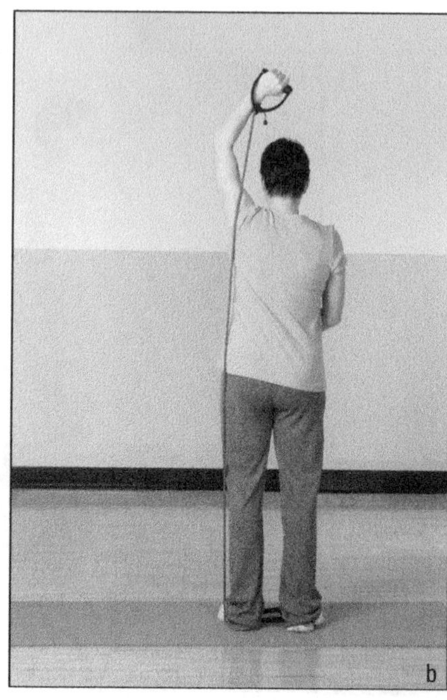

Figure 11-14: Tighten upper arms with the band tricep exercise.

3. **Slowly raise your hand until you've stretched the band straight up and your arm is fully extended, as shown in Figure 11-14b.**

   Remember to not lock your elbow.

4. **Return to your starting position and repeat. Start with 10 to 12 reps and gradually build up to 2 sets of 10 to 12 reps. Repeat with your right hand.**

Band shoulder exercise

You can get strong, sexy shoulder muscles by using a resistance band. Just follow these steps:

1. **Stand with the band under both feet. Grasp the ends of the band with both hands, palms facing out, and place your hands level with your shoulders, as Figure 11-15a shows.**
2. **Raise your hands by extending your arms up until they're straight and in line with your body, as shown in Figure 11-15b.**

   Remember to not lock your elbows.

3. **Slowly lower your arms to your starting position and repeat. Start with 10 to 12 reps and gradually build up to 2 sets of 10 to 12 reps.**

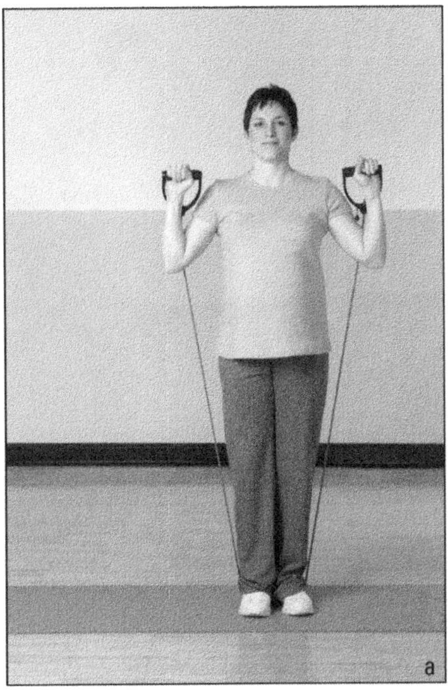

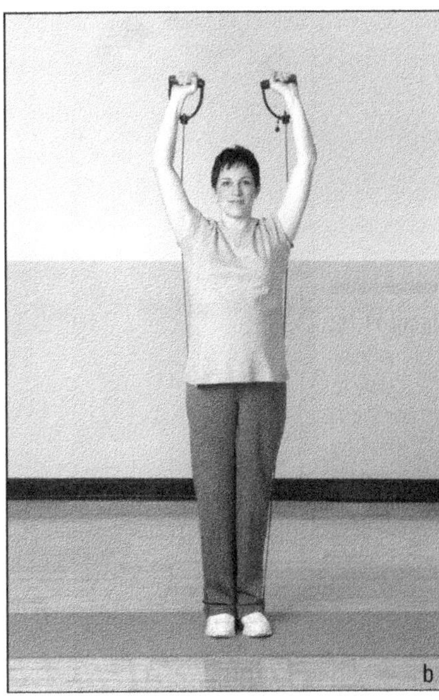

Figure 11-15: Work your shoulders with the band shoulder exercise.

Band row exercise

A *row* is an upright pulling motion, much like you use when rowing a boat. This row exercise works the upper arms.

1. **Stand slightly angled forward, with your left knee forward and bent, and your right leg extended with your foot flat behind your body, as shown in Figure 11-16a.**
2. **Place one end of the band under your left foot and grasp the other end with your left hand.**

   Make sure that you don't have any slack in the band when your left arm is straight.
3. **With your palm facing your side, slowly raise the band toward your shoulder by bending your left elbow. Pull your elbow up until it is level with your shoulder, as shown in Figure 11-16b.**
4. **Slowly return to your starting position and repeat. Start with 10 to 12 reps and gradually build up to 2 sets of 10 to 12 reps.**

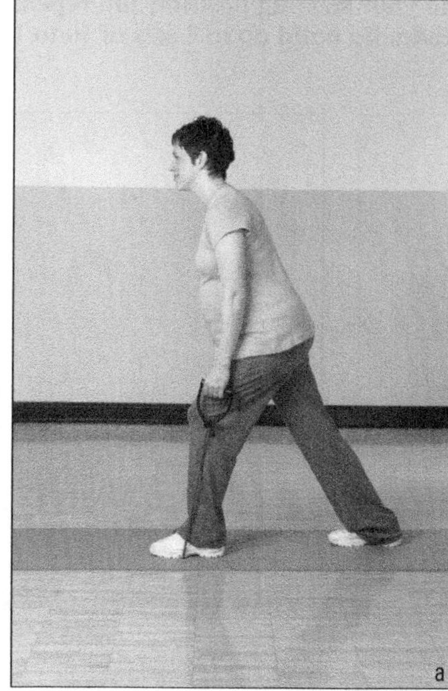

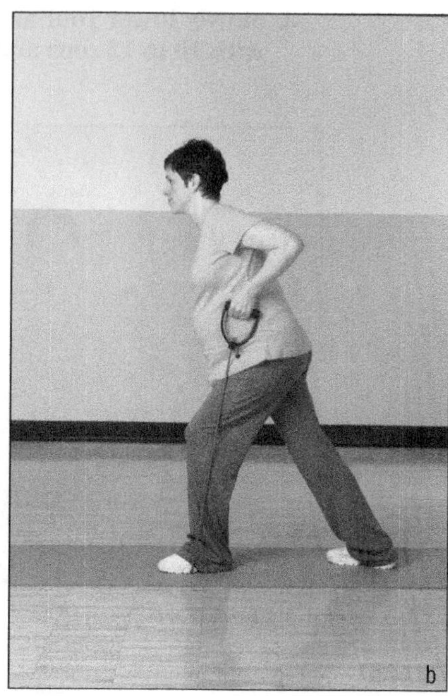

Figure 11-16: Row your way to stronger arms by using a resistance band.

Band deltoid exercise

The following exercise works your *deltoid* (upper back and shoulder) muscles.

1. **Stand with the middle of the band under your feet and one end of the band in each hand. Keep your palms facing your sides and your arms extended and parallel with your sides, as Figure 11-17a shows.**
2. **Slowly raise your arms out to your sides and up towards your shoulders until you feel the band become difficult to raise any farther, as shown in Figure 11-17b.**

   Try to keep your arms moving up in a straight line as you raise them, and only go to the point where you feel firm resistance.
3. **Slowly relax back into your starting position and repeat. Start with 10 to 12 reps and gradually build up to 2 sets of 10 to 12 reps.**

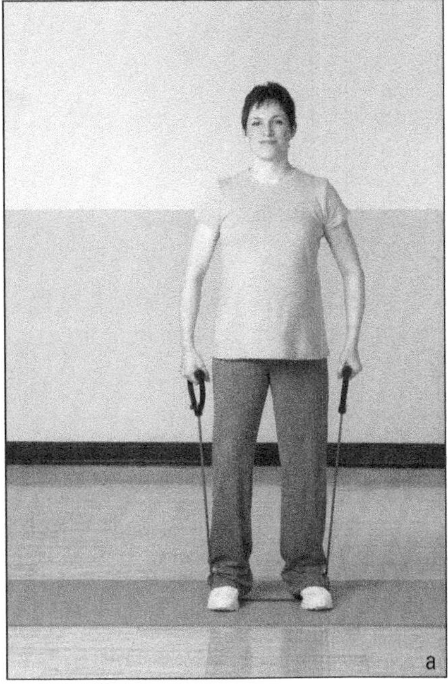
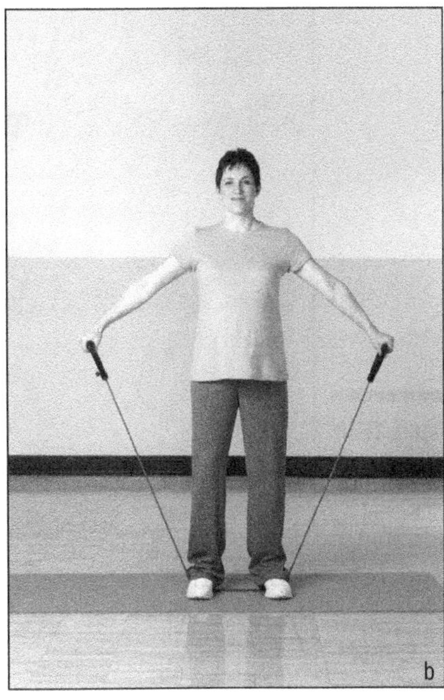

Figure 11-17: Strengthen your upper back and shoulders with the band deltoid exercise.

Band pectoral press exercise

The following exercise works your *pectoral* muscles (or *pecs*), which are your upper chest muscles.

1. **Stand with your elbows back at shoulder level and your palms facing your sides.**
2. **Place the band behind your back and grasp one end in each hand.**
3. **Adjust the band so that you don't have any slack in the band, as shown in Figure 11-18a.**
4. **Slowly stretch the band to a count of 3 by pulling your elbows forward, as shown in Figure 11-18b.**
5. **Return to your starting position, concentrating on pulling your shoulder blades together. Start with 10 to 12 reps and gradually build up to 2 sets of 10 to 12 reps.**

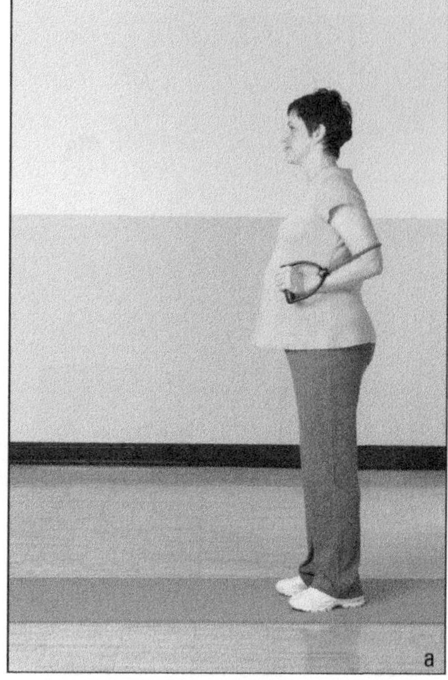

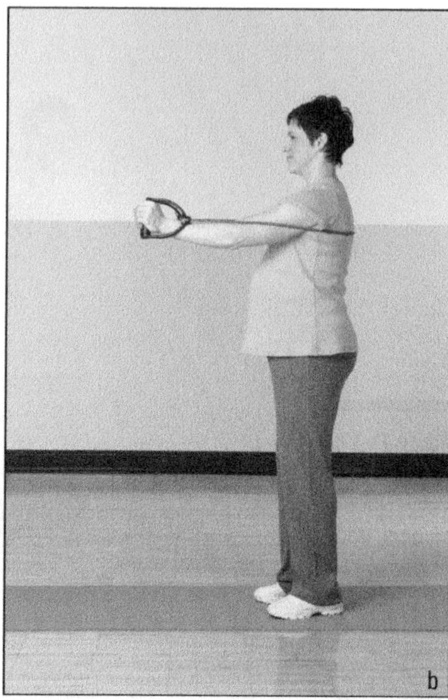

Figure 11-18: Work your upper chest muscles with the band pectoral press exercise.

Combining the ball and the band

You can use an exercise ball and resistance band together in the following unique lower-abdominal exercise. This exercise helps you contract and strengthen your lower abdominal muscles without putting stress on your low back.

1. **Sit on a workout ball and place a resistance band under your left foot, as shown in Figure 11-19a, grasping one end of the band in each hand.**

   Hold the band securely. You should feel some tension on the band in this position.

2. **Take a breath and slowly lean back as you exhale, keeping your back straight and bending from your hips (Figure 11-19b). Lean to the point where you feel your abdominal muscles start to contract and hold the contraction for 5 counts.**

3. **Slowly return to your starting position and repeat in the same position 10 to 15 times. Repeat with your right foot.**

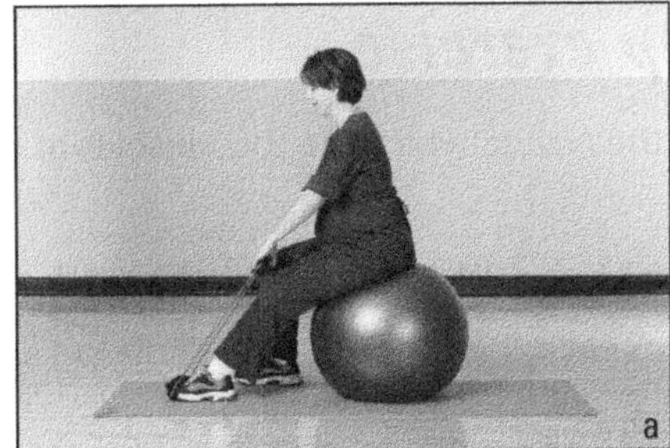

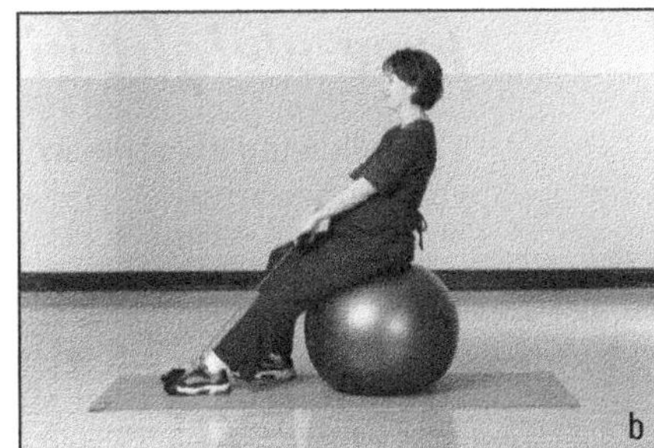

Figure 11-19: Using a band and ball together to strengthen your abs.

No Holds Barred: Bars and Hand Weights

When shopping for hand-held weights or a weight bar, look for vinyl-covered or cloth-covered equipment that feels comfortable in your hands. If you can't get a good grip on the bar or the bar cuts into your hand, you won't be comfortable as you work out. Also, find a table or other elevated surface on which to place your weights so that you're not constantly bending over to pick them up from and set them down on the floor.

Start with low weights, but keep in mind that if you're working out with weights that are too lightweight, you may not get very much out of the workout. You're generally using the proper weight if you can do 10 to 12 repetitions (reps) and the last one or two reps feel challenging, but still do-able. If you aren't able to do 10 repetitions with a weight, then the weight is too heavy: Choose a lighter weight. Monitor your body closely and discontinue any exercise that causes pain or discomfort during or after exercise.

The exercises in this section use hand weights (for which you can almost always substitute a weight bar, which we discuss in the "Introducing the Cheapest Exercise Equipment You Can Buy" section), but you can also purchase ankle weights that help you work out your legs. Expert opinions vary, but some people believe that leg weights during pregnancy put too much stress on the hip and knee joints, so you may want to avoid using them or at least discuss it with your healthcare provider. To get a great leg workout without using weights, consider using resistance bands (see the preceding section) or doing a leg-intensive cardiovascular workout, such as walking (see Chapter 12), aerobics (see Chapter 14), or cycling (see Chapter 15).

Free weight bicep exercise

The following exercise works the *biceps,* which are the muscles at the front of your upper arms.

1. **Stand with your feet shoulder-width apart.**
2. **Grasp one hand weight in each hand, with your palms facing up and your arms at your sides, as Figure 11-20a shows.**

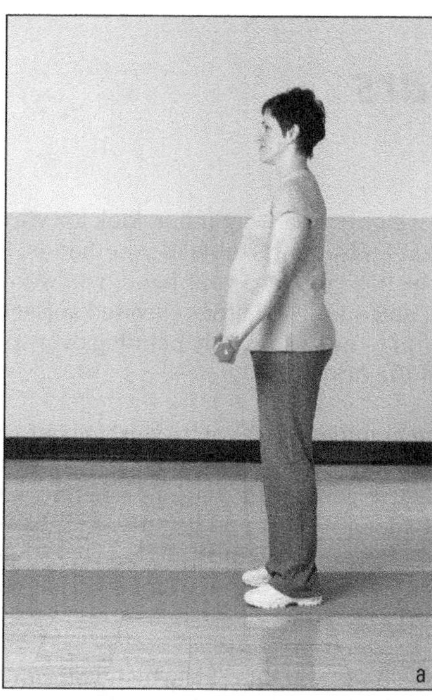

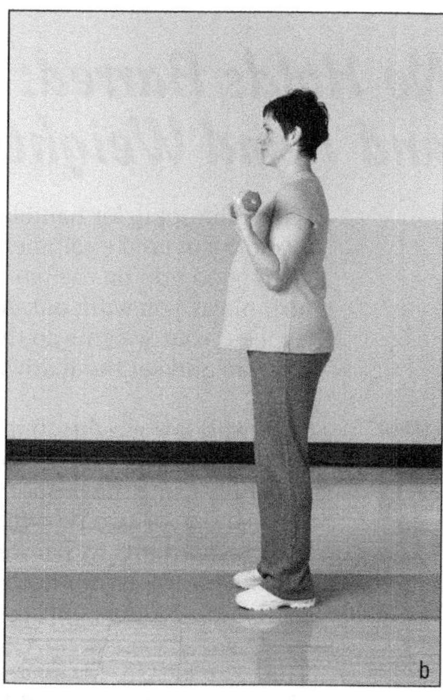

Figure 11-20: Lifting hand weights for the bicep exercise.

3. **Slowly curl the weights up toward your chest by bending your elbows, as shown in Figure 11-20b.**

   Make sure that you keep your elbows and upper arms stationary at your sides.

4. **Return at the same speed to your starting position and repeat. Start with 10 to 12 reps and gradually build up to 2 sets of 10 to 12 reps.**

Free weight tricep exercise

The following exercise works the *triceps,* which are the muscles at the back of your upper arms.

1. **In a standing or sitting position, hold a hand weight in your left hand and raise your left arm so that your elbow is in line with the top of your head.**
2. **Place your right hand under your elbow to support your left arm and bend your arm back until your elbow is at a 90-degree angle, as Figure 11-21a shows.**
3. **Lift the weight forward and up until your arm is straight, as shown in Figure 11-21b.**

   If you're unable to lift all the way up, the weight you're using may be too heavy. Choose a lighter weight and try again. Try to keep your elbow and upper arm as stationary as possible.
4. **Return to your starting position and repeat. Start with 10 to 12 reps and gradually build up to 2 sets of 10 to 12 reps.**

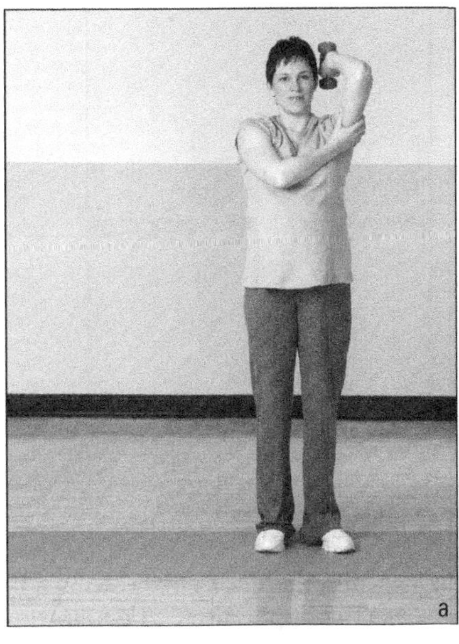

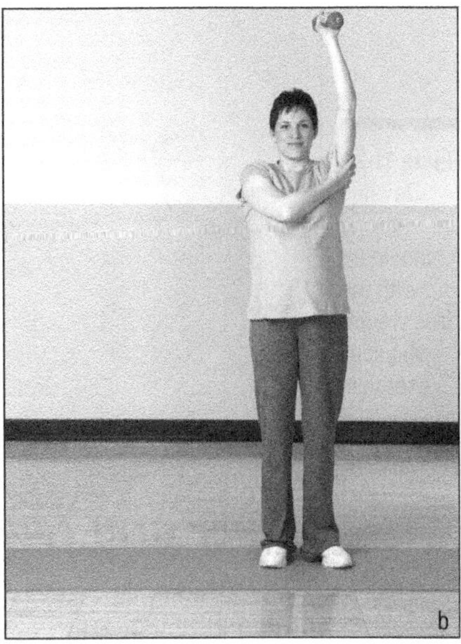

Figure 11-21: Tighten your triceps by using hand weights.

Free weight shoulder exercise

The following exercise works the shoulder muscles.

1. **Stand with a weight in each hand, bend your elbows, and hold your hands at shoulder level, palms facing forward, as shown in Figure 11-22a.**
2. **Slowly raise the weights until your arms are straight, keeping your arms close to a straight line above your shoulders.**

   Remember to not lock your elbows.
3. **Return to your starting position and repeat. Start with 10 to 12 reps and gradually build up to 2 sets of 10 to 12 reps.**

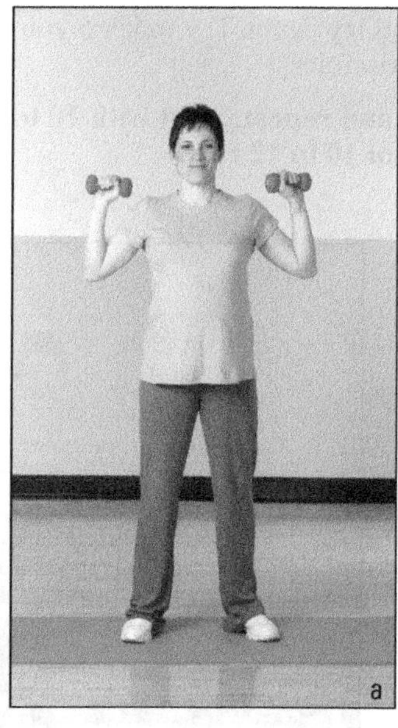

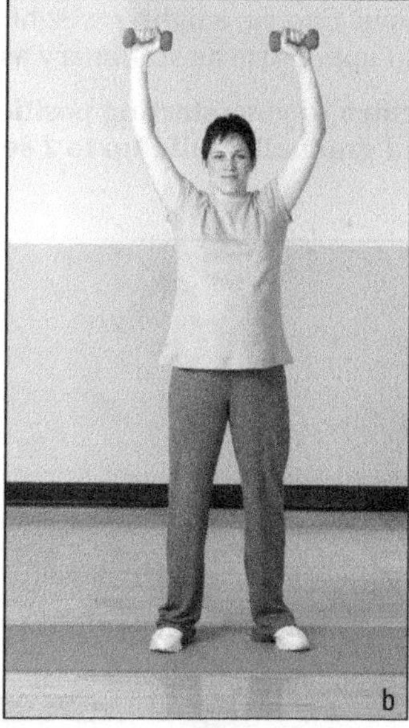

Figure 11-22: Develop strong shoulders with the free weight shoulder exercise.

Upper arm rowing exercise

In free weight exercise, a *row* is a motion that looks like rowing a boat — an upright pulling motion — that works the upper arms. The following exercise is one of the few that you can't do with a weight bar, but if you don't have free weights, try a can of soup to start, and gradually move up to a milk jug filled with sand or water.

1. **Stand leaning slightly forward, with your right knee forward and bent and your left leg extended with your foot flat behind your body. With your left arm nearly straight, grasp a hand weight in your left hand, as Figure 11-23a shows.**

   If you're more comfortable supporting your right knee by resting it on a chair or bench, go ahead. If you aren't using a chair or bench, press your right hand on your right thigh for support.

2. **Raise your elbow up toward your shoulder until your elbow is level with your shoulder, as shown in Figure 11-23b.**

3. **Slowly return to your starting position and repeat. Start with 10 to 12 reps and gradually build up to 2 sets of 10 to 12 reps.**

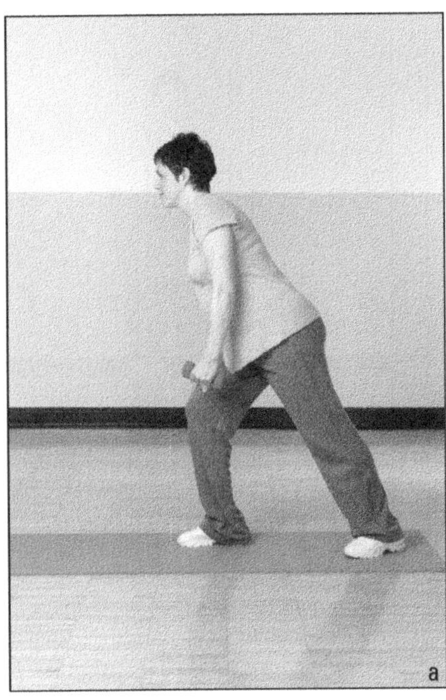

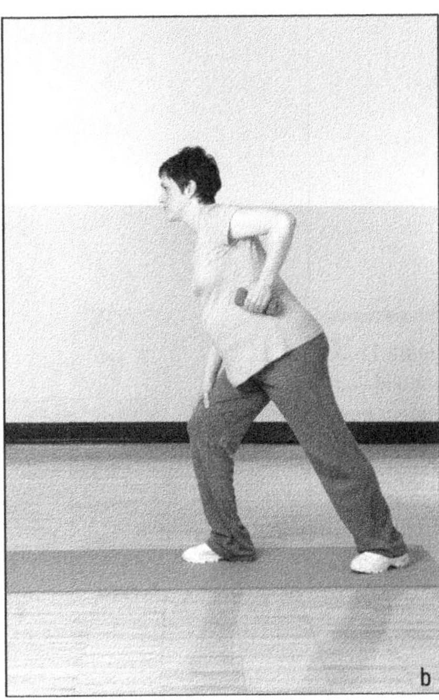

Figure 11-23: Row with free weights to tone upper arms.

Free weight deltoid exercise

The following exercise works your muscles, which are in your upper back and shoulder area. This exercise works only with free weights (not a weight bar) or with cans of soup or any other homemade free weight.

1. **Stand with a weight in each hand, with your palms facing down and your arms extended and parallel with your sides, as Figure 11-24a shows.**
2. **Slowly raise the weights out to your sides until your arms are level with your shoulders, as shown in Figure 11-24b.**

   If you feel any discomfort, you're lifting with too much weight. Choose a lighter pair of weights and try again.
3. **Return to your starting position and repeat. Start with 10 to 12 reps and gradually build up to 2 sets of 10 to 12 reps.**

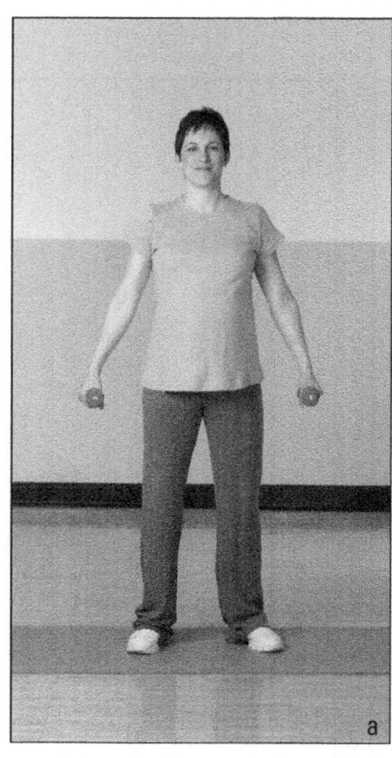

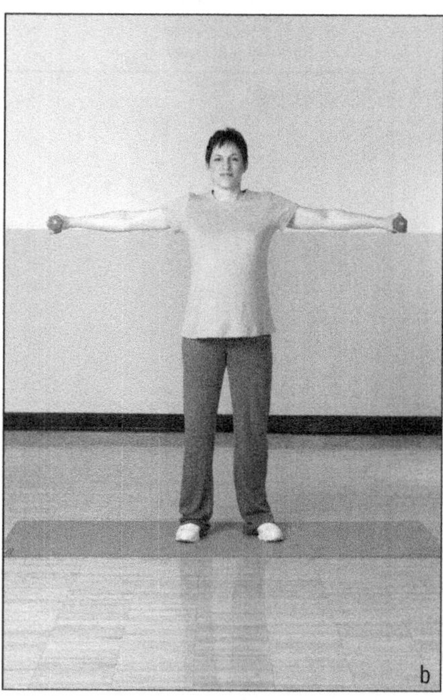

Figure 11-24: Build your upper back and shoulders with the free weight deltoid exercise.

Chapter 12

Fitness Walking and Running

In This Chapter

- Walking like you mean it
- Continuing a pre-pregnancy running routine
- Considering whether a treadmill is right for you

Walking is far and away the cheapest and easiest way to work out, and it's a favorite among pregnant women. You can walk outdoors on a sidewalk near your house or office, hike on trails, walk indoors in a mall or other indoor facility, or walk on a treadmill in your home or at a gym, which means you have plenty of options if the weather's bad or you need to work out in the dark. Walking is low impact, which means it's gentle on your body, yet this activity burns plenty of calories and gets your entire body fit if you do it with purpose. This chapter shows you how to begin a walking program, from knowing the techniques to creating a workout plan. You also find information on choosing a treadmill for either walking or running.

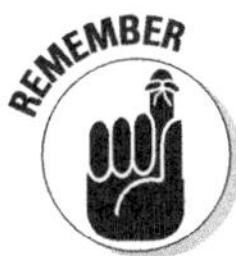

Running, like walking, is an excellent total-body workout, but it's a much higher-impact sport than walking and can be difficult to continue throughout your pregnancy. For that reason, healthcare providers usually recommend running only for women who are already experienced runners. By knowing what running feels like when not pregnant, pregnant runners can make adjustments to their workout schedules based on how well running and pregnancy mix. This chapter shares some tips for modifying your routine.

If you've never worked out before, check out Chapter 5 for four-day, five-day, and six-day-per-week workout plans that you can modify for any activity. The generic plans discuss activities in terms of minutes, not miles or laps, so you can use them for any activity.

Fitness Walking 101

Whether you've never exercised before or have been at it for years, walking is a great activity to develop and maintain fitness. You don't have to join a gym, sign up for classes, or master difficult techniques. And you can probably master proper fitness walking technique in a few minutes.

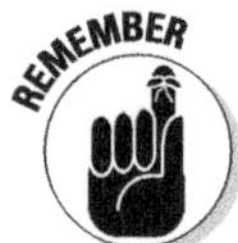

The term *fitness walking* differentiates walking with a purpose from meandering or strolling. Terms similar to fitness walking include plain-old *walking, power walking,* and *speed walking.* When walking for fitness, just make sure you're putting forth an effort and not window-shopping on Main Street.

Your biggest walking expense is in shoes, and you may need to get a new pair every trimester in order to keep your growing feet comfortable (see Chapter 7). Or, buy one size larger than usual: A bigger size not only leaves room for your swollen feet but also accommodates the permanent increase in foot size that comes after pregnancy. Many walkers choose to wear running shoes, which are usually quite comfortable for both activities. Although running shoes aren't any cheaper than shoes meant for walking, they come in a far greater number of styles than walking shoes do, which increases the likelihood that you'll find a pair that's perfect for your kickers.

Look for shoes that are flexible and breathable:

- To test flexibility, see whether you can fold the shoe in half (or nearly in half) when you have it in your hands.
- To determine whether a shoe is breathable, look for lightweight material that looks almost see-through in some areas. Shoes made of leather tend to get hot, but nylon shoes tend to breathe well.

Because bending down and tying your shoes becomes difficult as your pregnancy progresses, look for shoes with Velcro ties or other easy lacing systems. Also look for shoes with removable liners — you can pull them out and replace with thicker, gel-filled liners such as the ones Spenco offers (sold at sporting goods and discount stores).

Mastering the walking technique

Walking is so natural to humans that using it as a form of exercise almost seems like cheating. Without any difficult techniques to master, you can be out walking in no time.

Do pay attention to your technique, though. Simply by mastering a few basics, you can burn more calories and walk more comfortably and with less risk of injury (keeping in mind that walking has very little risk of injury to begin with) than if you neglect your technique.

- Stand with your back straight, your shoulders back but relaxed, and lean forward very slightly from your waist. Think about tucking in your butt so that you don't arch your back.
- Keep your eyes looking forward, not down at the ground. Your peripheral vision allows you to see what's happening on the ground in front of you.
- Don't allow your chin to fall forward (which is what happens if you're looking at the ground) or tip back (which often happens if you're fatigued). Don't move your head or let it bounce around as you walk.
- Keep your elbows tucked close to your body and your hands loosely cupped, as if holding a pencil, with your thumbs resting on your other fingers.
- As you walk, shoot one arm straight back with your elbow at a 90-degree angle and alternate with your other arm. Don't exuberantly push your arms too far back, however, or you may interfere with your perfect posture.
- Brush your thumbs past your hipbones as you walk, making sure the fingers on your forward hand never swing as high as your shoulder. Your concentration should be on the motion of your arm as it moves back.
- Land on your heel and quickly roll through your step from heel to toe, pushing off forcefully with your toes.

Increasing your need for speed

If you feel ready to increase your speed (and check out the discussion on intensity in Chapter 3 before you increase your walking pace during your pregnancy), keep the following tips in mind:

- To increase your speed, reduce your stride length (take a shorter stride) and take more steps per minute. If that seems like the opposite of what you've been taught, you've been yelled at by one too many high-school coaches who told you to "stride out" in order to speed up. The reality is that you want to shorten your stride (not lengthen it) in order to decrease your *turnover,* the time between when your foot hits the ground and when it leaves the ground again. A short turnover means a fast pace.

You can practice a one-minute *quick-feet drill* just after you finish your walk. Focusing on developing quick turnover, try to see how many steps you can take in 30 to 50 feet of space.

- Really push off as your toes leave the ground and push your knee forward, not upward.
- Drive your left arm forward as your right knee comes forward, keeping your upward arm movement to a level much lower than your shoulders.
- Move your hips forward, without any side-to-side motion. The more side-to-side motion in your hips, the less efficiently you walk.

In addition to watching your technique for opportunities to improve your speed, you can also do *speed workouts.* The basic idea behind any speed workout is that you warm up at an easy pace for 5 to 15 minutes, and then spend most of the rest of your workout playing with speed. You might walk faster for one minute (or walk faster to the next telephone pole or the next car in a driveway, and so on), slow down to your warm-up pace for one minute, speed up again for one minute, and so on. Follow any speed workout with a 5- to 15-minute cool-down, followed by stretches (see Chapter 8). Don't do speed workouts every day — always allow at least one day, preferably two days, of moderate walking in between any speed workouts.

Fitness Walking For Dummies, by Liz Neporent (Wiley), provides excellent information about technique, speed workouts, and other need-to-know information about walking.

Running for Your Life

If you were running before you became pregnant, you can probably continue to train through most if not all of your pregnancy. This section shares some tips for perfecting your running posture (which is especially important as your belly expands) and explains modifications to your training schedule that you may find necessary as your pregnancy progresses.

If you weren't running prior to becoming pregnant, don't start now. Running is a demanding sport that can quickly elevate the heart rate of the uninitiated. In addition, the changing center of gravity and the added weight of pregnancy can make running a difficult activity. Wait until you've delivered your healthy baby before getting into a running routine.

Perfecting your running technique

Because you're an experienced runner, you've been perfecting your running technique for quite some time. However, pregnancy can change your body enough that you may feel like a brand-new runner. This section provides a few reminders about running technique that may help you regain your comfort, in spite of your expanding abdomen.

Correcting your running technique takes time and may require several attempts on a number of runs. The good news is that, if you keep trying your new technique on every run, it'll soon feel completely natural.

Running posture

Running posture refers to how you hold your back, shoulders, and neck. To find out what your running posture looks like, have your partner take a video of you (straight on and from the side) or take a picture of you, from the side, as you run by.

To run with the greatest efficiency (which means you put forth the least effort), you want to lean just slightly forward from your waist. Note the word *slightly.* With just a slight lean, your arms, back, neck, shoulders, and diaphragm relax. Avoid leaning far forward when you run, which can happen as your pregnancy progresses, because leaning forward puts pressure on your lower back and can also interfere with your breathing.

You also want to avoid scrunching your shoulders up so that they're up near your ears. Instead, relax your shoulders and hold them slightly back, allowing your neck and shoulders to fully relax as you run. Finally, try to make sure your chin is neither tilted down toward your chest nor tilted up, as is common when runners get all tuckered out.

Arm carriage

Arm carriage refers to how you hold your arms when you run, and you want to hold yours so that your thumbs brush by your hipbones with each step. (To determine how you're holding your arms, run in place in front of a mirror or ask a friend to take a video or picture of you, from the front, as you run.) If you've been holding your arms too high, you'll think this position is too low, but it's not: You have far more power when you run with your thumbs brushing by your hipbones.

In addition, you don't want your arms to cross your *midline* (an imaginary line that runs down the middle of your body, from between your eyes down to your navel), or you'll be *crossing over.* Your legs follow the motion of your arms, so if your arms are crossing over, your legs are moving a little bit sideways on each forward step, and this makes for inefficient running. Practice brushing your thumbs by your hipbones and keeping your hips still, and you won't be able to cross your midline.

If you hold your arms too high or cross over, your arms may be weak. To make your arms as strong as your legs, consider cross-training with weights or a circuit routine (see Chapter 17).

You don't want to clench your fists when you run, and you also don't want to make your hands loose and floppy. To keep your hands loose but not too loose, imagine that you're carrying an invisible pencil or tube of lip balm in each hand. Then rest your thumbs on your fingers — your thumbs shouldn't stick straight up.

Modifying your workout plan

Because running is a sport that you continue from your pre-pregnancy days (as opposed to taking it up as a new sport while you're pregnant), we don't provide a basic workout plan here — a plan for beginning runners. Your running experience should be enough to guide you through these months of continued training.

That said, consider the following modifications that you may want to make as your pregnancy progresses:

- Be sure you're wearing a supportive sports bra, and move up to a larger size, as needed. Your breasts, which are likely already sore, can be subjected to a lot of movement and jostling while running, so you need to protect them.

  Some pregnant women find that wearing two sports bras provides better support and helps reduce skin friction.
- Reduce your mileage and/or pace, as necessary. You may find that you're able to continue your mileage, but at a slower pace, or that you don't need to adjust your pace, but do need to reduce your mileage. See Chapter 3 for more information.
- Keep in mind that your center of gravity is changing, and many women compensate by changing their running form, which can lead to injuries. Stay aware of your running technique, trying to use good, upright posture (that means not hunching your shoulders) and keeping your butt tucked under you as much as possible.
- On runs lasting 30 minutes or more, you may need to plan a bathroom break. Running on a treadmill is one way to ensure that you have access to a bathroom when you need it.
- Avoid running on trails starting at about your fourth month. If you're fatigued — or as a response to your weight gain — you may tend to shuffle your feet, and that may lead to stumbling over tree roots and other debris on a trail. Even if you're not shuffling, simply seeing roots and other problems on a trail can be difficult as your belly grows.

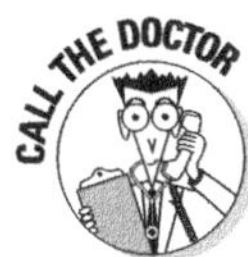

- If you're a competitive runner or walker, by the time your second trimester begins, stop all racing (marathons, half-marathons, 10Ks, and even a local 5K road race), speed workouts, and long runs. Your healthcare provider may want you to stop training for competition as early as when you first find out that you're pregnant. Training for racing and racing itself are very hard on your body, so even world-class runners take time off from racing to make sure their babies are growing normally.
- Between 18 and 24 weeks, you may experience *round ligament pain,* which is a pain or ache near your groin that comes from the ligaments on each side of the uterus stretching as the uterus grows. If you feel this pain while running, reduce your speed; if that doesn't help, walk until the pain stops and then start running again.
- As your uterus grows, consider getting a *maternity support belt,* commonly called a *belly brace* or *belly belt.* This support belt fits snugly under your belly and attaches around your back, stabilizing your abdomen as you run (see Figure 12-1). Some belly braces also fit around the top of your abdomen for additional support. A belly brace can also lift your belly enough to take pressure off your ligaments, which is especially useful if you're experiencing round ligament pain.

  To fit your belly brace correctly, wrap it around your back so that the center line of the belt hits the top of your hip. Tense your belly as you bring the brace together (to lift your belly a bit and give it more support), and then fasten it so that the top of the brace hits just below your belly button. When the brace is fastened, you should be able to breathe easily and shouldn't feel any tightness or *chafing* (rubbing that can cause raw skin). If you find that your skin is pinching or that you're experiencing chafing or a rash, you may want to put your brace over your workout pants or shorts — if you want to hide the brace, you can still put a shirt over your shorts and the brace. Baby powder under the elastic can also help reduce rashes.

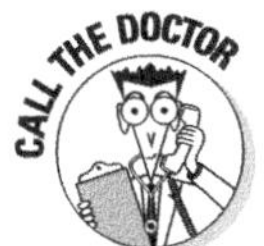

- If, during your late second trimester or beginning of the third trimester, you're out running and experience *Braxton-Hicks contractions* (false contractions that feel as though your stomach is balling up or tightening up), take the same approach as for round ligament pain: Slow down or begin walking, running again only if the pain stops. Also, check with your healthcare provider as soon as possible to make sure that you aren't experiencing true contractions.
- If the added weight of your baby makes running on land too difficult, consider running in water. Pool running is also an excellent alternative if you have any joint or muscle pain or if you're experiencing any swelling. See Chapter 13 for details.

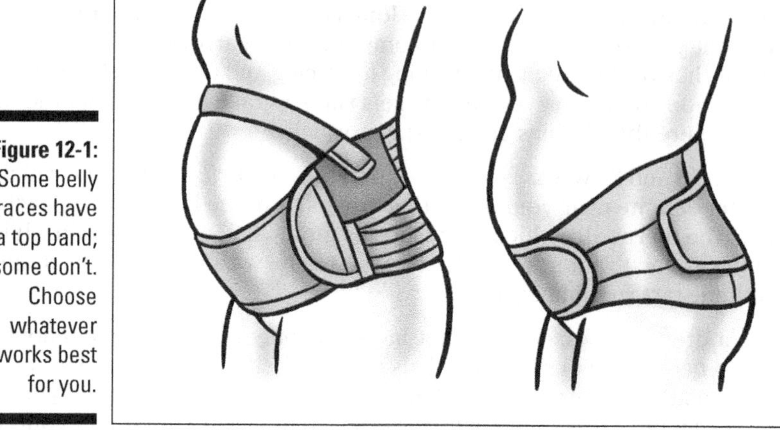

Figure 12-1: Some belly braces have a top band; some don't. Choose whatever works best for you.

When you run outside, always leave a note, explaining the route you're going and letting someone know when you plan to be back. Carry a cellphone with you, especially in your third trimester. If you're several miles from home and are too fatigued to finish a run or you experience any of the warning signs discussed in Chapter 3, you want to reach your partner or other contact immediately. If you don't have a cellphone or you train in an area without cellphone reception, run short loops around your home or car so that you're never more than a mile away from help at any given time.

Take plenty of water with you. Also, if you've experienced any blood-sugar problems since becoming pregnant, carry along a few sweets in case your blood sugar level bottoms out (and if that happens often, talk to your health-care provider about changes in when and what you eat).

Deciding Whether to Buy a Treadmill

If you live in an area with severe winters or your schedule requires you to walk or run in the dark, consider buying a treadmill to make your workouts convenient and safe.

We must caution you that, without a TV or other distraction, treadmill workouts can be unbelievably boring. (A radio does provide some relief, but that still leaves you staring at one spot on the wall for your entire walk or run.) If you're able to turn your TV loud enough to overcome the treadmill noise, you can watch your favorite TV show while working out and save yourself from agonizing boredom. Some people are able to read while walking on a treadmill; special book holders are available at many fitness stores. If you tend to get sick to your stomach while reading in a moving car, however, you may have the same reaction while reading on a treadmill.

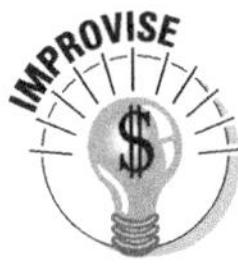

You can get a high-quality treadmill for around $1,000, which is what you'll need to withstand the pounding of running. For walking, you can get a much less expensive unit, some starting as low as $250. If that's still too much to spend at the moment, see whether a low-cost gym or the Y in your area has a treadmill you can use during the times of day you want to work out. (And keep in mind that, at a gym, someone may get to the treadmill(s) just a few minutes before you do, changing your workout plans for that day.) Also check classified ads in your area for gently used treadmills.

If you decide to buy a treadmill, look for the following features:

- **Size:** Some treadmills fold up when not in use, which means they take up much less space in your home. You still have to have enough space to use the treadmill when it's open (about two or three feet wide and five or six feet long), but a folding treadmill offers you more options than one that doesn't fold.
- **Speed:** Make sure the treadmill comfortably goes the speed you want it to go. This means that if you want it to go 7.5 miles per hour, you buy one that goes faster than 8 miles per hour, because otherwise, you'll be nearly maxing out the treadmill's top speed every time you use it. Plus, if you decide to increase the intensity of your workouts (see Chapter 3), you won't have much room to improve before your treadmill is pretty useless to you. If you're unsure about how many miles per hour you need the treadmill to go, see the sidebar, "What's my mph?"
- **Sturdiness:** A good treadmill doesn't move excessively when you're working out. Never buy a treadmill without first testing it in the store. Ask the clerk whether you can give the floor model a try, and then get on and start walking or running. After a few minutes, get the treadmill up to the speed at which you normally work out and check for excessive jiggling.

  The handrails of the treadmill should be as sturdy as the rest of the unit. If the floor model you're trying doesn't have the handrails attached, ask to have them attached before you try the model or start looking at a different model. Too many treadmills have handrails that aren't sturdy, which makes them even less sturdy and, often, louder as the handrails bang around.
- **Incline:** If you think you want to mimic the effort of walking or running on hills, be sure the treadmill you buy has an *incline* feature. And if you're using the treadmill for running and you're buying one with an incline feature, look for a treadmill that has a separate motor for the incline feature or a very large motor that controls both the speed and the incline. A treadmill with an undersized motor will slow down when you use the incline feature. When you're testing the machine before you buy it, set the machine on an incline and see whether the treadmill slows down, even temporarily. Any slowdown in the speed of the treadmill when put on incline indicates that the motor is underpowered.

- **Display:** The only guideline for what to look for in a display is that it doesn't annoy you excessively. If you want to focus on a TV or that spot on the wall and don't really want to know how fast you're going or how many miles you would've traveled had you been outside, look for a small, unobtrusive display without bells and whistles (literally — without sounds that keep you informed of your progress). If you like knowing every time you've gone the equivalent of one lap around a track (one-quarter mile) or some other distance, you can find treadmills that blink, beep, and otherwise broadcast how you're doing.

  Some treadmills also feature *handrail controls:* small, convenient switches on the handrails that control speed and incline. This feature means you don't have to lean forward and press on a large, awkward display area to change the speed or incline.

When using a treadmill, try to use the same walking or running technique that you use on land (see Figure 12-2). This means that you don't hang on to the handrails unless you feel extremely uncomfortable letting go of them. When walking and running on land, your arms get an excellent workout, so you don't want to waste the opportunity to keep your arms moving when using a treadmill.

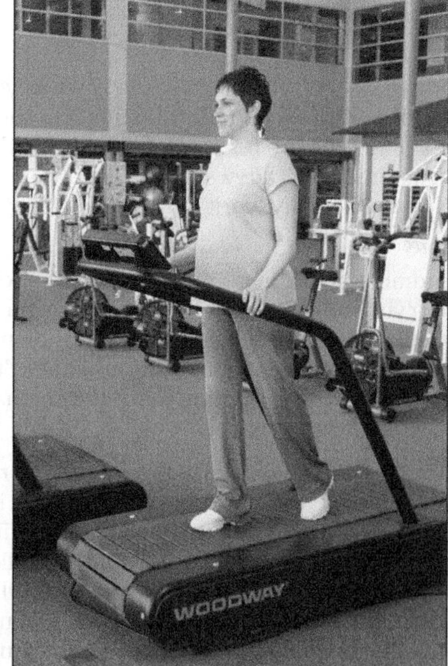

Figure 12-2: Use proper technique when walking or running on a treadmill.

In addition, keep the following safety tips in mind as you master your treadmill technique:

- **Always wear the *safety key*** (a plastic key that slips into a slot near the display — the treadmill won't run until the key is plugged in) on a cord that's slung over your neck or clipped onto your shorts. That way, if you fall or slip off the back of the treadmill, the unit will stop.

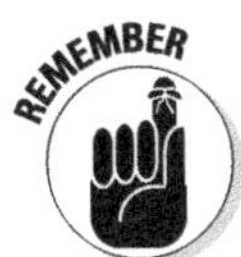

  Be sure the cord is the proper length for you. If it's too long, you may be sitting behind the treadmill on your butt before the unit turns off. If it's too short, the unit may turn off when you get a little farther back on the belt than usual, potentially causing an even bigger accident.

- **Keep yourself from getting too close to the back of the *belt*** (the portion of the treadmill that moves). Although this sort of accident is rare, slipping off the back of a treadmill is possible, especially if you walk or run very close to the back of the belt. Keep yourself in the middle of the belt as you walk or run.
- **Keep yourself from getting too close to the front of the belt.** Because some people fear slipping off the back of the treadmill, they walk or run as close to the front of the belt as possible. But if you get too close, you may step on a nonmoving part of the treadmill, which can interrupt your stride and cause you to stumble.
- **Don't get over to the far left or far right of the belt.** As in the preceding bullet, you may step on a nonmoving part of the treadmill, causing a fall.

  If you feel at all unbalanced, hold on to the handrails lightly as you walk or run.

- **Before focusing on a TV screen, make sure you're comfortable with how you're landing on the treadmill.** A TV introduces a distraction, which can be a blessing if you're bored but can also keep you from watching how and where you're landing on the belt. Focusing on a TV without frequently looking down at your feet and the treadmill's belt can lead to a fall.
- **Slow the speed down as you finish your run or walk, and then get off the treadmill slowly.** Be sure the belt comes to a complete stop before you get off the treadmill. When stepping off, hold onto the handrails until both your feet are on the ground.

If you're concerned about falling off your treadmill, surround the sides and back of the treadmill with pillows, exercise mats, or other soft items. Don't get them so close that they interfere with the belt or motor, though.

What's my mph?

Here's a formula for converting minutes per mile to miles per hour to help you know where to set your treadmill speed:

> 60 ÷ the number of minutes you take to run or walk a mile = the speed (miles per hour, or mph) at which you want to set the treadmill.

For example, if you walk a mile in 15 minutes, you do the following calculation: 60 ÷ 15 = 4 miles per hour. That's the speed at which you set the treadmill. If you run 9-and-a-half-minute miles, do this calculation: 60 ÷ 9.5 = 6.3 miles per hour.

Chapter 13

Swimming and Water Aerobics

In This Chapter

- Getting access to a pool
- Discovering swimming basics
- Demystifying water aerobics

If everyone had a pool next door, in the basement, or in the backyard, swimming and water aerobics would absolutely be the most popular ways to work out during pregnancy. Water sports (both swimming and water aerobics) are completely nonweight bearing, which means that you have very little risk of injury, yet you get a total-body workout that works your cardiovascular system and strengthens muscles. For pregnant women who experience swelling, exercising in a pool can reduce this swelling and discomfort. In addition, the regulated temperature of a pool makes becoming overheated almost impossible. And most people can pick up water aerobics techniques with very little practice and master basic swimming techniques with just a bit more time and training. In short, water exercise is an ideal way to get and stay fit during your pregnancy.

So what's the catch? Finding a pool and gaining access to it may be harder than doing the workouts themselves. In some states, every community — heck, every neighborhood — has a pool, but in other areas, you may go 100 or 200 miles with nary a pool in sight. This chapter gives you some ideas for getting pool time and also shows you how to begin a swimming and/or water aerobics workout program.

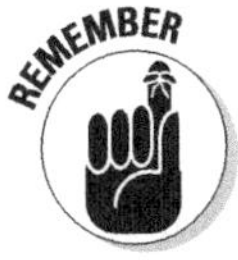

A pool is the only place you want to swim or do water aerobics. Working out in a lake or ocean while you're pregnant can cause an infection from unclean water entering your vagina. If you insist on swimming in the great outdoors, talk to your healthcare provider first to see if your can minimize your risk of infection.

For all the activities discussed in this chapter, you absolutely must have a comfortable swimsuit that fits properly and allows you to move freely. (No, this isn't an oxymoron — you really can be comfortable in a swimsuit during your pregnancy.) See Chapter 7 for details on maternity suits.

Finding Classes and Pool Time

If you're thinking of trying water workouts, but you aren't sure where the nearest pool is, consider the following locations that may have a pool that you can use:

- **YWCA or YMCA:** Many Ys built pools in the '70s and '80s, so if you have a Y in your area, it probably has a pool. YWCA and YMCA pools are often open very early in the morning (5:30 or 6:00) and remain open throughout the evenings and weekends, but the pool may also be quite busy during those times. Ys with pools also generally offer a wide variety of swimming and water aerobics classes and may even offer prenatal water-aerobics classes. To find the Y nearest you, log on to `www.ymca.com` and enter your Zip code on the home page. You can also visit `www.ywca.org`, click on Local YWCAs, and follow the instructions from there.
- **Fitness center or gym:** Although smaller, nonchain gyms usually don't offer a pool, the bigger chains, such as Bally's, often do. Call all the gyms in your area to see whether any offers a pool. When you find one that does, ask whether you can get a free pass to try it out — most gyms do nearly anything to get potential members in the door and will gladly grant your request. Anywhere from one-day to two-week free memberships are common. Also get a schedule of classes — a fitness center or gym with a pool is very likely to offer water aerobics classes several times a day.
- **Local community center or parks and recreation building:** Pools are so expensive to build and maintain that most community centers don't have one. However, the trend in community centers is to become more sophisticated and try to provide one-stop fitness shopping for the public, so some are adding pools in addition to their indoor tracks and fitness equipment, and they offer plenty of classes at those pools. Chances are, though, if your community center has a pool, you've already heard about it, because these pools, which are often available to the public all day long, are a Very Big Deal in most communities.
- **Boys' or girls' club:** Boys' and girls' clubs often have full gyms at which kids can play basketball, take gymnastics lessons, and so on. Once in a while, you can find one that has a pool, but because the boys' and girls' clubs are supposed to serve children, adults may have very limited pool hours. If you have a boys' or girls' club in your area, give it a ring and see what pool amenities it offers you.
- **Local high school:** This is the most common location for a community pool, but because of daytime use by physical education students and swim practices before and after school, the pool may not offer a lot of opportunities for you to work out.

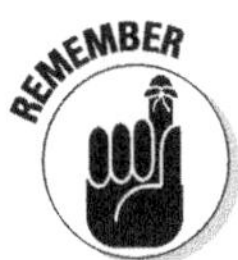

Just because your local high school has a swim team doesn't mean it has a pool. Some high schools rent pool time from neighboring schools so that they can field swim teams without the expense of building and maintaining a pool. This also means that if your local high school is renting its pool to other schools, the pool time available to you may be even more restricted.

- **Local college or university:** If you're fortunate enough to have a college or university in your area, find out whether the school has a pool and, if so, whether you're eligible to use it. Many small, liberal arts colleges don't have their own pools, but community colleges and large universities often do, and they make them available to the local public. Like high school pools, however, open swim times may be limited by the practice schedules of the men's and women's swim teams and by swim classes offered to university students.
- **Local hospital:** Because water therapy (also called *hydrotherapy*) is an excellent way to return injured and/or older patients to their full capacity, some hospitals have pools for this purpose. Although most aren't open to the public, if your hospital has a pool and an excellent prenatal program, you can bet that they'll let you use their pool for a fee. The times you can use the pool may be quite limited, however.
- **Hotels in your area:** Most hotels offer pools to their guests because people expect this amenity, yet few hotel guests ever use those pools. If that's the case at a hotel in your area, you may be able to convince the hotel manager to let you pay to use its pool during nonpeak hours. Peak hours vary: A business-class hotel gets the most use before and after the workday; a family-oriented hotel pool is usually brimming with kids from about 10 a.m. to 4 or 5 p.m. Few people tend to use hotel pools between check out and check in (usually noon to 3 p.m.), so if you're available during that time, you may be able to convince the hotel manager to let you use the pool then, unless, of course, that's when the pool is cleaned. Oh, and be prepared to sign a densely worded legal waiver, because a lifeguard will almost assuredly not be on duty.

  In some areas, hotels even offer low-cost membership programs to encourage the local community to spend time at the hotel. A hotel in your area may even allow more than one person to sign up on an account, which means that you can split the cost with a friend, or you and your partner can pay just one fee.
- **A friend's house:** If you live in a warm area (or, if you have a really, really rich friend with an indoor pool — lucky you!), you may be able to borrow a friend's pool for one hour, a few days per week. If your kind friend agrees to this arrangement, consider drawing up some paperwork that eliminates her liability if anything happens to you while you're in the pool. Also offer to clean the pool once a week to "pay" for your pool time, but do avoid exposure to heavy cleaning chemicals.

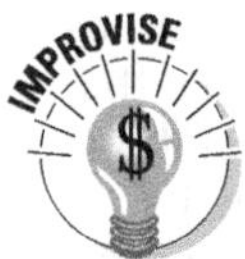

Most pools charge from $1 to $5 per session, although those $1 rock-bottom rates are harder and harder to find. You may have to join the pool for a year, at a rate of $150 to $300. Or, the pool may offer a punch-card pass that's good for a certain number of sessions. If you're unsure whether you'll like swimming or water aerobics, pay the single-use fee until you're hooked, and then buy the pass that results in the cheapest per-session rate.

After you find a pool that allows you to work out at times that fit your schedule, consider signing up for adult swimming classes, if offered (these are pretty rare) or a water aerobics class. Because water aerobics is very popular among pregnant women (and, incidentally, among the elderly — it's definitely not the hippest sport in the world), you may even find a prenatal water aerobics class in your area.

Swimming with the Current

Swimming is an excellent way to get and stay fit during your pregnancy, and after you master one or two swimming strokes (discussed in the following section), it's an activity that you can continue for the rest of your life.

Although swimming attracts people of all ages, you see more elderly people swimming than participating in any other sport. This is because swimming gets your heart rate up and tones your arms and legs, yet it's easy on your joints, doesn't require any special skills, doesn't subject you to endure harsh weather (unless you're working out in an outdoor pool during a tornado!), and is usually pretty inexpensive.

IM-ing in the water

In competitive swimming, swimmers compete using the four main strokes: butterfly, freestyle, breast stroke, and backstroke. An additional event, called the *individual medley* (or *IM*), utilizes all four strokes. Swimmers do one or more lengths of the butterfly (yep — they start out with the hardest stroke!), then do an open turn to the backstroke. They backstroke for one or more lengths, and do either a flip turn or open turn (depending on the length of the IM) to the breast stroke. They breast stroke for one or more lengths and do an open turn to the freestyle, which they swim for one of more lengths. Some IM events are quite short, but others are more like a distance event.

Swimming strokes: Like a duck to water

If you took swimming lessons as a kid, after a quick review of this section, you'll be ready for a swim workout. However, if you were never taught formal swimming *strokes* (the way you move your arms and legs as you swim), use this section to familiarize yourself with the basics and then see whether you can work with a swim instructor or coach to perfect your technique. Note that many swim classes are meant for kids, but you may be able to find a class that specializes in adult lessons.

The three main swimming strokes that most people use — crawl (or freestyle), breast stroke, and backstroke — are discussed in the following sections. Note that this section doesn't describe the *butterfly* (also called the *fly*), because it's just too darned hard. Your arms come out of the water together, go up and over your head, and then move powerfully back into the water, making a full circle. As your arms come out of the water, your head comes up so that you can take a breath; meanwhile, your legs are kicking powerfully and your hips are moving up and down. All in all, it's one of the most difficult and exhausting moves of any sport. Because many excellent swimmers never master it, and they're not pregnant, we've decided to leave that stroke out of this book.

Crawl (freestyle)

The most commonly used swim stroke is the *crawl,* which is known as *freestyle* in racing circles. So named because you look like you're crawling along the surface of the water, the crawl, shown in Figure 13-1, works like this:

1. **Place your face down in the water, with your tummy facing the bottom of the pool and your back toward the ceiling.**

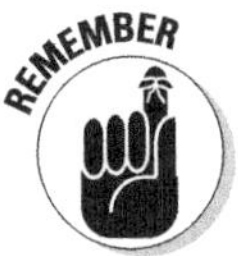

   As you swim, keep your face in the water, but look upward, in the direction you're moving. Most swimmers like to wear goggles (discussed in Chapter 7), because they allow for clear vision without the burning that comes from keeping your eyes open in chlorinated water. If you're wearing goggles, you want the top of your goggles to be at the water's surface. Just a bit of your head should show above the water's surface.

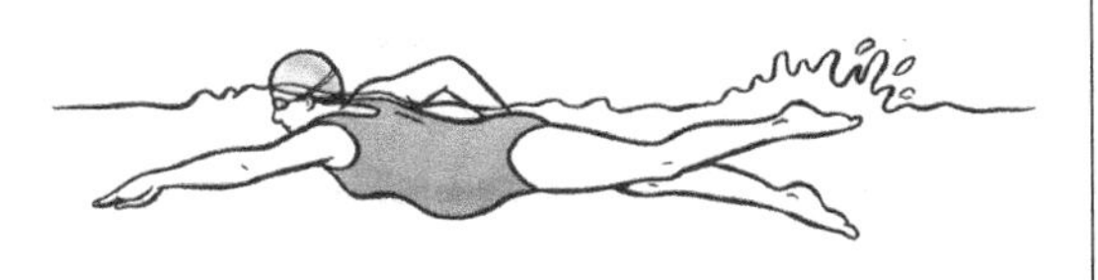

Figure 13-1: Crawling down your lane.

2. **With your elbow slightly bent, bring your right arm up out of the water, next to your ear, and then reach that arm as far forward as you can.**

   Cup your hands slightly so that your hands move easily through the water. And make sure your elbows come high out of the water.

3. **Use a flutter kick continuously as you reach your arm forward.**

   A *flutter kick* is a serious of small, rapid, up-and-down kicks with your legs. You're supposed to move your legs much faster than you move your arms, and with a little practice, you'll quickly become coordinated enough to do these two different paces at the same time.

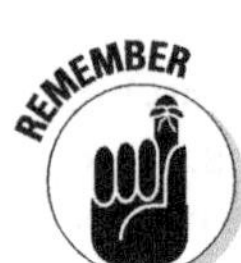

   Don't kick too much. If you're getting a lot of water spray from your kick, chances are, you're overkicking. Let your hips do the work, not your feet and lower legs.

4. **Repeat Step 2 with your left arm.**

   As your left arm is coming out of the water and moving up next to your ear, your right arm is moving downward through the water.

   Never cross your *midline* (an invisible line that runs down the middle of your body, from the top of your head to between your two feet). Instead, each arm should come right up to — but never cross over — your midline. This is the most efficient way to move forward with the least effort.

5. **Every two to four strokes (a *stroke* in this sense is one arm's motion through the water and air), lift your mouth out of the water by turning your head to one side or the other. When your mouth is out of the water, take a deep breath.**

   Breathe the air out slowly while your face is fully immersed in water.

Breast stroke

The breast stroke, which is done in the same facedown position as the crawl, is, for some people, an easier stroke than the crawl. For other people, it's next to impossible. The motion is quite different from the crawl, as you see in the following steps:

1. **Place your face down in the water, with your tummy facing the bottom of the pool and your back toward the ceiling.**

   Keep the top of your goggles at the water's surface, with your face in the water. Just a tiny bit of your head should show above the water's surface.

2. **Push both arms forward as far as possible, with straight elbows, keeping your arms next to your ears.**

   Your fingers should nearly come together in a point, far above your head, completely elongating your body.

   Although your elbows are straight, they shouldn't be locked. Never lock your elbows with any swimming stroke.

3. **At the same time, straighten your legs, point your toes, and put your toes as close together as possible, lengthening your body as long as possible.**

   See Figure 13-2.

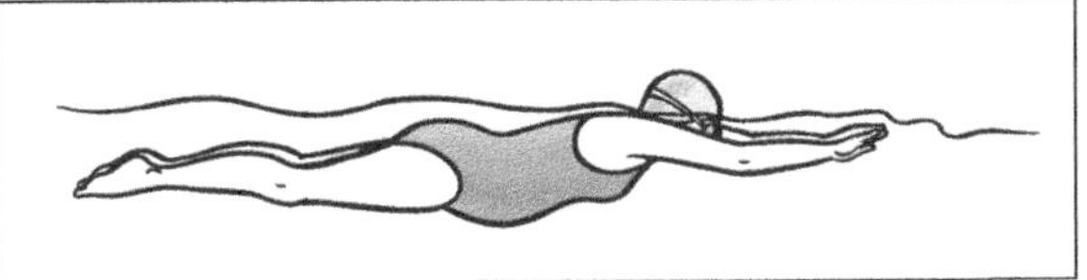

Figure 13-2: Elongating before the breast stroke.

4. **Keeping your toes pointed, your legs straight, and your elbows straight, cup your hands (palms down) and begin to pull them around your body in the direction of your legs, until your arms form a large Y.**

   See Figure 13-3. This motion is the first half of what's called the *pull* (the second half of the pull is in Step 5). Don't think of yourself as pushing your arms back; instead, you're making an inward sweeping, pulling motion.

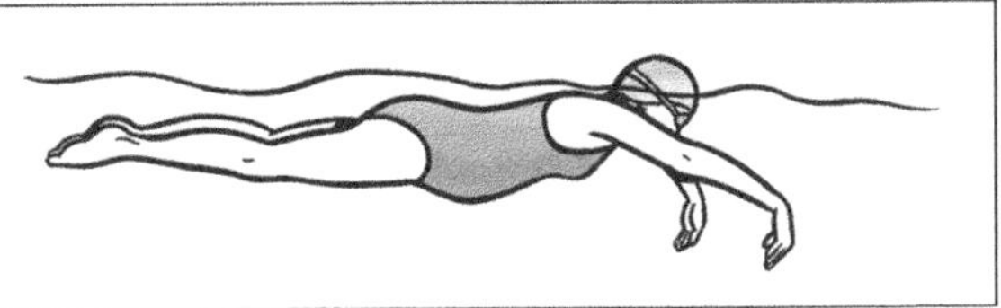

Figure 13-3: Forming the Y.

   Keep your face in the water, in line with your spine.

5. **When your hands reach the Y position, bend your elbows slightly and lift them out of the water, until your elbows reach about the height of your eyes. Then pull your hands toward your chest until your fingertips touch.**

   You're pulling your arms toward your breastbone, which is how this stroke got its name.

   Steps 4 and 5 happen without any break in between. Pull your hands into the Y, and then immediately push your hands toward your chest and begin lifting your chest and head out of the water (see the following step).

6. **At the same time, thrust your chest and hips forward, elevating your hips and bringing your head out of the water.**

   Keep your hips as high in the water as you can. Your hips are the power behind the breast stroke.

7. **When your head and chest come out of the water, take in a deep breath, letting the air out throughout the rest of the stroke.**

   See Figure 13-4.

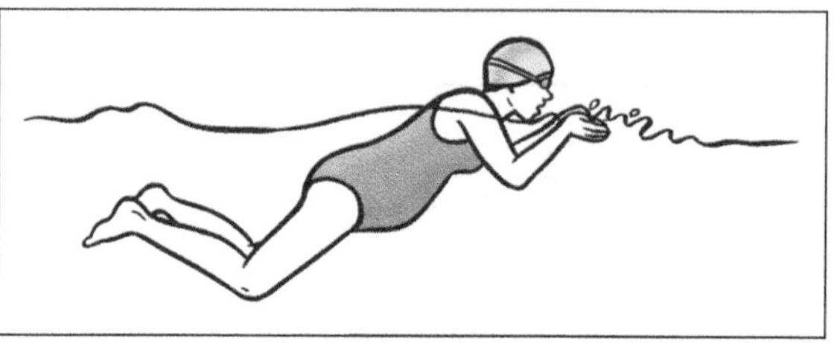

Figure 13-4: The breast stroke.

8. **Begin to thrust your arms forward as far as you can. As you push your arms forward, bend your knees in a *frog kick* to push you forward again.**

   See Figure 13-5. This portion of the breast stroke, including the frog kick, is called the *push.*

   Don't snap your legs as you do the frog kick, or you may hurt your knees. Glide your legs gently through the water.

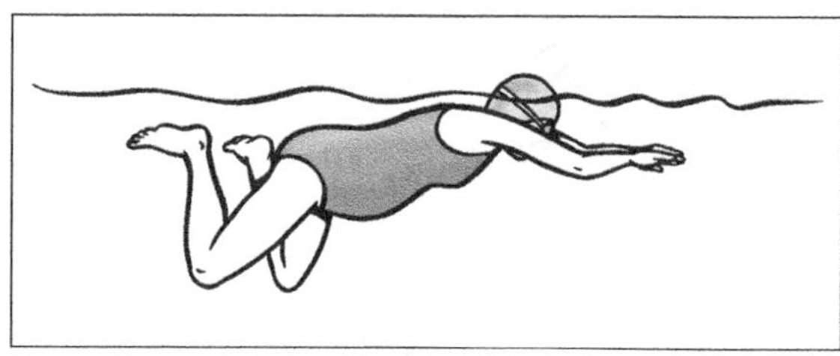

Figure 13-5: The frog kick.

9. **Push your legs into a Y (straight, unbent legs), and then bring your toes back together as they were in Step 2.**

Granted, it sounds pretty complicated, but doing the breast stroke is a great whole-body workout, and when you do all the steps together, it's not as hard as you may think. Keep trying the stroke and you'll begin to nail it. If possible, get some feedback from anyone at your pool who you think is knowledgeable, even if it's just some guy who seems to be doing the breast stroke pretty well. And try not to giggle when you say, "breast stroke" — swimmers have heard all the jokes already.

Backstroke

If you can't seem to master the intricate breathing techniques of the crawl and breast stroke — or if you're new to swimming — you may have the most success with the backstroke, which is really simple to master. Just follow these easy steps:

1. **Begin on your back, with your tummy pointing toward the ceiling and your arms at your sides.**

   With the backstroke, you keep your face out of the water at all times, simplifying the breathing process.

2. **Using a flutter kick (a serious of small, rapid, up-and-down kicks with your legs), swing your right arm — straight, but not with a locked elbow — up out of the water, past your ear, and back into the water behind you.**

   See Figure 13-6. You're rotating your right shoulder as much as you can. If your body turns or rotates as a result of your rotating shoulder, that's perfectly okay. Don't try to keep your body perfectly flat, or you won't get the power you need from your shoulders.

3. **Pull your right arm back underwater, bend your elbow, and bring your right arm to your right hip bone as you swing your left arm out of the water and behind your head.**

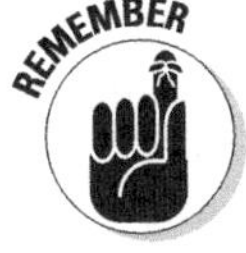

   Don't forget to breathe throughout each stroke. Thankfully, because your face is above water the entire time you're swimming, you don't have to breathe only at certain times.

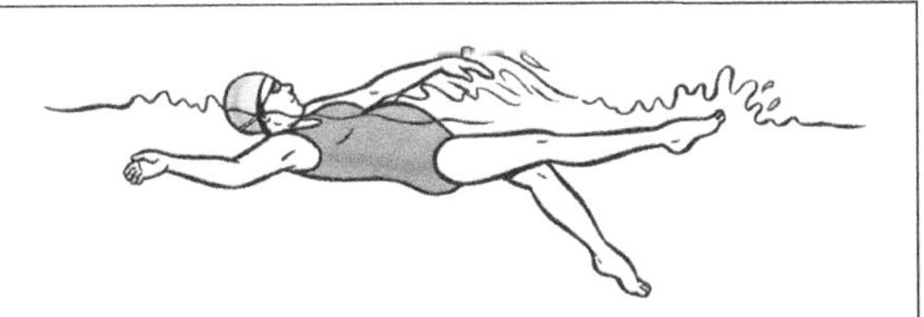

Figure 13-6: The backstroke.

Getting in the water and making turns

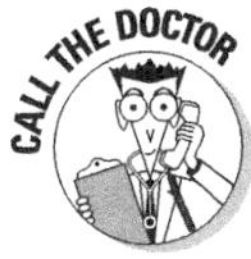

When you're pregnant, you get in the water by walking down the ladder provided on the inside walls of the pool or by sitting on the edge of the pool and lowering yourself in. Use common sense, which for most pregnant women means avoiding diving. If you're used to diving, ask your healthcare provider whether that's a good idea for you.

After you're in the water, begin swimming laps. (Swimming the length of the pool and back is known as a *lap,* and because you'll probably do this more than once, you're swimming *laps,* plural.) The problem is that, to complete a lap, you have to get yourself turned around and headed back in the opposite direction. And with a large abdomen, changing your momentum isn't always easy. You basically have three ways of turning around:

- **Do a flip turn.** This is the kind of turn you see during the Olympics. A *flip turn* involves doing a half forward somersault in the water, kicking your feet off the pool wall, twisting your body around in a halfway rotation, and then beginning your stroke again.

  Here's a reality check: Somersaults? Twisting rotations? Pregnancy? Suffice it to say that a flip turn isn't a great idea if you're past your first trimester. Sure, those turns look super streamlined and cool, but even if you're an experienced swimmer, as your abdomen grows, you're likely to crash into the wall as you flip. Save flip turns for after your baby is born.
- **Do an open turn.** Ah, this one is much easier, especially when you're sporting an ever-growing belly. With an *open turn,* you approach the pool wall, touch it with one or both hands, pull yourself into a *tuck position* (knees pressed as close to your chest as possible), swing yourself around, and push off the wall with your feet. No flipping, whatsoever.
- **Stand and turn.** That's right: Forget about how competitive swimmers turn, and just stand on the bottom of the pool (assuming you aren't in the deep end) and turn your feet around until you're facing the opposite way. You're not going to win any awards for gracefulness, but if you're at all nervous about making an open turn, just stand up and turn around.

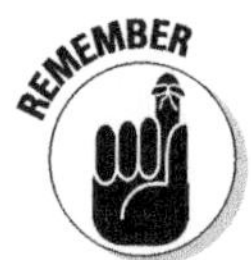

If you choose the stand and turn method, don't stand for too long before turning unless you absolutely need to take a break. You improve your cardiovascular system by swimming continuously, not by taking frequent breaks.

Dousing yourself in a workout plan

If you've never worked out before, check out Chapter 5 for generic four-day, five-day, and six-day-per-week workout plans that discuss activities in terms of minutes so you can modify them for swimming or water aerobics.

Plan to work out 3 to 5 days per week, starting with 15- or 20-minute workouts and working up to anywhere from 30 to 60 minutes per session. Vary your swim sessions so that you're not swimming the same distance, at the same speed, using the same stroke, day in and day out. (This is a surefire recipe for getting bored and quitting your workouts.) In fact, you can vary your stroke throughout your workout, for example, starting with ten minutes of freestyle, then five minutes of breast stroke, and then ten minutes of backstroke.

See Chapter 3 for information on monitoring the intensity of your workouts. During pregnancy, you don't want to overwork yourself, but you do want to work out hard enough that you feel as though you're putting in a good effort. Always monitor how you're feeling as you work out — as long as you continue to feel good, your baby is growing normally, and you're gaining weight as your healthcare provider wants you to, you can probably continue your workouts.

If you're getting a little bored with swimming or just find any of the three strokes too difficult to master, consider combining or replacing it with water aerobics, which we discuss in the following section.

Aerobicizing Underwater: The Ultimate Low-Impact Aerobics

Water aerobics, also called *aqua aerobics,* is a fairly new activity that's very popular among women, pregnant or not. Think of it as an aerobics class conducted in water, and because you're floating as you work out, you put absolutely no pressure on your feet, legs, and joints. Your body is partially submerged (that is, your chest and shoulders are completely out of the water, and the rest of your body is underwater), and your head never gets wet, which is a godsend for women who tend to get all nasal and stuffed up after swimming and for those who hate wrestling with nappy, chlorinated hair.

In addition to *deep-water aerobics,* in which your legs never touch the bottom of the pool, you can participate in *shallow-water aerobics,* in which you stand on the bottom of the pool — usually in special shoes. Deep-water aerobics has the obvious advantage of being non-weight-bearing, so it's easier on your body. However, you need less special equipment to do shallow-water aerobics, because you don't have to keep your body afloat.

Water aerobics offers a number of benefits. Like land-based aerobics, it offers a cardiovascular workout that also tones muscles throughout the body and improves your balance and coordination. Because the water provides a warm, gentle environment, water aerobics can also improve your flexibility. Finally, water aerobics is a lot of fun, especially if you're able to work out with a friend or become friends with the people you meet in class. Even a difficult workout just doesn't seem as hard as, say, running or biking, because the atmosphere of the class and the variety of the aerobics moves tends to make the workout more interesting and makes the time pass quickly. Some instructors even use music during water aerobics workouts, further increasing interest.

Gearing up

To begin a water aerobics workout program, you need some or all of the following. Aside from your swimsuit, much of this equipment may be available at the pool where you're taking classes. (See Chapter 7 for details and illustrations of this equipment.)

- **Buoyancy belt:** Also called a *water vest* or *flotation vest*, this belt keeps you afloat and in the vertical position as you work out. Note that if you're doing shallow-water aerobics, you don't need a buoyancy belt.

  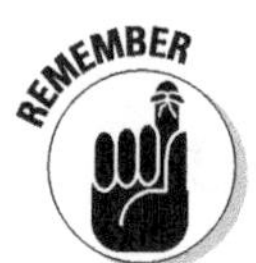

  Some instructors prefer that you not wear a buoyancy belt, keeping yourself afloat instead by treading water or using some other method. If you're naturally buoyant enough, this approach can give you a great workout, but for most people, we don't recommend it. Working to stay afloat *and* doing aerobics moves is just too difficult. If your instructor insists on shedding your buoyancy belt, look for another class.

  Another alternative to a buoyancy belt is a *noodle,* which is a long, thin, buoyant tube that keeps you afloat, but not as well as a buoyancy belt. Most pools have noodles available for use during your class.

- **Footwear:** If you're doing shallow-water aerobics, you need something to protect your feet, because the bottom of most pools is nubby and, occasionally, has sharp points. This footwear can range from a clean pair of running or aerobics shoes that you use only in the pool (to limit dirt and other impurities from getting into the pool) to special footwear, called *aqua socks,* similar to what scuba divers use. If you're taking a shallow-water aerobics class, ask your instructor what type of footwear he or she recommends.

  If you're doing deep-water aerobics and want to increase the intensity of your workout, consider using a pair of water shoes (also called floatation shoes, aqua runners, and aqua cuffs).

- **Water hand weights:** Water hand weights (also called dumbbells), are the cornerstone of most water aerobics classes. Shaped like regular hand weights (although they're sometimes substantially larger), water hand weights are made of buoyant material that provides resistance during your session.

- **Webbed gloves:** Webbed gloves (also called water mitts) provide additional resistance as you move your arms through the water. Many water aerobics enthusiasts love webbed gloves, but some instructors discourage their use because they can encourage you to push so hard against the water's resistance that you injure yourself.

Keeping your head above water: A few water aerobics moves

Just as in land-based aerobics (see Chapter 14), water aerobics workouts may include up to a hundred different moves. Rather than give you a smattering of moves, which doesn't do the overall activity justice, we leave water aerobics techniques up to your class instructor. However, in the interest of showing you a little of what water aerobics is all about so that you can determine whether you want to take up this activity, take a look at Figures 13-7 and 13-8, which show some common moves.

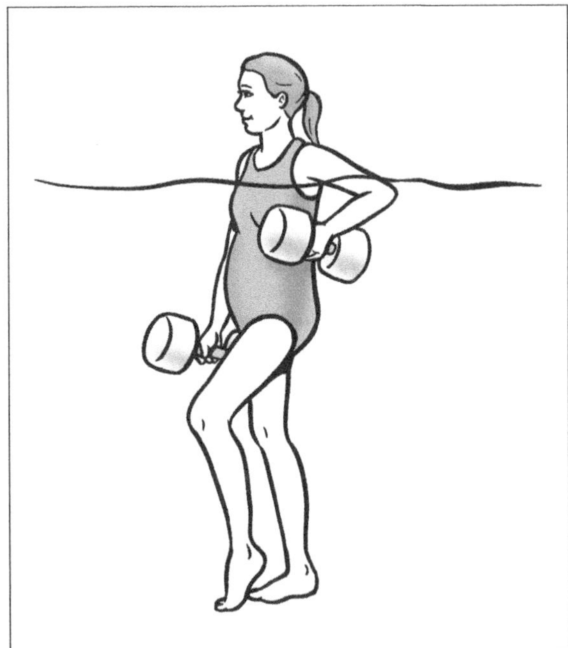

Figure 13-7: Lifting water hand weights underwater.

Note that an advanced form of water aerobics is called *pool running* or *water running*. Instead of doing the aerobics-based motions described here, you use the running motion, creating a workout that's very much like running on land. Check out the next section for more info.

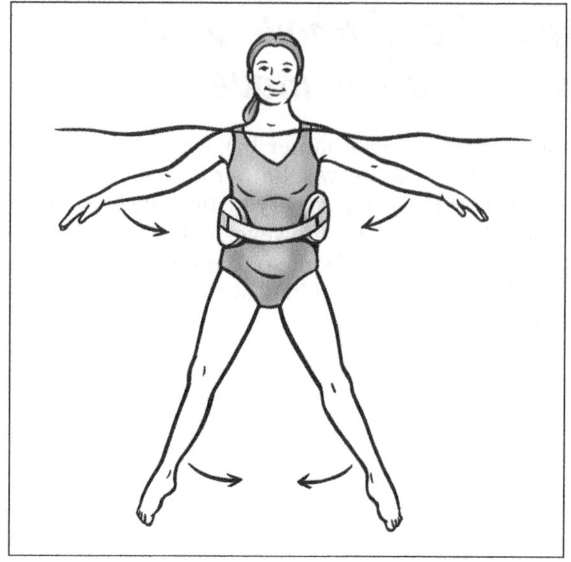

Figure 13-8: Doing full-body scissors.

Pondering pool running

If you're looking for a no-impact way to achieve a high-energy workout *and* run throughout your pregnancy, consider pool running. *Pool running* (also called *water running*) starts with a buoyancy belt that keeps you afloat in water so that your feet never touch the bottom of the pool. With your head and the tops of your shoulders above water level and the rest of your body submerged in an upright, vertical position, you move forward — very slowly, because of the resistance of the water — using the exact same running motion as you use while you run. You move your arms back and forth just as with land running, lifting one knee and fully extending the other leg on each "step." See Figure 13-9 for details.

Most people need to use the deep end of a pool or the diving well in order to avoid touching the ground while running. If you're using a traditional swimming lane, always run in water that's at least a foot deeper than you are tall.

In order to stay vertical, keep your back completely straight, without any forward lean. If you try to do a combination of running (in which your body is vertical) and swimming (in which your body is horizontal), you won't get the benefits of either running or swimming. Taking this approach results in a workout that's easier than swimming because of the buoyancy belt, and easier than running on land because the angle of your upper body cuts down substantially on the resistance the water is supposed to create against your body. (The resistance you should feel is similar to the feeling of running into a very strong wind — you're doing a lot of work, but you're not going forward very fast.) Always use a running motion with your arms and legs, and never cup your hands the way a swimmer does; instead, keep your hands in the same position you use while running on land.

One more note about pool running: Because you're running against the resistance of the water, the first time you run in the pool, your arms may feel really fatigued by the workout — far more than you'd feel running the same amount of time on land. If this happens to you, try using your legs more aggressively to move you forward. Chances are, you're letting your arms do a lot of the work, and your legs are getting off easy.

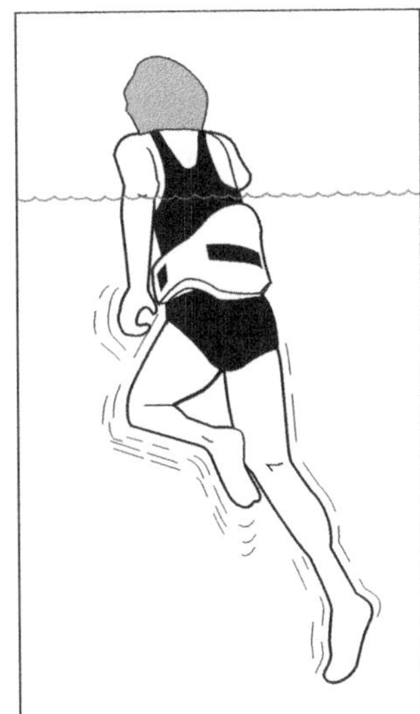

Figure 13-9: Good pool-running technique.

Chapter 14

Yoga, Pilates, and Low-Impact Aerobics

In This Chapter

- Relaxing — and building strength — with yoga
- Complementing your pregnancy fitness routine with Pilates
- Taking home a few tips about aerobics
- Determining whether a video or a class suits you best

Ever wonder what all the yoga and Pilates hype is about? This chapter gives you a basic rundown of both types of workouts, along with their close counterpart, low-impact aerobics. Because each of these topics is a book all its own, this chapter gives you only a brief overview of these three activities so that you can decide whether these are activities you want to pursue.

Yoga, Pilates, and low-impact aerobics share the following similarities, which is why we group them together in one chapter:

- You can do all three activities in your home with a video.
- You can find all three activities as classes at gyms, YMCAs, community centers, schools, and so on.
- You need approximately the same gear for all three activities: an exercise mat and comfortable clothing.

These three forms of exercise do have some differences, however:

- **Yoga** is a quiet, meditative activity that relaxes you completely while strengthening and toning your body. Yoga also greatly improves your flexibility. It is not, however, a cardiovascular workout that gets your heart pumping and your lungs working hard.

- **Pilates,** like yoga, doesn't focus on cardiovascular fitness, but instead on developing power and flexibility in muscle groups throughout the body. However, Pilates tends to be more difficult than yoga and, therefore, isn't especially meditative or relaxing.
- **Low-impact aerobics** is a cross between fitness walking and dancing, creating an excellent cardiovascular workout that revs you up instead of feeling relaxing or meditative.

We briefly discuss each of these activities in this chapter. If you decide to pursue one (or more) of them, check out Chapter 5 for four-day, five-day, and six-day-per-week workout plans that you can modify for these activities. The plans in Chapter 5 are generic, because they discuss activities in terms of minutes (versus miles or laps), so you can use them as a model for nearly any activity.

Yoga: Soothing Your Mind and Body

Yoga is a unique blend of *poses,* or body positions, that improve flexibility, balance, and strength. A pose may be one position or a series of positions, and each pose offers specific physical benefits that may also help you through some of the discomfort you're experiencing in your pregnancy, including back pain, nausea, tension, and so on.

One of the major benefits of yoga is that you can continue practicing the poses right up until you deliver your baby and can resume your workouts shortly after labor, so your workout routine may suffer less disruption than with other activities.

What about power yoga? Only if you're experienced!

Power yoga is a cross between yoga and aerobics. Unlike traditional yoga classes, a power yoga class may leave you feeling physically drained and very sweaty, because it consists of a demanding cardiovascular workout that also incorporates yoga poses meant to increase flexibility and strength. As a result, if you've never taken a power yoga class, wait until you deliver your baby, and then give it a try.

Power yoga can be an excellent workout after you deliver your baby, although we recommend taking a class instead of using a video, because the number of injuries among untrained participants tends to be high. If you've been doing power yoga for years, you can certainly continue your routine, with your healthcare provider's okay. (Keep a close eye out for signs that the activity may be too demanding for you — see Chapter 3.)

If you're not taking a class or watching a video made specifically for pregnant women, be sure to avoid poses that require you to lie on your stomach or on your back for several minutes if you feel lightheaded or dizzy in that position. If any pose feels painful or uncomfortable, or if any part of the yoga routine just doesn't feel right, skip that move and try the next. Avoid jumping into poses, instead going into each pose gently.

Yoga offers another benefit: its meditative qualities. Although walking for 30 minutes or taking an aerobics class gives you a great workout and helps relieve tension, nothing quite matches yoga's ability to calm and soothe. If your pregnancy is creating physical or emotional stress in your life, consider doing yoga once or twice per week to reap the benefits of its calming powers.

Yoga requires only the following:

- Comfortable, stretchy clothing, such as sweat pants, shorts, or a unitard (see Chapter 7)
- Bare feet, saving you the cost of shoes, although you can always purchase special yoga soft shoes
- A mat (preferably one that's a little sticky so that your bare feet don't slip), towel, or blanket
- A quiet, restful place to work out

The following sections describe four basic yoga poses, just to give you an idea of what a yoga workout is like. These step-by-step instructions are for demonstration purposes only: A book, video, or class tells you how long to hold these poses, how often to repeat them, and how to combine them with other poses to create an entire workout. Georg Feuerstein and Larry Payne discuss most of the poses in *Yoga For Dummies* (Wiley). Taking a yoga class is another way to master the many yoga poses that make up a yoga workout; if you can find a prenatal yoga class in your area, all the better. And look in the "Going solo with a video" section later in this chapter for details about an excellent video that incorporates many different poses into a relaxing workout.

Easy pose

The easy pose is a simple sitting pose in which many workouts begin. Simply do the following:

1. **Sit on the floor.**
2. **Bend your knees, keeping your feet flat on the floor, and then wrap your arms around your knees.**
3. **Press your knees to your chest to straighten your spine.**

4. **Release your arms when you no longer feel any stretch in your spine, cross your legs, and let your knees drop to the floor, as shown in Figure 14-1 (what's very politically incorrectly called *Indian style*).**

   Be sure to keep your head and body in a straight line.

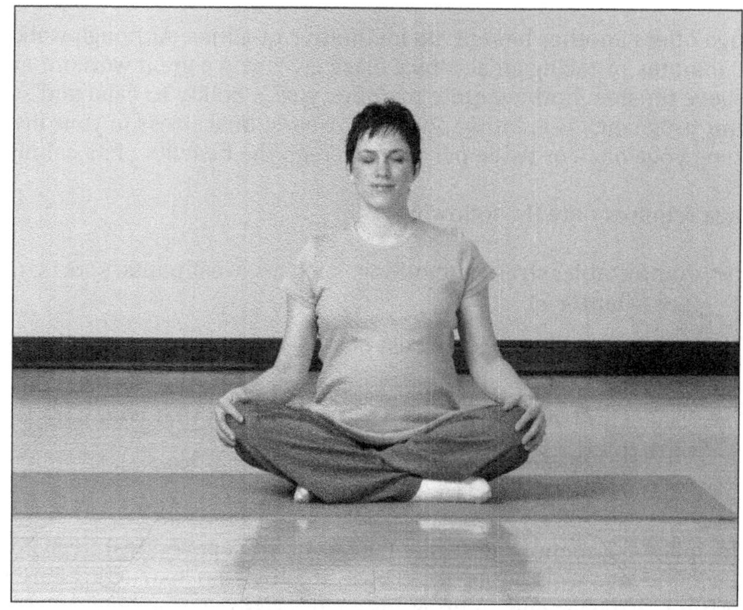

Figure 14-1: Many yoga workouts start with the easy pose.

Forward bend

The forward bend can be very relaxing during pregnancy, because you loosen your back and legs. Keep in mind, however, that this pose may become increasingly difficult to perform as your pregnancy progresses.

1. **Start in a sitting position, with your legs out in front of you in a V (whatever width of V is comfortable for you), toes pointed up toward the ceiling.**
2. **Pull up on your butt so that you're resting on your pelvic bone.**
3. **Stretch your arms straight up, trying to lengthen your spine as you stretch, and inhale.**

4. **As you exhale, lean your chest forward, keeping your back straight.**
5. **Try to bring your chin to your ankles and your chest to your thighs.**
6. **Hold onto your feet or ankles without bending your knees, as shown in Figure 14-2.**

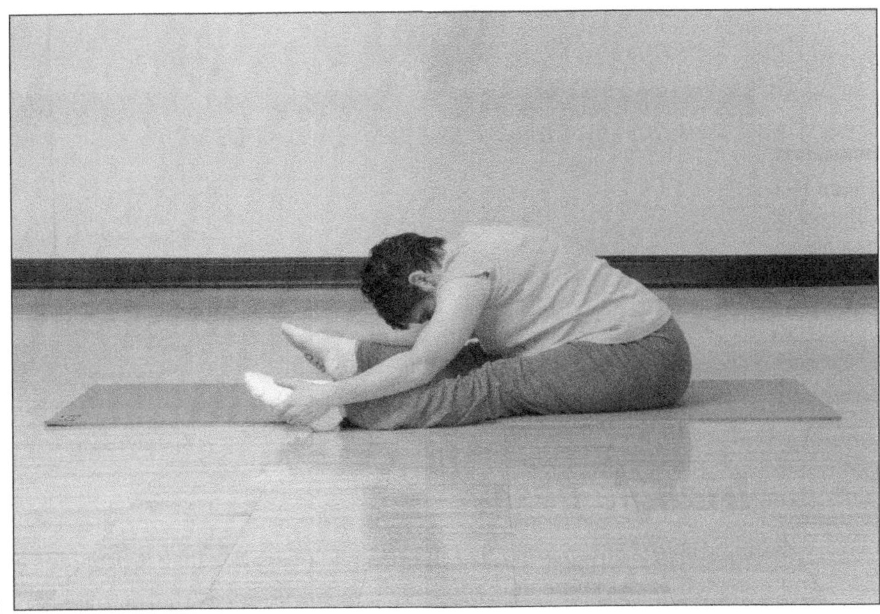

Figure 14-2: The forward bend is great for relaxing during pregnancy.

Cat tilt pose

The cat tilt helps alleviate pressure on your back and elongates your spine.

1. **Rest on your hands and knees, with your belly facing the floor.**
2. **Inhale deeply.**
3. **Exhale and pull in your abdominal muscles, tailbone, and butt.**
4. **Pressing down on your hands, press your back toward the ceiling so that your spine rounds, as shown in Figure 14-3.**

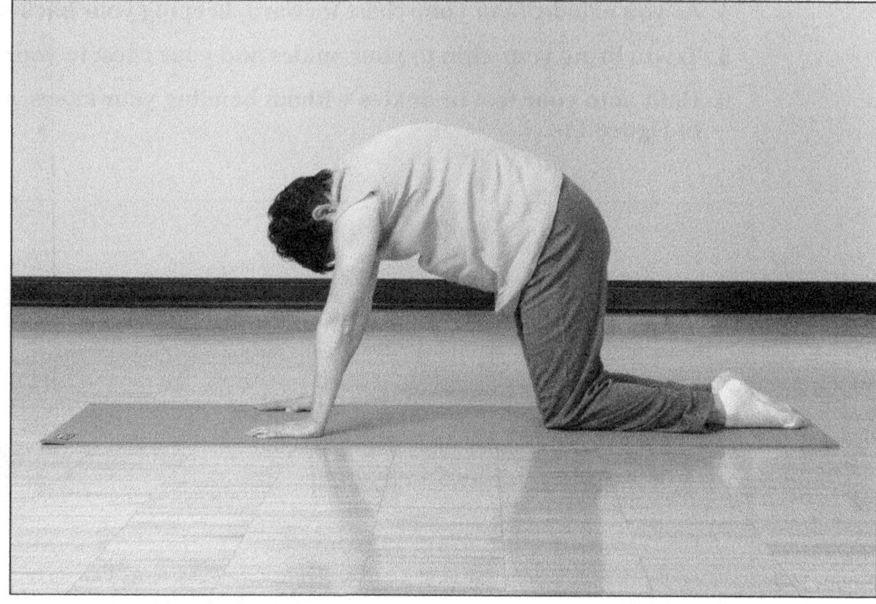

Figure 14-3: The cat tilt pose is perfect if your back muscles feel tight.

Triangle pose

Yoga classes frequently use the triangle pose, because it provides an excellent stretch of the spine and abdomen.

1. **Stand with your feet much wider than your shoulders, with both arms straight out to the sides, parallel to the floor, and palms facing up.**
2. **Inhale deeply.**
3. **Exhale and bend to the right, as shown in Figure 14-4.**

   Keep your knees straight and your hips facing forward. Don't twist your lower body; simply bend at your waist.
4. **Slide your right arm down your right leg as you bend, and then hold your leg or ankle.**
5. **Hold this position, slowly breathing in and out several times.**

   If you're able to, now lift your left leg off the floor, anywhere from 3 to 18 inches, keeping your knee straight.

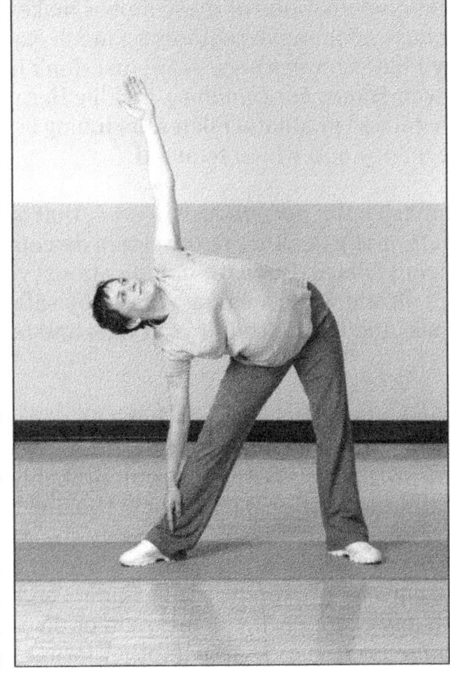

Figure 14-4: Stretch your spine and abdomen with the triangle pose.

Pilates: Strengthening with Concentration and Control

Pilates, named for its founder Joseph Pilates, has been around for nearly 100 years, but didn't become mainstream until the turn of the 21st century. To get a sense of what Pilates is like, picture yoga poses combined into a workout, with slow lifting and rolling movements to get into and out of poses. This activity combines elements of yoga, of course, with gymnastics and martial arts, all done in slow, controlled movements, accompanied by deep breathing.

Like yoga, Pilates stretches and strengthens the body and can also be quite meditative after you master the moves. Because you do the movements slowly, however, the moves require a great deal of strength, which is why Pilates takes months to become skilled at. The activity has hundreds of movements and exercises, and each has anywhere from three to ten steps, all requiring a great deal of explanation — different combinations of these moves make up varying overall Pilates workouts. Because each move requires so much explanation, we don't try to show you any Pilates moves here — we just don't have the space to give it justice. However, *Pilates For Dummies,* by Ellie Herman (Wiley) has an entire chapter on prenatal and postnatal Pilates, including lists of which exercises are safe during pregnancy and which to avoid.

Because Pilates tends to emphasize the *powerhouse* or *core,* that is, the lower abdomen, back, and butt, many healthcare providers discourage pregnant women from practicing Pilates. But with modifications, you can keep your abdominal muscles strong while keeping your baby safe. You can also strengthen your legs, arms, and back, stretch your hips and back, and improve your balance.

In general, steer clear of any movement that has you lying on your belly or on your back after your fourth month. You also don't want to do any exercise that resembles a sit-up during pregnancy, as much as you probably want to keep your tummy firm and flat — a traditional sit-up puts too much pressure on both your low back and abdomen and doesn't effectively strengthen your lower abdominal muscles. Be careful when doing Pilates moves that involve deep stretching, because you can easily overstretch ligaments and tendons and even injure them. As with any exercise, if you feel pain or discomfort or something just doesn't feel quite right, move on to another form of exercise.

Low-Impact Aerobics: Big Results with Little Joint Stress

Chances are that you're familiar with aerobics, which exploded in popularity in the 1980s and is still a good way to work out today. Generally, aerobics involves moving to music in a choreographed way, is more structured than dancing, yet is too fun and invigorating to ever be boring. Sometimes, aerobics classes also involve using hand weights (see Chapter 11) or working out on a step (see the sidebar, "Step it up? Not until you deliver"), which increases the difficulty and intensity of the workout.

Notice that we put an emphasis on *low-impact* aerobics, as opposed to power aerobics or any other high-impact aerobics workout. Higher-impact aerobics, such as Tae-Bo and other martial-arts-based workouts are just too intense for most pregnant women. If you can do the workouts at half-time and substitute low kicks for high kicks, you may be able to continue a high-impact routine if your healthcare provider agrees. But if you're an aerobics novice, stick to low-impact, which means you won't do any steps, jumps, hops, or kicks. (See the "Step it up? Not until you deliver" sidebar for more on step aerobics.)

Step it up? Not until you deliver

Step aerobics isn't for beginners, so if you're just starting out and past your first trimester, a step aerobics class may not be a good idea. If you've been doing step aerobics and your healthcare provider agrees that continuing isn't a problem, keep in mind the following:

- Limit your step aerobics workouts to two days per week.
- Keep the step at no more than four inches high, double-check its stability, and make sure your entire foot (not just the front part of your foot) is on the step when you're using it.

As your pregnancy progresses, you have a harder time seeing your feet and may have difficulty placing your foot safely during step aerobics.

Also consider the following precautions when doing aerobics during your pregnancy:

- Do the entire workout with gentleness in mind. Warm up slowly and move gradually into more difficult cardiovascular work.
- Keep your intensity at a level that feels moderate to somewhat challenging — in the 12–14 range on the rate of perceived exertion scale that we describe in Chapter 3.
- To avoid falling, steer clear of quick turns and don't cross your feet, shuffling them, instead.
- Use small steps and rise up onto the balls of your feet slowly.
- Avoid any deep knee bends or unsupported squats (a *supported squat* is one in which you use a chair or other heavy object to support you as you squat).
- Breathe normally as you work out (don't hold your breath).
- Although the entire workout including warm-up and cool-down can be longer, try to keep the aerobics portion to 30 minutes or less.

Your best bet is to purchase a video or attend a class specifically geared toward pregnant women. If you feel that a class is more appropriate for you than a video (see the following section) but can't find a prenatal aerobics class in your area, talk with your instructor about your pregnancy and ask for alternate moves. If your instructor is unable to tell you how to modify your workout for your pregnancy and he or she isn't trained to work with pregnant women, find an aerobics video specifically for pregnant women.

Deciding Between a Class and a Video

Taking a yoga, Pilates, or aerobics class can be a great way to get a workout while meeting new people. But following the instructions in a video is convenient and far less expensive than a class. Either way, you get good workouts, so the choice of whether to enroll in a class or follow an exercise video is strictly up to you. Let your personality be your guide.

Joining a class

You'll probably prefer a class if

- You enjoy working out with others.
- You tend to perform best with personal attention from an instructor.
- The structure of working out at a set time is motivating for you.
- You can afford to pay the fee for each class or for each month's membership at a workout facility.

If you decide to attend a class, call your local YMCA, YWCA, hospital, community center, high-school community education office, fitness center, or dance studio. Ask specifically about classes for pregnant women and see whether you can sit in on any class before signing up. Before committing to a class, look for the following features:

- The class is either specifically for pregnant women or can be modified in light of the demands of pregnancy.
- The instructor has a background in prenatal fitness, actively supervises the class, and monitors the participants.
- The facility is climate controlled and has mats, well-maintained equipment, and restrooms.
- The class is offered at a convenient time. (***Note:*** If you're not a morning person and the class is offered at 5:30 a.m., chances are, you won't stick with it very long. If you always work late, and the class is at 5:00 p.m., you'll have plenty of excuses to skip.)
- The class is offered at a convenient location. (***Note:*** If you have to drive ten miles out of your way to get to the class, you'll probably skip the class just as often as you attend it.)

Going solo with a video

Chances are that a video is appropriate for you if

- You like the flexibility of working out on your own schedule, by yourself.
- You tend to be self-motivated and will actually work out, as you've planned, without the structure of a class starting time.
- You can stay focused and get through the entire workout without stopping for distractions in your home.
- You catch on quickly and can pick up the technique without any personal instruction.
- You have a comfortable space in your home with a TV and VCR or DVD player, where you can work out without bothering other household members.

You can find literally hundreds of videos about yoga, Pilates, and aerobics, and you should choose the one that suits you best. (If you can, borrow videos from your library or rent them from a video store before making a purchase, but do plan to buy them eventually so that a video is available to you at a moment's notice.) For videos that aren't specific to pregnancy, be sure to avoid any poses or techniques that cause pain or just don't feel right.

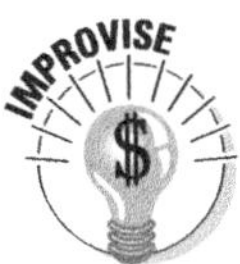

Consider forming a workout group with friends and workout partners, using one video (sharing the cost) or alternating different videos from each group member for each workout. You can meet at one location or rotate the group from house to house. This way, you get the benefits of working out at a set time (and not bagging the workout at the last minute) without the expense of paying for a class.

We recommend the following videos, but this list isn't anywhere near exhaustive:

- *Yoga Journal's Prenatal Yoga* with Shiva Rea (distributed by Gaiam) is a relaxing video that uses three different models, one in her first trimester, one in her second, and one in her third, each modifying the poses just a little. You can follow whichever model best meets your needs.
- *Basic Yoga Workout For Dummies,* a video by Sara Ivanhoe (Wiley), presents 12 basic poses and additional modifications to those moves.
- *Beyond Basic Yoga For Dummies,* another video by Sara Ivanhoe (Wiley), extends the first video with additional poses and challenges.

- *Pilates Workout For Dummies,* a workout video by Michelle Dozois (Wiley), demonstrates Pilates techniques for beginners but also offers challenging workouts as you advance.
- *Denise Austin's Pregnancy Plus Workout* (aerobics; Just For Kids Home Video) features fitness guru Denise Austin, who is arguably the most upbeat aerobics instructor on the planet. Austin is pregnant with her first child on this video.
- *Kathy Smith's Pregnancy Workout* (aerobics; Sony) features a pregnant Kathy Smith sharing her well-rounded pregnancy workout. Not as upbeat as some videos, but an excellent workout without a lot of hype.
- *Stepping Through Pregnancy,* a video by Nancy Anderson (aerobics; Collage Video), is — in spite of its name — a low-impact aerobics video that features three levels of difficulty, allowing you to adjust the workout to match your experience and goals.

Chapter 15

A Bicycle Built for Two

In This Chapter

- Deciding which type of bike is right for you
- Making safety a top priority
- Adjusting your bike and riding it effectively
- Getting started in your cycling workouts

Cycling is a fun, easy-to-master activity that is ranked as one of the best all-around ways to stay fit. It's extremely popular among pregnant women because it has almost no impact on your joints, yet cycling helps you develop muscle strength and also gives you an excellent cardiovascular workout. (Note that although running, cross-country skiing, and rowing are often listed ahead of cycling as some of the best ways to burn calories and get a great all-over workout, many pregnant women find that those three other activities are just too difficult during pregnancy.)

In this chapter, you find out which bike is best for you, discover a few safety pointers, come to understand the ins and outs of cycling techniques, and get some tips on how to handle your first few workouts. For the lowdown on cycling get-up, see Chapter 7.

We understand that you may not be ready to include all the following cycling tips into your pregnancy fitness routine, but if cycling is a sport you want to continue throughout life, come back to this chapter after your pregnancy to take your cycling fitness routine to the next level.

If you're thinking of continuing to ride after your baby is born, keep in mind that some women find that cycling during the days and weeks after delivering a baby is just too uncomfortable. Generally, this discomfort lasts from six to eight weeks and then clears up on its own as your body heals. Start with short rides and purchase a gel seat to ease the discomfort.

Investing in Cycling Equipment

Bikes come in two basic forms: outdoor and indoor. This section gives you tips on buying either bike so that you can begin working out right away.

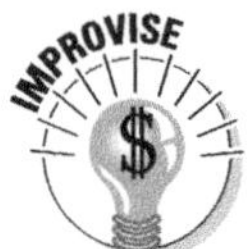

If you aren't sure that you want to take up cycling, see whether you can get a temporary membership at a gym before spending money on a bike. Often, local gyms offer a two-week membership for a low price, allowing you to try the equipment before making a yearlong commitment. And if you're looking for other ways to save money on buying a bike, always shop the classified ads in your area to see whether anyone's selling a used bike. You may also want to try Internet auction sites, such as eBay (`www.ebay.com`), but if you go that route, be sure to factor in the shipping costs for a heavy item like a bike.

Taking it outdoors

The price range for outdoor bikes is tremendous; expect to pay between $200 and $1,500. If you really want to fork out some cash, consider getting a *recumbent outdoor bike* (somewhat like the La-Z-Boy of bikes in that you sit very comfortably — yet you still get an optimal workout).

Recumbent bikes haven't yet caught the public's eye (or maybe they're just too steep for the average pocketbook), but they're far more comfortable than upright outdoor bikes. Instead of perching your tush on a skimpy seat, moving the pedals down below you, and leaning over to grab the handlebars, you simply lean back in a seat with a back (like a chair), pedal with your legs straight out in front of you, and hold onto handlebars that are comfortably designed at about chest height. On most recumbent bikes, you also sit lower to the ground, which makes falls less likely. However, outdoor recumbent bikes take some getting used to; balancing, especially, can be difficult at first, so be sure you're comfortable riding on an outdoor recumbent bike before venturing out. You can also find recumbent indoor bikes — they're quickly becoming the most popular indoor bikes available and are already the favorite of many pregnant women — see the following section.

Finding a bike that fits you best

Outdoor bikes range from traditional 10-speed road bikes to 15- to 20-plus-speed mountain bikes (also called *trail bikes*). The tires may be thin (for riding on smooth, paved roads) or wide (for off-road trail riding), and many pregnant women find that the fatter tires make for a softer, more stable ride and make switching between different road surfaces a little easier. The bike's frame may be very low to the ground (which is very hip right now, although riding on a low-frame bike isn't very comfortable) or it may be what you think of as a more traditional size.

We suggest looking for a *hybrid bike* (a traditional bike crossed with a mountain bike; ten speeds with wide tires) or a *beach bike* (a one-speed bike with very upright handlebars, a wide seat, and cushy ride), both of which tend to have wide tires and are comfortable on a variety of surfaces. Within these styles, look for a model that lets you sit in a very upright position and allows room for your abdomen to grow.

Ask a salesperson to help you find a bike that fits you perfectly, and plan to shop around at a variety of stores until you find the best one. If you're planning to share a bike with your partner, but the two of you are built quite differently (especially in terms of height), forget that plan, because you need a bike that fits your frame perfectly — otherwise, neither of you will ever be comfortable! And because your height and leg length don't change when you're pregnant, whatever bike you buy will fit you the rest of your life.

Settling on a seat

Look for a bike with a good seat — one that feels cushy and comfortable and isn't too narrow for the shape of your butt. The bike seat (also called a *saddle*) is the equivalent of your shoes when walking or doing aerobics: It's the only thing between you and the road, and it has to fit you perfectly. You want a seat that's specifically made for women — a wider and shorter model than the ones made for men. Make sure you feel well cushioned and well supported when you try out any seat. Some women also find that a *split saddle* (in which the back half of the seat is split apart lengthwise, leaving a hole between the two split-apart portions) helps reduce pelvic pressure and numbness that sometimes accompanies cycling. A *gel seat,* one that's padded with a gel substance like that in running and walking shoes, cushions your tush even more.

As you try different bikes at a bike shop or sporting goods store, keep in mind that you can swap out the seats. If you love everything about a bike except the seat, just ask for a different seat when you discuss the price. If you're buying a bike at a discount store, you have to take the bike as is, but you can still swap out the seat later by going to a bike shop and asking about its cushy seats. Replacing a seat is super easy — you may need a screwdriver, but that's it — and takes less than ten minutes.

Don't forget the helmet!

Never ride — even a short distance — without a helmet that fits you perfectly. A helmet can make the difference between surviving an accident and not surviving it, and unlike your baby's body and brain, your brain isn't cushioned by layers of fluids and body fat that protect you when you fall. See Chapter 7 for more on cycling helmets, including the optional windscreens or sports shields that attach to certain models.

Considering toe clips

Although your local bike shop may try to sell you *toe clips* or *snap-in clip/shoe* combinations, avoid these accessories while you're pregnant. The idea is to secure your foot to the pedal with a strap or other device, giving you quite a bit more power as you ride. However, because toe clips lock your foot into place, just imagine what happens if you need to put your foot down quickly and don't have time to unlatch the strap — you fall right over! After you deliver your baby, you can add toe clips to your bike or buy cycling shoes that clip in to special pedals; for now, your changing center of gravity and inability to see your feet as your abdomen grows make this type of gear dangerous.

Moving it inside

For some women, the ability to balance becomes so impaired — especially in the second trimester — that an indoor bike is their only option. Another plus of indoor bikes is that they're adjustable, so one size fits all. The seats are generally pretty cushy, too.

Indoor bikes generally come in two varieties, both shown in Figure 15-1:

- **Traditional stationary bike (also called an upright bike):** This type of indoor bike is shaped quite a bit like an outdoor bike, with a small seat, pedals that are located well under the seat (between the seat and the floor), and handlebars.

  Although traditional stationary bikes are easy to find in most discount stores and sporting goods stores and may be the lowest-cost option, you may find that, by the third trimester, your belly is so large and heavy that this type of bike causes low-back pain.

- **Recumbent indoor bike:** A recumbent indoor bike looks quite different from an outdoor bike: The main difference is that a large, comfortable chair (with a back on it) replaces the puny seat. This means you can sit back in the chair and pedal in front of you, taking pressure off your abdomen and pelvis. Recumbent indoor bikes generally don't come with handlebars, but some come with bars that you can move forward and backward, just to give your arms a workout.

  For an excellent whole-body workout, keep a few hand weights within reach of your recumbent bike as you ride. At a specified time (say, every 10 or 15 minutes), do a short weightlifting routine (see Chapter 11) as you continue to ride. Although lifting hand weights and riding at the same time may feel a little awkward at first, you'll quickly get the hang of it. (Lifting while riding is a lot harder on a traditional indoor bike, though: You're sitting up higher, which means that you can't reach the hand weights as easily, and the seat is smaller, which means that you have to concentrate harder to stay on it.) Combining two different activities in this way is called *cross-training* — check out Chapter 17 for more ways to mix up your workouts.

Expect to spend between $100 and $400 on an indoor bike, depending on the quality, design (recumbent tends to be more expensive than traditional), and features, such as large displays that tell you how fast you're riding, extra-cushy seats, and so on.

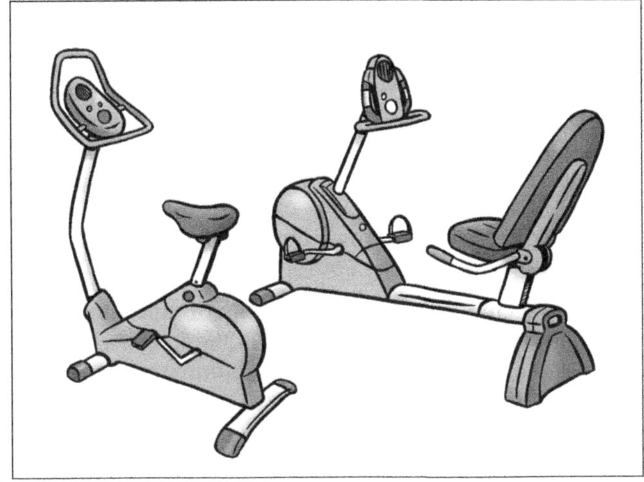

Figure 15-1: A traditional stationary bike and a recumbent bike — recumbent bikes are usually more comfortable during pregnancy.

Taking a Few Outdoor Safety Precautions

If you're riding outside — and this is a decision to make with your healthcare provider, who may ask you to begin cycling indoors after your first trimester — you need to take a few safety precautions. This section tells you how to keep your tires and chain in good condition, take precautions in case of a blown tire or bad weather, stay well hydrated, and keep yourself from getting injured in a fall.

Sending clear turn signals

Did you memorize cycling turn signals when you were a kid? In case you never knew or have forgotten them, here we show you the universal hand signals for giving drivers and other cyclists a hint about your next move:

- **Left turn:** Left arm straight out to your side and parallel to the road
- **Right turn:** Left arm in the shape of an *L*, with your fingers pointing to the sky
- **Stop:** Left arm in the shape of an upside-down *L*, with your fingers pointing to the ground

Common-sense cycling safety tips

Most cycling safety tips are really common sense, but if you haven't ridden before, some of the following information may be new to you. Before heading out the door and while you're getting your bike ready to ride, keep the following tips in mind:

- **Make sure your tires are properly inflated.** If you don't have a hand- or foot-operated pump that you can attach to your bike, consider getting one, looking especially for one that also measures tire pressure. Check the pressure before every ride, using the information stamped on the tire wall (usually, "Inflate to 90 PSI max") as your guide. Then at any stop (such as at a stoplight), do a quick visual check of both tires to make sure they're holding air. If you're not sure how much to fill your tires or what properly inflated tires look like, stop by your local bike shop for help.
- **Make sure your chain has the proper tension and looks well oiled.** Also, know how to fix a chain that has derailed. If you don't know how, ask someone at your local bike shop to demonstrate or pick up a book on cycling.

If you're riding on a dirt road or crushed-rock trail (as opposed to a paved road), go to your local bike shop and have your chain lubricated with a paraffin dip, which doesn't attract dirt, avoids the greasy mess of most bike chains, and is easier to maintain.

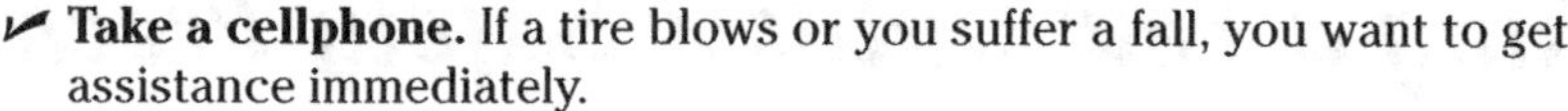

- **Take a cellphone.** If a tire blows or you suffer a fall, you want to get assistance immediately.
- **Tell someone your route.** If no one is home when you leave the house, write a note detailing which direction you're going and when you expect to return home. And if you're not exactly sure where you're going, take a map with you and leave a note about the general vicinity you'll be in.
- **Take two full water bottles with you on each ride.** Cycling can dehydrate you, and those bottles may be your only water source along the way. Ideally, you want water bottles that you can open and close with your tongue and teeth — if you don't have to use two hands to get water, you're more likely to drink the amount you need during the ride. Also take a snack — fruit, crackers, or juice — for a quick snack along the ride.
- **Wear bright and reflective cycling gear to make sure you're seen.** See Chapter 7 for more on specific types of gear, and then go hunting for colors like lime green, brilliant yellow, bright orange, and so on.
- **Take foul-weather gear, in case a storm surfaces.** Many nylon and GoreTex jackets fold up into tiny square pouches that fit in nearly any bike pack.

Avoiding pitfalls that lead to falls

Cycling during pregnancy is less jolting to your body than many other sports, but it isn't without risks if you ride outdoors.

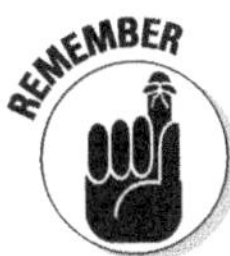

Almost none of the information in this section applies if you're cycling indoors. The risks involved in cycling all have to do with the potential for falling or crashing, and given that indoor bikes are designed such that they're nearly impossible to fall off of, falling isn't a major issue when you're riding indoors.

From the time you were a tot, chances are you've heard warning after warning about falling when riding outdoors. If you're already a cyclist, you understand that falling is very uncommon among the cycling elite. By nature and by training, cyclists tend to have excellent balance, so with just a bit of training, you too can keep yourself from careening your bike into a street sign, bench, or other bike.

Three situations, however, tend to make falling inevitable, so novice riders should take the utmost caution during pregnancy:

- **Cycling on trails:** Often called *trail biking, off-road biking,* or, most commonly, *mountain biking,* this type of cycling means encountering tree roots, downed tree limbs, slippery rocks, rushing streams, and so on. Although these elements make mountain biking exciting, they also make falling a pretty sure thing.
- **Your shifting center of gravity:** This adjustment is probably causing you balance problems, which means that at times during your pregnancy, you may have trouble staying upright while walking, much less riding. If you don't feel comfortable riding outdoors or your healthcare provider asks you to stop riding outside, switch to indoor cycling.
- **Riding on roads that require intense concentration:** Roads with sharp drop-offs, sharp turns, and roads that need repair can lead to serious falls. The same can be said for high-traffic areas, which require careful maneuvering and close attention.

For the reasons noted in the preceding list, you want to ride on the wide, smooth shoulder of a paved road that has little or no traffic (always ride *with* traffic) or on a bike trail that's paved or lined with crushed rock (not a dirt trail), and only if you are *not* experiencing any balance problems as a result of your pregnancy. Also, keep a close eye on drivers so that you can identify potentially dangerous drivers before they get too close. Anyone who's talking on a cellphone, eating, or swerving on the road is a giant red flag for you. Chances are, that person isn't paying close attention and may not even know that you're on the road. That leaves you in charge of getting out of the car's way.

If you ride in the country on narrow roads, use caution as you head up hills, because you may not see a car that's speeding toward you. If you ride in the city, avoid areas with a lot of cars — the excess exhaust isn't good for your baby and will almost certainly make you feel nauseated.

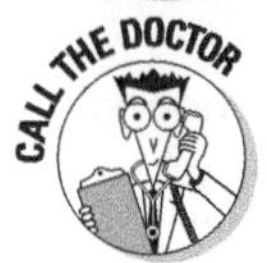

If you do fall, get up slowly, using the technique in Chapter 18 for getting up from a lying position. If anything feels amiss, call your healthcare provider immediately.

Basic Cycling Techniques: No Training Wheels Required

Cycling technique isn't much different from what you mastered as a kid, but instead of using your bike only to get to your best friend's house and back, you're now using it for fitness, so take note of a few pointers. This section helps you adjust your bike, know how fast to pedal to get the best results, and find out how to take on hills (assuming you're on an outdoor bike) with a growing belly that makes doing so tough.

Adjusting your bike

Properly adjusting your bike makes you more efficient, which means that you can work out with as little wasted effort as possible. Your best bet is to get your bike fitted by experts at your local bike shop and to have those experts show you how to tweak the bike yourself, especially to accommodate your growing abdomen.

However, if you don't have that option, here's what you need to know (see Figure 15-2):

1. **Adjust the seat so that when you're sitting on it and the pedal is as low as it goes, your foot rests comfortably on the pedal and your leg is nearly straight, but not fully extended.**

   Place the seat too high, and your hips will do most of the work (which isn't healthy for your hips). In addition, you'll probably get some *chafing* (rubbing that results in raw skin) on your inner thighs. Place the seat too low, and your knees will do too much of the work (which isn't healthy for your knees). If you've adjusted your seat to what you think is the proper height, but then feel pressure in your hips or knees, lower or raise the seat, as needed.

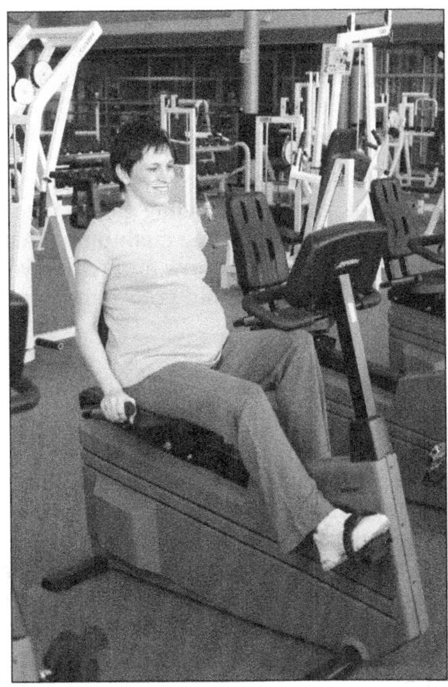

Figure 15-2: Sitting comfortably on a bike.

Most seats come with clamps that are easy to release, allowing you to adjust the seat height. You may have to get on and off the bike a few times, though, as you make adjustments. If you're using a recumbent bike, adjust the seat by moving it forward or backward — closer to or farther from the pedals — so that you're using a straight but not fully outstretched leg.

2. **Ensure that the seat is parallel to the floor and not tilted at all.**

   If you tilt the seat forward or back, most likely, you'll have all sorts of chafing problems.

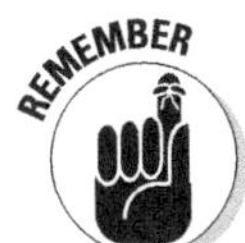

   Occasionally, pregnant women find that if the bike is putting too much pressure on the pelvis, tilting the seat forward helps. Use caution as you do this, though, and put the seat straight again if you start to develop chafing or back pain.

3. **If you're using a bike with handlebars, adjust the handlebars as many times as you need to in order for them to be comfortable.**

   For maximum back comfort, you want the handlebars to be the same height as — if not much higher than — the seat. Note that this is a different adjustment than elite cyclists use: They generally place the handlebars lower than the seat.

If you're using an indoor traditional bike or an outdoor bike, as your belly grows, you want to sit up as straight as possible, which may mean continuing to raise the handlebars throughout your pregnancy. If you just can't seem to raise the handlebars high enough, call your local bike shop to see whether the bike experts can help.

To avoid numbness and potential nerve damage that can come from gripping handlebars for long periods, purchase cycling gloves (see Chapter 7) or handlebar covers, both of which offer some cushioning. As you ride, move your hands from time to time to vary how and where you're gripping the handlebars — you don't want to hold your hands and wrists in one position for a long period of time.

Pedaling like a pro

The secret to efficient riding is to pedal fast and consistently, using the lowest gears you can in order to continue pedaling consistently, regardless of the terrain. Elite cyclists turn the pedals 90 times per minute (referred to as *revolutions per minute,* or *RPM*), which is about 3 times every 2 seconds, regardless of whether they're going uphill, riding downhill, or going on flat areas. (This pace or speed is also called a *cadence.*) Unless you're a world-class cyclist who's having the easiest pregnancy in history, though, you're not going to be cycling at that pace.

Keep your gear low so that you can turn the pedals easily, and then work on pedaling faster than seems normal — you may even want to time yourself, just to see how many RPM you're turning. If you're able to turn 60 to 70 RPM while pregnant, you're getting an excellent workout. Just keep in mind that the faster you turn the pedals, the better you're working your heart, lungs, and muscles. Yet, you never want to exceed your abilities — be sure to read Chapter 3 for details about adjusting the intensity of your workouts while you're pregnant. So, although you want to strive to pedal quickly at low gears (whether you're training indoors or out), you also want to slow to a more moderate cadence whenever you feel that you've overexerted yourself.

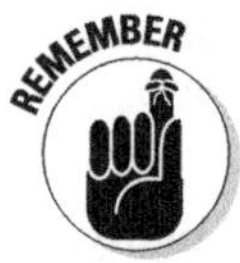

Spinning is a type of cycling workout, usually done indoors at a gym during a spinning class, which uses low gears and quick pedaling to get a good workout. It tries to mimic the way world-class cyclists pedal (a fast cadence in low gears), but most pregnant women find that spinning is too intensive, because you can get very hot (without the wind that you get when riding an outdoor bike) and you may not take breaks as often as you need them, given the structure of the class and the continued encouragement of the instructor. If you've been spinning and your pregnancy is progressing well, you can probably keep up the activity, with modifications, although you want to discuss it with your healthcare provider.

Riding uphill

For obvious reasons, you can ignore this section if you're using an indoor bike. If you ride outside, though, keep the following tips in mind:

- **As you approach a hill, downshift to a lower gear and pedal faster.** This saves wear and tear on your knees and makes going up the hill much easier.
- **Try not to stand on the pedals to climb a hill.** Cycling efficiently while standing is very difficult, and it usually slows down your cadence (when you want to do just the opposite — increase your cadence). That said, some people can get their hips into the uphill, standing-pedal process and although they look goofy, can get pretty efficient at it.
- **If scaling the hill's just too darn tough, get off your bike and walk up the hill.** There's no embarrassment in this!

The key is to ride with an easy rhythm when going up hills and to not try killing the hill — or yourself.

Wheeling through a Cycling Workout Plan

Most women find that starting with 15 to 20 minute rides, 3 or 4 times per week, feels challenging but isn't overly strenuous. From there, gradually build up your speed and distance, keeping the rate of perceived exertion (RPE) scale that we discuss in Chapter 3 in mind at all times. If you're looking for some idea of what pace to choose, most women find that 12 to 15 miles per hour is a good place to start, but if you find that's too much, back off until you feel comfortable.

Start with a short ride at a slow cadence, and if you continue to feel good, your baby is growing normally, and you're gaining weight as you should, gradually increase your speed and distance, cutting back if you no longer feel great. Don't overdo your first few rides, even if you feel like you could ride a hundred miles (or an equivalent number of minutes if you're riding indoors). Chances are, all you'll do is make yourself very sore.

If you ride outside, vary your workouts as much as possible. Riding the same route for the same amount of time, day in and day out, will likely make you bored beyond belief. But if you have four or five different routes — all of varying distances — you'll likely look forward to reexploring each route. In the same way, ride easy on some days, and a little harder on others. You can vary your workouts in other ways, too, from whether you ride on flat roads or hilly ones to whether you use mostly low gears or higher ones. And, as Chapter 5 indicates, you want to take at least one day completely off each week.

Ride short loops near your house or office, repeating them to build your mileage. That way, you can always add another loop or two if you feel good, but you can also stop your workout if you're feeling fatigued. Keeping your loops close to home means you'll never be stuck several miles from home while not feeling good enough to continue your workout.

If you've never worked out before, check out Chapter 5 for generic four-day, five-day, and six-day-per-week workout plans that you can modify for cycling.

Cross-training that complements your cycling

If you're not able to cycle (for example, if your tush is just too sore right now), the following activities use the same muscles as cycling:

- Cross-country skiing (and cross-country ski machines, which we discuss in Chapter 17)
- Rollerblading and speed-skating (probably not a great idea when you're pregnant, though, given the risk of falling)

Strange as it seems, skiing and skating really do use a lot of the same muscles as cycling; in fact, many elite cross-country skiers and speed-skaters train on bikes during summer months. This means that, if you want to continue to train for cycling (for example, if you've been interested in entering a local cycling race after you deliver your baby) but aren't able to while you're pregnant, using a cross-country ski machine will keep you in excellent cycling shape.

On the other hand, running or walking (jog back to Chapter 12) and swimming (see Chapter 13) use very different muscles than cycling does, so if your goal is to cross-train in order to use as many different muscles as possible, alternating cycling, running or walking, and swimming gives you an excellent overall fitness routine. See Chapter 17 for more on cross-training.

Chapter 16

Weightlifting and Indoor Machines

In This Chapter

- Getting the scoop on indoor machines
- Facing a weight machine without fear
- Climbing to new heights with a stair-stepper
- Gliding along on an elliptical machine
- Cross-country skiing even in summer
- Rowing for the water-phobic

No workout book would be complete without at least a little info about all those fancy machines that you see at your local gym or on TV infomercials. So, this chapter covers the basics of using exercise machines, whether you want to lift weights on a weight machine or use other indoor equipment, such as a stair-stepper, cross-country ski machine, elliptical trainer, or rowing machine. We cover them roughly in order from those machines requiring the least exertion to the most demanding.

Two machines that aren't discussed here are covered in other chapters: For more on treadmills, check out Chapter 12; for the lowdown on indoor bicycles, see Chapter 15. In addition, for information on using simple hand-held dumbbells and other free weights (as opposed to a weight machine), see Chapter 11.

If you're new to exercise, see Chapter 5 for four-day, five-day, and six-day-per-week workout plans that you can modify for any activity. The plans listed in that chapter discuss activities in terms of minutes, not miles or laps, so you can use them for any of the exercise machines in this chapter.

Indoor Machines: The Pros and Cons

Using indoor machines offers some obvious advantages over exercising outdoors (being able to work out in the middle of winter or early on a dark morning, for example), but the news isn't all good. This section shares both the pros and cons of using indoor machines.

The pros

Working out on indoor exercise machines can be both fun and convenient. Here's why:

- **You can work out in a climate-controlled environment, any time of year, even when it's pitch black outside.** This benefit is especially helpful during those short winter days.
- **You may be able to multitask,** watching the news or your favorite TV show, or listening to the radio or a book on tape.

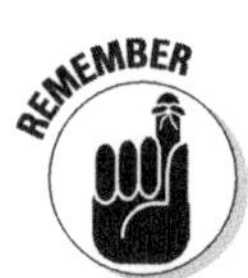

  Stay safe! If a machine requires your full concentration (an elliptical trainer is one example), don't watch a TV show while working out and risk injuring yourself.

- **You can be much more aware of — and control — your speed.** Ultimately, however, you want to monitor your workouts not by the number on the machine display but by your perceived rate of exertion (see Chapter 3).
- **If your machine is in your home (as opposed to a gym), you have an ultimately convenient workout.** No messing with frustrating traffic — all you have to do is stroll on down to the basement or some other room.

  Don't use a dark, dank basement for your exercise space. Instead, choose a cheerful and easily accessible space. If your basement is dark and musty and it's all you have available, spruce it up with lots of light, carpeting, and a TV or CD player.

- **If you're using the machines at a gym, you have a great variety of machines to choose from;** in fact, you can use a different machine every day. Gyms may have also have weight machine stations and other types of machines set up for circuit training (see Chapter 17).

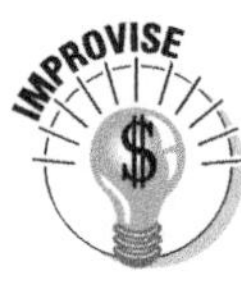

  If you shop around and have enough space, you can set up a minigym in your own home. For example, if you buy a used indoor bike and rowing machine through your local classified ads (see the "Saving money on exercise equipment" sidebar for information), buy an elliptical trainer on sale at your local sporting goods store, and use resistance bands and hand weights for weight training (see Chapter 11), you may be able to set up your own cross-training minigym for around $400, which is what some gym memberships cost. For another $300 to $400, you can also add a treadmill.

Saving money on exercise equipment

If you buy a new piece of equipment from a shop that specializes in exercise equipment, you'll probably get great service during and after you hand over your credit card. You may also pass out when you actually see the receipt. Exercise equipment can be very expensive, so take note of some ways to save money:

- **Buy through the want ads.** The sad truth is that people like the thought of working out and getting fit a whole lot more than they like working out. For this reason, people buy a lot of exercise equipment that they either never use or use only for a few days before they abandon it. But someone else's decision to abandon a piece of exercise equipment can be a tremendous cost benefit to you. Scan the want ads every day, and plan to spend from 25 to 75 percent of retail costs, depending on how much the item has been used. Remember to always try before you buy — a machine that sounds great in an ad may not be in great working order.
- **Ask your local gym, YMCA, community center, or local college** how often it replaces its equipment and whether it sells old machines to the public. The equipment at these facilities tends to be the sturdiest and most expensive equipment available — the best of the best — and even if they've been used for years, they still have plenty of life left in them.
- **Consider going to garage sales and auctions,** where you may see machines that cost only 10 or 20 percent of what new ones cost. If you choose either option, however, insist on trying out the equipment before you make an offer.

  Warning: Avoid buying exercise equipment over the Internet: You'll pay so much in shipping costs that you won't save money.
- **Ask friends and relatives.** You don't want to spend $300 on an elliptical trainer, and then discover that your sister-in-law has one she never uses.
- **Check discount stores.** Costco, Sam's Club, and other discount stores sometimes carry limited quantities of exercise equipment at substantial savings. Stay on your toes and check back often, because they may not have any exercise equipment at all, and then have a few dozen rowing machines that sell out fast. As always, try before you buy.

Remember: If you buy used equipment, first check the U.S. government's Web site at `www.recall.gov` (click Consumer Products, and then select Product Search to search by product type or Product Description Search to search by keyword) to obtain a list of equipment that has been recalled. Print out the list and take it with you so that you can easily identify potentially dangerous equipment. Also, for all used equipment, choose a machine that has an owner's manual over one that doesn't. Sometimes, the only way to get the right parts and accessories is by calling a number that appears only in the owner's manual.

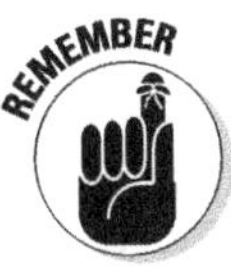

Before buying any piece of exercise equipment, put it to use. Don't buy any equipment that you can't try first, even if the salespeople tell you that they can't bring the display unit down from a platform or take it out of the box. If that happens, go to another store. Be sure to wear workout clothes when you go to look at any machine and spend at least five minutes working out, just to see what kinks are in the equipment.

The cons

Indoor machines do, admittedly, have a few disadvantages. The chief complaint is that you lose the scenery that makes the time go by so fast while working out outdoors. You may find that, while exercising outdoors, 10 or 15 minutes goes by without you even thinking about the time. Indoors, that number may drop to 2 or 3 minutes. Other drawbacks, especially if you keep an exercise machine in your home, include the following:

- **Exercise machines are expensive to buy.** Although you can always buy used machines and look for sales, buying high-quality, long-lasting, easy-to-maintain equipment and the extended warranties to cover future problems can break even the most liberal budget. One alternative is to look for inexpensive equipment and buy new every year or two. If, for example, a low-cost stair-stepper with a one-year warranty costs $120, while the top-of-the line stepper with a three-year warranty runs $450, you can afford to buy three lower-quality stair-steppers (a new one every year) for less than one high-quality stepper.

  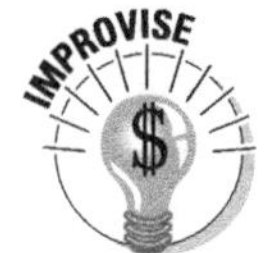

  If you can't afford to buy exercise equipment or join a gym, check out Chapter 11, which shares several low-cost ways to build strength, and Chapter 12, which discusses perhaps the cheapest of all activities: walking.

- **Although most exercise equipment is simple to maintain, you're responsible for some maintenance.** At just the basic level, you need to make sure your equipment is well dusted to keep dirt, dust, and pet hair from affecting the lubrication of parts. You also need to keep equipment away from extreme heat and out of any area that may leak water (such as a basement). You may even need to grease or lubricate some equipment every year — or have a professional do it for you. Have the salesperson or technician where you purchase the equipment run you through basic maintenance before you take your equipment home.

- **Exercise machines take up space,** so unless you have a lot of extra space in your house, you may be stubbing your toe on it throughout the rest of your day. Some machines fold up when not in use, however, so you can store them in a closet or other out-of-the-way area. If you choose a fold-up model, be sure that you can fold and unfold the machine on your own, or you'll be stuck asking for help before and after every workout.

- **You may waste your money.** As evidenced by the high number of exercise machines listed for dirt-cheap prices in classified ads, having a machine in your home doesn't necessarily mean that you'll use it. Although an at-home exercise machine is convenient, if you're not motivated to use it, the machine may end up being only a convenient place to hang your laundry.

- **If you keep only one machine at home, you may get bored with that one form of exercise.** If you add variety by occasionally switching to another activity that doesn't require a machine or by purchasing more than one machine, you'll be less likely to succumb to exercise boredom.

If you decide to join a gym in order to use the machines there, keep in mind that several other people may have the intention of using the same machine at the same time, which means that you have to wait in line. Before buying a membership, stop by the gym on a few different days at the exact time you plan to work out, just to see how many people are waiting to use the machines that interest you.

Weightlifting: We Want to Pump You Up!

Working out on a weight machine (sometimes called a *home gym*) won't make you develop bulky muscles, but it will tone and strengthen muscles all over your body. You need toned muscles to carry your baby around after he's born —after all, the average newborn weighs eight pounds when born and doubles his weight by six months. And you'll be lifting and carrying your baby throughout every day of his young life. No doubt about it: You need a strong upper body!

Weight machines like the one shown in this section's figures work only the arms. Other machines also have leg attachments that allow you to lift with your leg muscles, but most women get a lot of lower body work with other forms of exercise (walking, cycling, doing aerobics, stair-stepping, and so on) and not much upper body work (unless they take up swimming or rowing), so you want to concentrate on strengthening those upper body muscles, which will prepare you for lifting and carrying your baby.

Weight machines come in two varieties:

- **Machines that use *free weights*,** which are disks of varying weight that you attach to the machine. You adjust the weight you're lifting by adding to or taking off weighted disks from the machine. Free-weight machines can be dangerous, because you have to lift the weighted disks off of the floor or a table and attach them to the machine. Also, if you *bench press* (lay a bar with these weighted disks across your chest and lift the bar up and down), the weights can fall on you.
- **Machines that have fixed weights** and may have the brand names Universal, Nautilus, and Cybex, to name a few. On these machines, the weights are permanently affixed to or even stored inside the machines, and you adjust the weight by turning a dial or sliding a key into the weight level that you want to lift. Fixed-weight machines are very safe, but they're also quite expensive. Chances are that the only way to afford these weight machines is by joining a gym.

Whether you're buying your own machine (and you can find some pretty cheaply — as little as $60 for free-weight machines; see the sidebar, "Saving money on exercise equipment") or deciding to use one at a gym, make sure that all the weights are adjustable in small increments and that the lowest weight isn't too heavy for you. Also look for lots of padding anywhere your body touches the machine.

In this section, you get to see a few weight-machine exercises in action, but we're only giving you a taste, to help you see whether weightlifting is an activity you want to pursue. For excellent information about taking up weightlifting, which may be very useful if you want to expand your weight training after you deliver, get a copy of *Weight Training For Dummies,* 2nd Edition, by Liz Neporent and Suzanne Schlosberg (Wiley). And check out Chapter 11 in this book for additional exercises that build strength by using a resistance band or handheld weights, which are less expensive than a home gym. Most women don't need any fancy weight equipment to improve strength — even soup cans do the trick.

A few weightlifting pointers

To get started on the right foot (or arm, or whatever), you want to make sure that you're being safe and getting the most out of your workout. The info in this section helps you do just that.

Whenever you weight train, keep the following tips in mind:

- **Always warm up before you start lifting.** Take a short walk, work out on a stationary bike, or do any other activity that elevates your heart rate. You want to feel a little sweaty before you begin your workout. Afterward, always stretch, using Chapter 8 as your guide.
- **Start with low weights.** Don't try to set any Miss Universe records; instead, use the lowest weight the first time you lift, and increase the weight until you find one that allows you to do 10 to 12 repetitions (reps) without discomfort, but is also challenging to lift by the last few reps. If you feel fatigued after the first few reps, you're lifting too much weight. As you increase your fitness, you can increase the weight when you feel that you're no longer being challenged, or you can add another set of 10 to 12 reps. Just be sure to progress slowly and use caution.
- **Lift deliberately.** You build strength by lifting weights, not by holding them, so concentrate on the lifting portion and do so carefully and deliberately. You don't have to lift excruciatingly slowly, as some people

recommend. Just move carefully through each lift of the weights, using a count of 3 to lift and a count of 3 to return to your starting position.

- **Never hold your breath as you lift weights.** Instead, exhale as you lift and inhale as you slowly return the weights to your starting position. *Breathing correctly is extremely important.* If you hold your breath and bear down as you lift, you can increase your blood pressure and put stress on your abdominal wall.
- **Avoid exercises that involve lying on your back, holding your breath, or using a tremendous amount of effort during the exercise.** Maintain an upright or semiupright (inclined) position during all exercises.
- **When lifting, use good form.** To check your form, follow instructions in a book, watch a video, or ask the advice of a trainer at your gym. Poor form can lead to injuries.
- **Most experts recommend weightlifting only every other day, because your muscles need at least 24 hours of rest between weight-training bouts to recover.** If you weightlift too much, too fast, and/or too often, you risk getting injured. Because weightlifting usually isn't a cardiovascular workout, alternate weightlifting with walking, cycling, or swimming to give you a total-body workout routine.

Some simple exercises

The exercises in this section get you started with a basic weightlifting routine. For each exercise, build up to 10 to 12 repetitions. After you can do one set of 10 to 12 without fatigue, build to 2 sets of 10 to 12 repetitions.

Seated bench press

The seated bench press exercise works the *bicep* muscles, which are on the inside of your upper arm.

1. **Take hold of both handgrips and pull them back toward your chest so that your elbows are fully bent. Keep your back pressed against the backrest and the backs of your thighs pressed down on the seat. See Figure 16-1a.**
2. **Without moving your back or thighs, slowly press outward until your arms are almost fully extended, as shown in Figure 16-1b.**
3. **Slowly pull back to your starting position and repeat.**

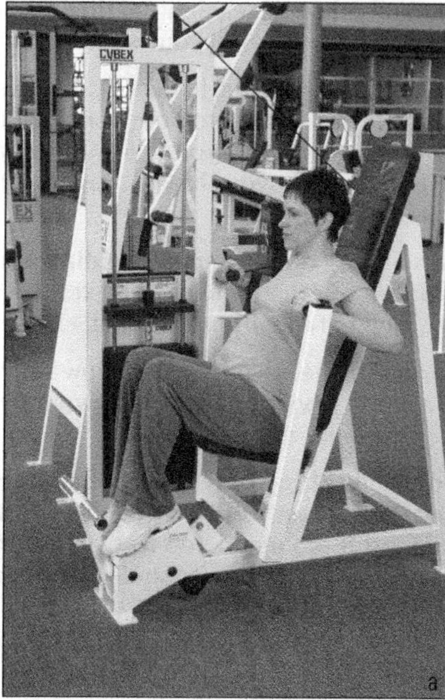

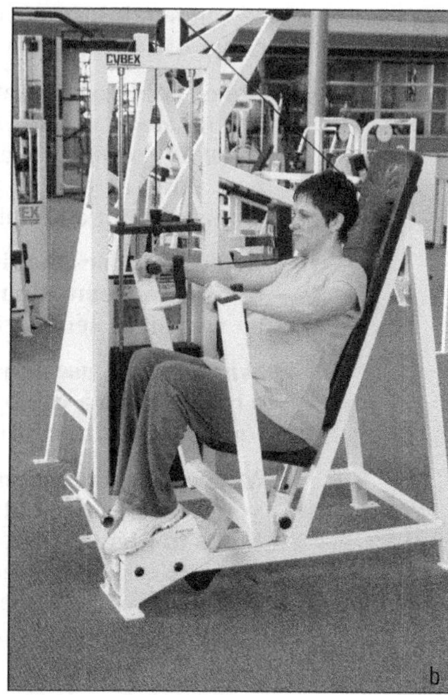

Figure 16-1: Work your biceps with the seated bench press.

Bicep curl

Bicep curls are another way to work the biceps.

1. **Grasp the handgrips with both hands and extend your arms almost completely. Keep your back pressed against the backrest and the backs of your thighs pressed down on the seat. See Figure 16-2a.**
2. **Slowly curl the weight toward you by pulling your hands toward your chest until your elbow is completely bent (refer to Figure 16-2b). Keep your back pressed against the backrest.**
3. **Slowly return your arms to the fully extended position and repeat.**

Shoulder press

Shoulder presses work many of the muscles in your upper body, including your *triceps* (the muscles on the back of your upper arms), shoulders, upper back muscles, and chest muscles.

1. **Grasp the handgrips with both hands and pull the weight toward your shoulders so that your elbows are fully bent. Keep your back pressed against the backrest and the backs of your thighs pressed down on the seat. See Figure 16-3a.**

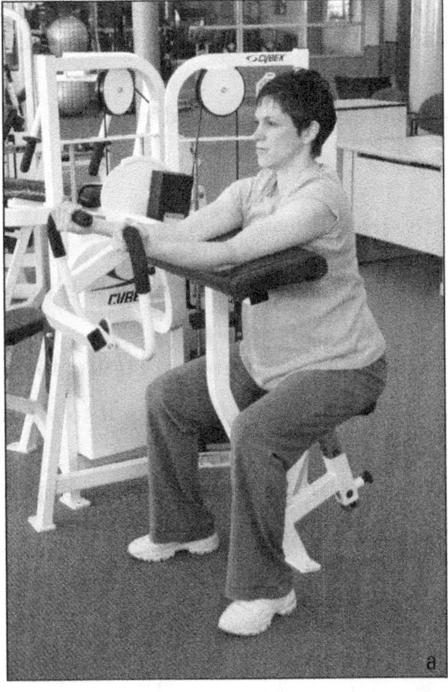

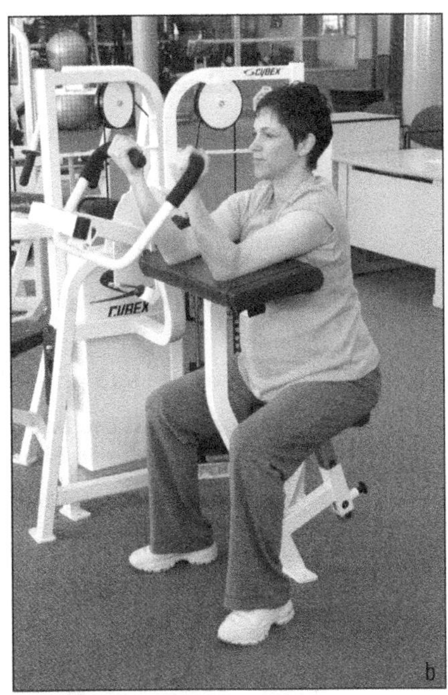

Figure 16-2: Get those biceps ready for lots of baby lifting!

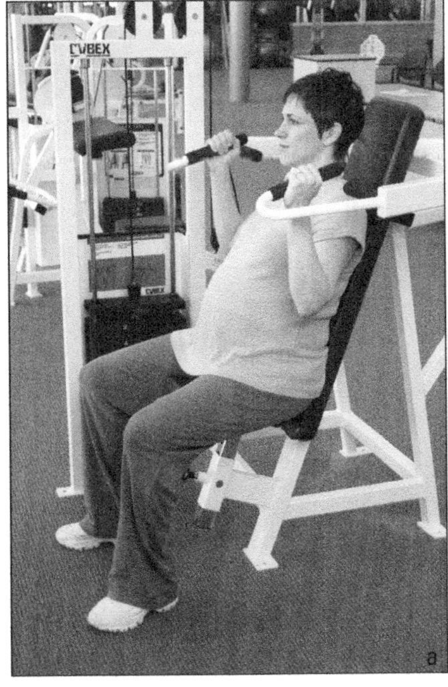

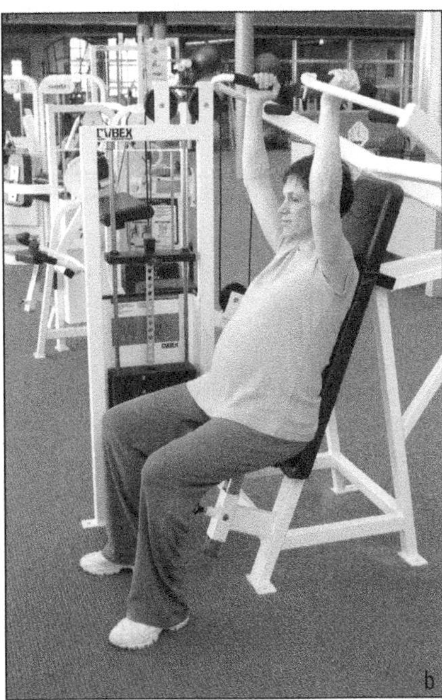

Figure 16-3: Work several upper-body muscles at once with the shoulder press.

2. **Slowly push your arms straight up until they're almost fully extended, as shown in Figure 16-3b. Your back should still be snug against the backrest.**
3. **Slowly pull down to your starting position and repeat.**

Lat pull

Lat pulls are an excellent way to strengthen your triceps.

1. **Sit on the seat at the lat-pull station and plant both feet firmly on the floor.**
2. **Reach up and grasp the handgrips, as shown in Figure 16-4a.**
3. **Slowly pull the bar down in front of you, bringing it to about chest height. Refer to Figure 16-4b.**
4. **Slowly allow the bar to return to its starting position. Repeat.**

   A lat-pull bar tends to snap back a little as you return it to its starting position. Be sure to let the bar up slowly.

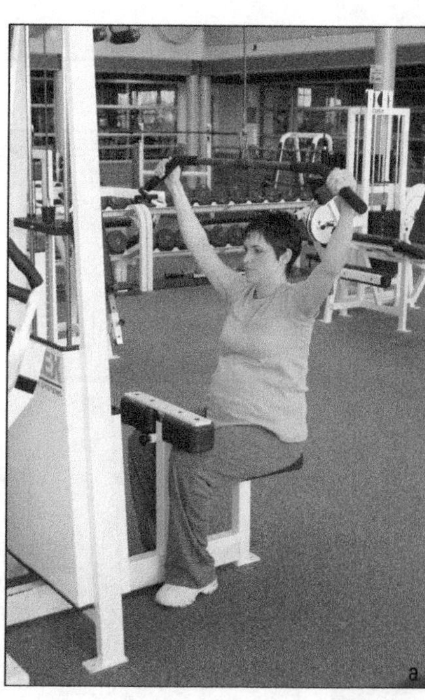

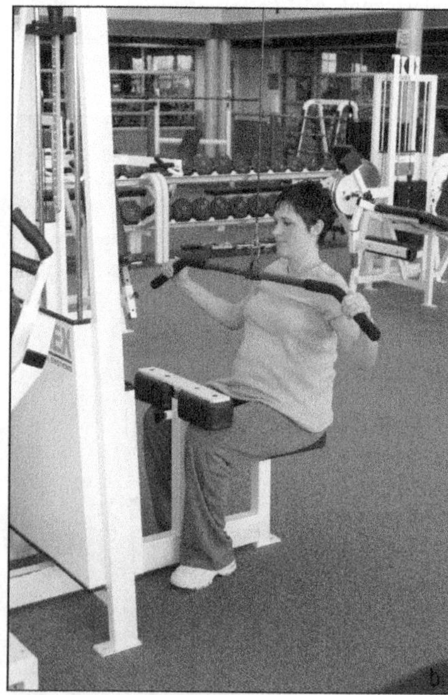

Figure 16-4: Tone troublesome triceps with the lat pull (and then say that three times fast).

Tricep extension

The following exercise also works the triceps.

1. **With your hands near your ears and your elbows resting on the pad, grasp the handgrips with both hands, as shown in Figure 16-5a.**
2. **Keeping your back pressed against the backrest and the backs of your thighs pressed down on the seat, slowly extend your arms forward until they're almost fully extended (refer to Figure 16-5b).**
3. **Slowly return your arms to the starting position and repeat.**

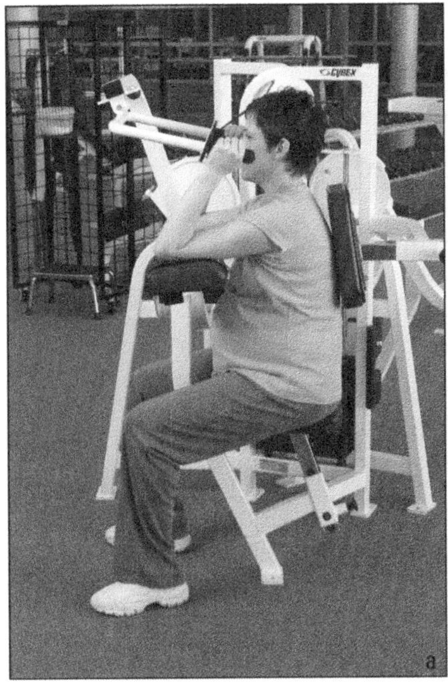
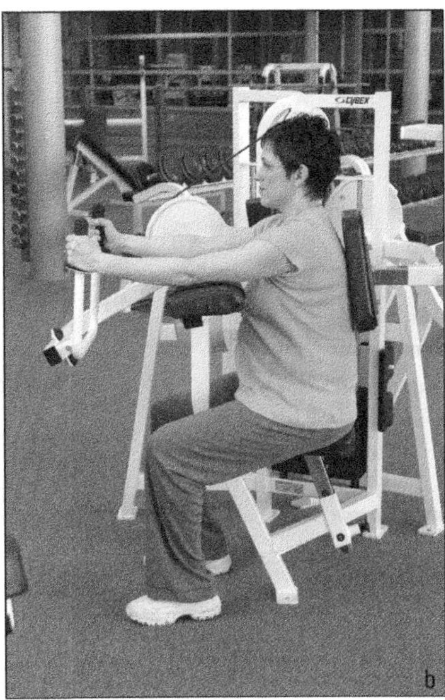

Figure 16-5: The tricep extension works — you guessed it — your triceps.

Stair-Stepping to Heaven

A *stair-stepper,* also called a *stair-climber,* is a machine that mimics climbing stairs, but instead of going up and down the stairs, you stay in one place, as shown in Figure 16-6. A stair-stepper works many of the muscles in the lower body, especially your butt, which makes it a great cross-training workout with an arm-intensive workout, such as swimming, tennis, or weightlifting. You can also buy a stair-stepper that has an arm attachment, although you have to concentrate pretty hard to coordinate your steps and the movement of the arm attachment.

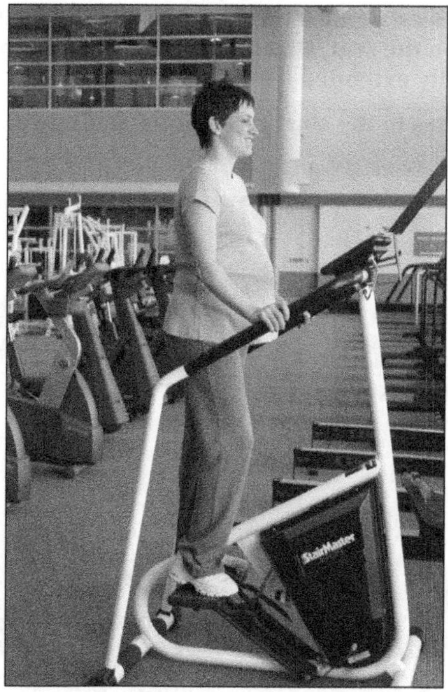

Figure 16-6: A stairway going nowhere.

Start stair-stepping slowly, because this activity can offer an intensive, rigorous workout. Work out only to a 12 or 14 perceived rate of exertion, which we discuss in Chapter 3. Also, keep the following tips in mind:

- **Keep the resistance low (if your stepper has a resistance setting) and step quickly.** As with most aerobic workouts, you get a better workout when you have *quick turnover* — taking small, quick steps with low resistance.
- **Try to keep your feet flat while stepping.** Staying on your toes means that your calves will get a better workout than the other muscles in your lower body, and you want a total-body workout, not a calf-intensive one. Staying on your toes may also bring on shin splints, which can be quite uncomfortable.

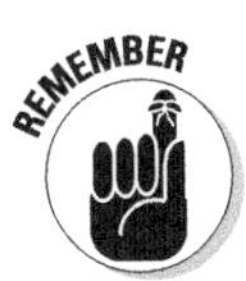

- **Hang on tightly to the handrails and be sure that the machine has come to a complete stop before you get off the steps.**

  If you're buying a stair-stepper, look for padded handrails that are at a comfortable height.

- **If you aren't using an arm attachment, consider watching TV while stepping.** The design of the machine makes watching a TV at eye level pretty comfortable and generally safe.

Elliptical Trainers: Combining Cycling, Skiing, and a Whole Bunch of Other Stuff

Elliptical trainers are so called because the motion of your legs follows the shape of an *ellipse,* which is a flattened circle. A recent addition to the list of standard exercise equipment, elliptical machines have become popular because they're fun and give you a great workout. You especially tone your quadriceps (your thigh muscles), but all your lower-body muscles benefit. In addition, because nearly all elliptical trainers come with arm attachments, you can get an excellent upper-body workout at the same time.

Think of an elliptical trainer as a combination of running, stair-stepping, cross-country skiing, and cycling (see Figure 16-7). You can adjust the resistance on the machine: *Low resistance* means that you can move your feet easier; *high resistance* means that the trainer is harder to move. No matter what resistance you choose, you can also increase the intensity of your workout by increasing the speed at which you move your feet back and forth. And you tend to get a better cardiovascular workout by moving your feet quickly on low resistance than moving more slowly on high resistance. By keeping your feet flat on the pedals, you get a very low-impact but extremely effective workout.

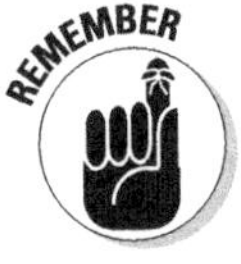

The concentration that an elliptical trainer requires to properly move your feet and work the arm attachment at the same time is mind-boggling. You may find, especially as your speed increases, that you have to concentrate completely on just getting your feet and hands to go the right way, although the motion does become more comfortable with time. For this reason, we don't recommend watching the morning news while using an elliptical trainer!

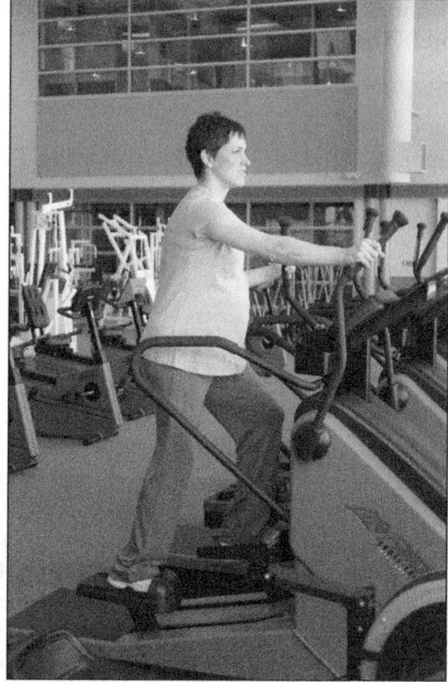

Figure 16-7: Going around and around on an elliptical trainer.

Skiing, Cross-Country Style

If you examine a list of the most demanding exercises or a rundown of the activities that burn the most calories, cross-country skiing is always among the top two or three. Thankfully, you don't have to brave snowy, windy trails to get the benefits of a cross-country ski workout, because indoor ski machines bring the outdoors into your home. In an almost no-impact activity, you get a total workout — legs, butt, arms, shoulders, low back, you name it! And the workout is very cardiovascularly intensive (meaning, it gets your heart pumping!).

The idea is pretty simple: The machine simulates outdoor cross-country skiing, so you glide on a wooden or metal frame that makes you feel like you're moving skis back and forth. Meanwhile, you hang onto attachments or rails that simulate ski poles. Most machines allow you to control the resistance: Less resistance means that you can move your legs faster and easier; higher resistance means that your feet are harder to push. By moving your legs fast on low resistance, you make this already difficult workout even harder and more effective!

Cross-country skiing outdoors: What you need to succeed

If you work out on a cross-country ski machine while you're pregnant and live in a cold winter climate, you may want to try outdoor cross-country skiing after you deliver. (Unless you've been skiing outdoors and your healthcare provider approves, don't ski outdoors while pregnant. The risk of falling is too great, and you don't want to mess with the chances of being stuck in a remote area in cold weather when you go into labor or otherwise need medical attention.)

To make the switch from skiing indoors to out, you need the right equipment: skis, poles, boots, *bindings* (the device that attaches your boots to your skis), and outdoor workout gear (see Chapter 7). You may also need a lesson or two to master the technique, which is a tad more difficult than using an indoor ski machine. Finally, you need *groomed trails,* which means that some wonderful person has used a machine to create a two-track trail for you to follow as you ski. Skiing on an ungroomed trail is possible, but it's so difficult that you may never ski again.

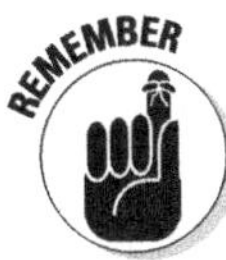

Some women have found cross-country ski machines to be just too uncomfortable to use during pregnancy. The intensity that these machines require can be too demanding. In addition, the way the front supports of the machines are designed and the motion that you use during the exercise can put too much pressure on the abdomen. Before buying a machine, which can run from $450 to over $1,000, try one out first.

Cross-country ski machines can be tough to find. Most gyms don't carry them, and only a few specialty fitness stores have even one model for sale. But people's garages and basements are filled with barely used models (the machine is harder to use than people think, which is why so many people abandon them), so watch the classified ads in your area. Look for the NordicTrack brand name; it was the inventor of the indoor cross-country ski machine and still makes models that last a lifetime.

Row, Row, Row Your Boat

We save rowing machines (or *rowers*) for the last section in this chapter because — and we want to be on record for telling you this — rowing is *not* easy, so you want to start with a short duration (just a few minutes) and build up very slowly. Rowing nearly always ranks at the top of the most-calorie-burning exercises. In return for taking up rowing, however, you can develop amazing fitness in your arms and shoulders, certainly, but also in your butt, back, *quads* (the front of your thighs), and abdominal muscles. Rowing is probably the best total-body workout you'll ever find and is basically no-impact because you glide along rails on the machine.

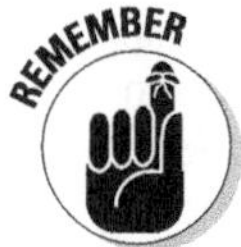

Some women find that using a rowing machine during pregnancy causes back soreness, which is usually due to using improper technique and may also be from having weakened abdominal and back muscles. If you notice back discomfort, avoid extending too far back as you pull, which puts stress on your low back. Also cut back on your duration until your back pain subsides. If back pain or discomfort continues, stop rowing and find another form of exercise.

To work out on a rower, you do the following:

1. **Strap your feet into the stirrups near the front of the machine.**
2. **Beginning with your seat as far forward as possible (see Figure 16-8a), push yourself back until your arms and legs are fully extended.**
3. **When your seat goes as far back as possible, pull yourself forward, using both your arms and legs, as Figure 16-8b shows.**

   Start with a low number of strokes per minute and build up over time (a *stroke* is one complete forward and backward motion). If your rower allows you to increase or decrease the resistance, initially use the very lowest resistance available and row as quickly as you can.

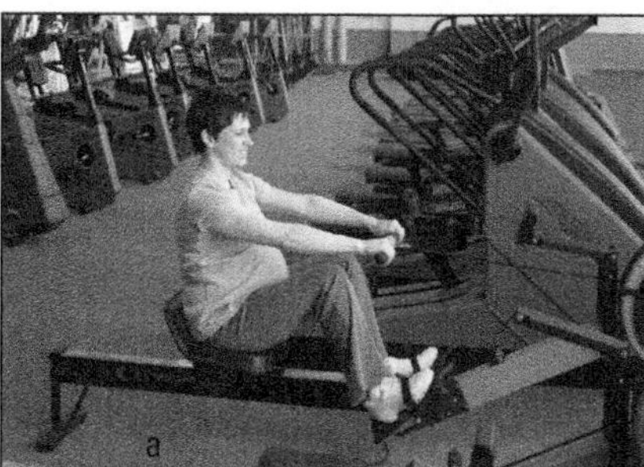

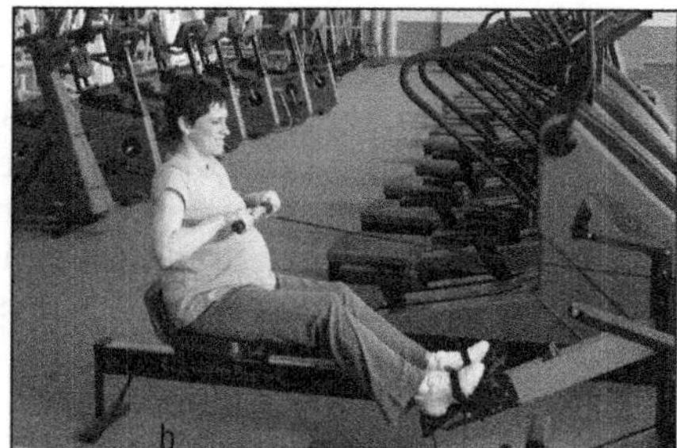

Figure 16-8: Pushing yourself back and pulling yourself forward.

Rowing machines are available at many gyms, and you can purchase one for your home. They start at about $500 and go up from there, but if you maintain them as spelled out in the owner's manual, you can own one machine for life. Look for a smooth, comfortable seat, because that's where you'll spend all your time on a rowing machine. Although the seats on older rowers are just flat, padded cushions, newer rowing machines come with comfortable backs on the seats. If you're tall, also make sure that the machine is long enough for you — some are so short that you can't stretch out fully.

Chapter 17

Mixing It Up: Combining Different Exercise Routines

In This Chapter

- Getting a feel for how cross-training works
- Finding great reasons to cross-train
- Working cross-training into your exercise routine

Cross-training is a pretty simple concept: You use more than one activity, for example, walking and weightlifting, to get fit and stay in shape. Putting cross-training into practice can also be pretty easy, after you understand the basics. For example, do you do two different activities, alternating each one on opposite days, or do you do six different activities, one for each of your workout days during the week? Or do you do two or three different activities on *one* day, and do the same workout the next day? The answer is "yes," because cross-training takes a number of forms. This chapter helps you understand the various ways that you can cross-train and also explains why cross-training invigorates your workouts, from alleviating boredom to reducing your risk of injury.

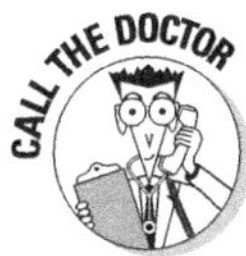

As with all exercise during your pregnancy, when cross-training, you need to monitor your body — not just during a workout, but until the next workout, too. Specifically, keep track of the following:

- Whether your baby is growing normally
- Whether you're gaining weight normally
- Overall, whether you feel good or bad

If your baby is growing normally, you're gaining weight the way you should, and you feel good throughout the day, your cross-training activities are working for you. But if you stop gaining weight, you no longer feel good, or your baby stops growing normally, you and your healthcare provider need to review your cross-training routine.

Finding Great Reasons to Begin Cross-Training

If you're just getting comfortable regularly working out with one activity, the thought of adding one or more other activities to your workout routine may be overwhelming. If so, stop reading right here and focus on your one chosen activity. You're doing so much good for you and your baby by incorporating that one activity into your daily routine, you don't need to complicate your life with cross-training.

However, if you've ever experienced any of the following, cross-training may be right for you:

- You're interested in another workout activity and aren't sure how to incorporate it into your current training routine.
- After several weeks or months of exercise with your chosen activity, you don't think it's getting certain areas of your body as fit as you want — think tank-top-exposing arm muscles or great calves.
- Your workouts aren't as challenging as they were a few months ago (and we understand that this situation is unlikely, given your growing baby and the challenges that come with continuing to exercise into your second and third trimesters).
- You're getting bored and/or unmotivated to work out.

If any of these situations apply to you, cross-training may be able to help you add another activity that interests or challenges you, exercise more of your body, and make your workout routine less boring. The following sections tell you how cross-training gives you these benefits.

Keeping boredom at bay and staying motivated

A popular reason to cross-train is that you get to test drive — and even get good at — more than one activity. Suppose you've been walking six days per week for the last few weeks or months. During that time, you've built up your endurance by walking a little farther during some of your workouts, and you've found that, in spite of your growing abdomen, you're walking faster than you were when you started. Your baby is growing normally, you feel great, and you like the way the muscles in your legs are getting more defined. However, you keep seeing ads on TV for the Gazelle elliptical trainers, and it looks like they're a lot of fun — and with winter coming on, having a machine to use indoors on really cold days is beneficial. In addition, you've overheard people talking about weight training, and after reading Chapter 11, you're thinking that using some light hand weights isn't a bad idea. But you don't want to give up walking.

Your workout routine doesn't have to be an either-or proposition, such that you work out *either* by walking *or* by using an elliptical trainer *or* by lifting hand weights. By cross-training, you can try a variety of activities and incorporate the ones you like best into your routine.

As you try additional activities, you find that a tremendous benefit of cross-training is that exercise becomes much more fun and interesting. Fun? Sure! Working out is always supposed to be fun, and altering your routine tends to keep it that way. Consider what recess would've been like if, every day, you jumped rope with the same friends — no hopscotch, no monkey bars, no swings, no slide, no kickball, no Red Rover — just jump-rope. After a while, jumping rope may have become as appealing as eating lima beans or cleaning the toilet, instead of being the enjoyable activity it was meant to be. Cross-training expands recess to include all the fun activities at hand, and it keeps you from getting bored in the process. And when you're having fun doing interesting activities, you're motivated to go at it again the next day.

Getting optimum fitness results

Although most exercises work several of the muscles in the body, they tend to leave other parts of the body untouched. For example, running works the arms, shoulders, legs, and buttocks, but tends not to do much for your abdomen. Like running, walking works the legs and butt, but it doesn't work the arms as well as other exercises can. Swimming works the arms and shoulders intensely, but it doesn't work the legs, abdomen, and back as much. Cycling can have an amazing benefit on your legs, butt, and back, but it doesn't do as much for your arms and abdomen. The answer to this partial-body workout conundrum is to cross-train with two or more activities, which allows you to work a variety of muscles throughout your body.

In the same way, some workouts raise your heart rate, but others don't. *Cardiovascular workouts* raise your heart rate, thus getting your heart in good shape. Generally, a good cardiovascular workout is one that keeps your heart rate elevated constantly (without breaks) for 15 minutes or longer (see Chapter 5); examples include running, walking, cycling, swimming, aerobics, some types of yoga, cross-country skiing, rowing, using an elliptical machine, stair-stepping, and other activities. Although cardiovascular workouts are excellent for improving your overall health and fitness and they burn plenty of calories (see Chapter 10), they may not always tone your arms and legs as much as you want them to. We're not talking about developing Miss Universe–type muscles, but many people turn to exercise to get well-toned muscles, and that's where adding weightlifting (see Chapters 11 and 16), resistance-band and exercise-ball training (see Chapter 11), and yoga (see Chapter 14) can make a difference in your overall fitness level.

So when you combine a couple of cardiovascular activities that work out different muscles and also do one or two days per week of strength training, you're getting it all: great heart workouts that use most of the muscles in your body combined with strength work that tones and sculpts.

Working a variety of muscles in the body has the added benefit of reducing your risk of injury. When you repeatedly work only certain muscles, the balance between two muscles that work together (such as the abdomen and back, front of leg and back of leg, front of arm and back of arm) gets off kilter because one group becomes stronger than the other, and this imbalance is one of the major causes of athletic injuries. The same is true of joints and *ligaments* and *tendons* (the tissue that joins muscle to muscle and muscle to bone), so when you work all your joints, ligaments, and tendons, you reduce the risk of injuring those areas. When you do a variety of activities that work a variety of muscles, joints, ligaments, and tendons throughout your body, you substantially reduce your risk of injury. Also, the repetitive stress on joints and muscles from doing only one activity can increase your risk of injury and fatigue.

Incorporating Cross-Training into Your Routine

You won't find a national cross-training association that sets rules for cross-training and decides exactly how to incorporate various activities into your routine. Instead, cross-training is a loose idea that you can apply to your own exercise routine however you see fit.

People tend to cross-train in one of four ways, which we describe in the following sections. Although you don't need to follow any of these four methods of cross-training, we present them to give you an idea of how to design a cross-training routine that works for you. The first two are the most common ways to cross-train, but they're also the most serious (and, in our opinion, least fun) ways. We included them anyway for all you fitness buffs out there. If you're not a fitness buff and aren't interested in anything but fun, however, skip the next two sections and concentrate on the last two in this chapter.

Targeting different muscle groups

The most common way to cross-train is to do one activity that targets a particular set (or group) of muscles one day, and the next day, do an activity that targets a different muscle group. The idea is to get a whole-body workout and use a variety of muscles by engaging in two or more very different activities, each one working different muscles.

So, one workout may focus on arms (weightlifting, swimming, rowing, tennis), but the next workout focuses on legs (walking, cycling, stair-stepping), and so on.

Figuring out which workout uses which muscles doesn't have to be rocket science. Simply use your common sense and think about how various muscles feel during and after a workout. Common sense tells you that, for example, swimming works your arms and shoulders more than it works your legs, because your arms and shoulders are powering you forward as you swim laps. Although swimming does work your legs, it places far more emphasis on your upper body than on your lower body. In addition, if your aerobics workout tends to fatigue your arms, shoulders, and back but doesn't feel like it works your legs as much, it's probably an aerobics routine that focuses on the upper body (and not all aerobics workouts do — see Chapter 14) that you can balance with a more leg-intensive workout, like walking.

On the other hand, some people exercise the front (bicep) muscles of the arms one day and the back (tricep) muscles of the arms the next day. Or, the front (quadricep) muscles of the legs one day and the back (hamstring) muscles of the legs the next day. Same with the upper back and lower back. This approach to exercising each specific muscle group, however, requires a pretty detailed knowledge of both your body's muscle groups and the exercises that work those exact groups, so we don't recommend bothering to take a specific muscle approach unless a knowledgeable coach or personal trainer is supervising you.

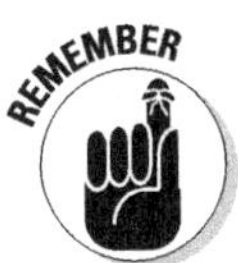

Some activities use different muscles groups in one activity, giving you a total-body workout without having to cross-train. For example, rowing uses the arms, back, buttocks, and legs all in one workout, as does cross-country skiing. So, if you're looking for a total-body workout, you don't necessarily have to cross-train to get it. Also, if you like a particular activity that doesn't necessarily use the entire body (for example, working out on an indoor bike doesn't usually involve exercising your arms), you may be able to alter the workout by adding another activity simultaneously, such as lifting light hand weights while cycling indoors. And to get the ultimate total-body workout when cross-training, try doing circuits, which we discuss in the "Mixing several activities in a workout: Circuit training" section at the end of this chapter.

If your ultimate goal (after you deliver a healthy baby and get through those first months of sleepless nights) is to get in shape for a particular event, such as a bike race or a marathon, cross-training by using different muscle groups each day generally *is not* a great way to train. Instead, if you want to compete, you need to train specifically for the activity in which you want to excel: In other words, you can't successfully run a marathon by doing most of your training on a bike or with an aerobics video! Cross-training by using different muscle groups gets you in great overall shape, but it usually doesn't prepare you to compete in one specific activity.

Using the same muscles through different activities

If you love one particular activity or are competitive in a sport, you can still cross-train by mimicking your one sport with similar activities. If bad weather keeps you from participating in your chosen sport (and that's usually the reason people take this cross-training approach), you may be able to find a substitute activity that uses those same muscles and keeps you in shape for your chosen sport. Here are some examples:

- If you're big on walking or hiking outdoors, in winter, you can switch to snowshoe walking, which is a slightly different, but similar enough activity. Throughout the long months of winter, you can continue to keep those walking muscles in shape so that, come spring, you can go back to your walking routine without skipping a beat.
- If you run or walk and don't have access to a treadmill and don't live in a snowy enough climate to snowshoe run in the winter, you can run in the pool (wearing a floatation vest) during the winter and switch back to running in the spring. More on pool running in Chapter 12.

  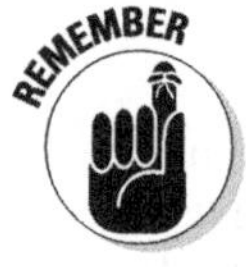

  Although pool running isn't identical to running on land — in pool running, you don't strike the ground with each step, you don't encounter any hills, and you breathe a very pure, humid air that's unlike the air outdoors — many world-class runners have trained in a pool while injured and have come back to race on the track or roads without skipping a beat.
- Cycling, speed skating, and rollerblading all use the same muscles. So, a speed skater can rollerblade in the summer, or a cyclist training in a harsh winter climate can switch to speed-skating in winter. Okay, not many recreational athletes have access to a world-class speed-skating facility, but we're just trying to make a point here that you can switch to very different activities and still maintain your high level of fitness in one activity.

Sometimes, the issue isn't weather; instead, you may want to stay fit for one activity, but you're getting bored training for that activity. Or, you may not be able to train at a particular sport because the pool isn't open before and after work or the reduced amount of daylight in winter makes going outside impossible with your schedule.

Whatever the reason for not wanting to or not being able to train in the activity you like best, here are some tips for finding similar activities:

- **Always consider the obvious indoor alternatives to outdoor sports.** You can walk on a treadmill at any time of day or night, and you use the exact same muscles as if you walked outside. An indoor bike works the same muscles as an outdoor bike does. Ditto with an indoor cross-country ski machine and an indoor rower.
- **Brainstorm activities that mimic your chosen sport.** Does a particular aerobics routine feel like your outdoor walking routine in terms of the muscles you're using? Can you do an activity in a pool, while wearing a floatation vest, that uses the same muscles as your sport?
- **After doing the alternative activity once or twice, notice whether you're sore in new places.** Are you sore in different muscles than those muscles you usually work? This soreness is a sign that the two activities really aren't working the same muscles. Try another activity and see whether you can more closely match the muscles you use.
- **Pay careful attention to how tired you feel and adjust your workouts accordingly.** Are you more fatigued or less fatigued than you normally are? If the two activities are very similar, you shouldn't see any difference in how tired you are after the activity. If you do see a difference, consider reducing the duration or intensity of your activity if you feel particularly tired during or after a workout (see Chapter 3).

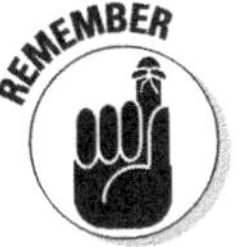

Keep in mind that an alternate activity may actually be harder (or easier) than your chosen activity. Suppose you're used to running, and during winter, you switch to snowshoe running, figuring the activities are similar enough. So, you try to snowshoe run at the same speed for the same length of time that you actually run, but you feel completely drained after your first snowshoe outing. The difference may be that snowshoe running — which requires you to move relatively heavy snowshoes through thick, damp snow with each step — is actually more difficult than running. By comparison, running in a pool, which doesn't offer any hills and doesn't require you to push off the ground with each step, feels easier than running on land, which means that you may be able to spend *more* time running in the pool and feel the same after the workout as if you ran less time on land.

Alternating activities without the muscle-group mumbo jumbo

Another way to cross-train is one that we like to advocate and that most people enjoy: Just do an activity every day, and don't worry about muscle groups at all. You may decide to do a different activity every day of the week, like this:

- **Monday:** Swim laps after work
- **Tuesday:** Power walk with co-workers at lunch
- **Wednesday:** Lift weights at home before breakfast
- **Thursday:** Day off
- **Friday:** Take a yoga class after work
- **Saturday:** Take an easy bike ride with a group of friends in late morning
- **Sunday:** Do an hour-long aerobics video in the afternoon

Or, you may want to do fewer activities and repeat them more often, like this:

- **Monday:** Swim laps after work
- **Tuesday:** Take an easy walk with co-workers at lunch
- **Wednesday:** Do an hour-long aerobics video early in the morning
- **Thursday:** Day off
- **Friday:** Swim laps after work
- **Saturday:** Take an easy walk with your family in late morning
- **Sunday:** Do an hour-long aerobics video in the afternoon

The idea behind alternating activities without any thought of which muscle groups you're using or not using is to think of exercise as fun activities that you do alone or with friends, at varying times of the day, and at varying levels of intensity (see Chapter 3). Exercise then becomes like recess: You look forward to it, do it every day (but take at least one day off each week while you're pregnant, just to give your body a break), find a new game to play each day, and have a great time doing it.

People who cross-train in this way almost never get bored with exercise, and they rarely think of what they do as "exercise"; instead, it's just a fun way to get outside or hang out with friends or have time to think. In addition, because the focus is on having fun and being active and not on doing one particular type of workout, conditions don't have to be perfect for you to exercise. If you want to swim but find that the pool is closed, go on a walk, instead. If you were going to walk at lunch but encounter a heavy rainstorm, forgo the walk and stop by an aerobics class after work.

Cross-training with randomly alternating activities can have a few disadvantages, but most people find these potential problems easy to overcome:

- Because you may not stick to any sort of a schedule (such as working out every morning at a gym or going to aerobics class every Monday, Wednesday, and Friday), you don't have the built-in support from the people who work out with you — those people you don't want to let down by not showing up. However, you're probably having so much fun exercising that getting motivated to work out isn't much of an issue.
- If you can change your planned activity at the drop of a hat (like deciding against walking in a rainstorm), you may also find that you can drop the activity altogether and not work out at all that day. Again, however, because exercise is really a fun playtime and not a chore, opting out is unlikely.
- You won't be able to compete in any one activity, because you aren't spending time training your body to do one activity very well. If you're the kind who likes to have a lot of fun, though, competing probably doesn't hold a strong attraction for you. Instead, you can walk or bike over to the local road race, cheer on the competitors, and walk or bike back home.

Mixing several activities in a workout: Circuit training

Lean in closely — we have a secret for you. We know of a fun, interesting way to get your body into great shape, and it isn't very complicated, expensive, or time consuming. Interested? Read on.

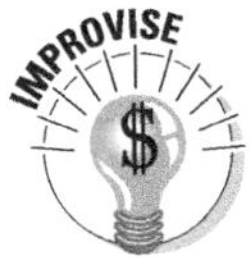

Circuit training (or just plain *circuits*) includes several exercises, set up at several *stations* (areas ready for you to work out), in between which you walk briskly or, if you're used to it, run. You can set up circuit stations in your own backyard, basement, garage, or other area, and at each station, you can do whatever exercises you choose — we suggest some here, but you can be creative!

Setting up stations

You need only the following inexpensive equipment, but you can improvise with the common household items you find in parentheses:

- **Station #1:** A resistance band (any stretchy, elastic fabric that also offers some resistance) and a pair of two-pound or three-pound weights (a pair of half-gallon or smaller orange juice or milk jugs filled partway with water, flour, or sand — weigh them on your bathroom scale to be sure of the weight; also look for sales on hand weights, which often include a buy-one-get-one-free offer)

- **Station #2:** An exercise mat (one or two thick towels)
- **Station #3:** A sturdy chair or bench — not a folding chair (borrow one from your dining room); you can also use a resistance ball, discussed in Chapter 11
- **Station #4:** A plastic step of varying height — we mean a "step" as in step aerobics (or the bottom step of a stairway), something that's roughly four to six inches high.
- **Station #5:** A pair of five-pound or eight-pound weights (a pair of gallon or larger orange juice or milk jugs filled all or partway with water, flour, or sand — weigh them on your bathroom scale to be sure of the weight)

Place these items around the room or other area in which you'll be working out, putting the mat anywhere from 10 feet to 20 yards from the light weights, putting the light weights 10 feet to 20 yards from the chair, and so on. Setting up the stations in a circle works well, but if you don't have space for a circle, you can situate the stations more randomly.

If you have other equipment that you can use as a station, including a weight bench, a pull-up bar, or a rowing machine, include those pieces, as well. And after you deliver your baby, consider adding a jump-rope station, because jumping rope is an excellent tool for getting fit but usually is too intense and involves too much movement when you're pregnant.

At each of these stations, choose exercises that use what you have there. Here are some suggestions, all detailed in Chapter 11:

- **Station #1 (band and lighter weights):** Triceps strengthener, chest pull, upright row, lat pull
- **Station #2 (exercise mat):** Core stabilization, Sahrmann exercises, diaphragmatic breathing, transverse abdominis raise, oblique exercises, pelvic rock, side-lying abdominals
- **Station #3 (chair):** Chair dips, pelvic tilt, lunge, squat, dip, plie, hip abductor strengthener, hip flexor strengthener, gluteals strengthener
- **Station #4 (step):** Single-leg squats, toe raises, step-ups
- **Station #5 (heavier weights):** Biceps curls, one-arm row, shrugs

You can pick and choose which exercises you want to do or do them all, for example:

- Triceps strengthener (at Station #1)
- Core stabilization (at Station #2)
- Chair dips (at Station #3)
- Single-leg squats (at Station #4)

- Biceps curls (at Station #5)
- Chest pull (at Station #1)
- Sahrmann exercises (at Station #2)
- And so on. . . .

Try to separate stations that use similar muscles so that you give those muscles a rest in between. For example, try to do an exercise for your legs, then arms, then your back, then legs again, then arms, and so on.

After you decide which exercises you're going to do at each station, place a sheet of paper at each station that lists, in order, the one, two, three, or more exercises that you're doing there. That way, you won't forget which exercise you're supposed to be doing at each station.

Timing yourself

You're going to need some sort of a timer that can time for 20 to 45 seconds (many timers can do only increments of one minute, so watch for this) and can keep repeating that countdown over and over. The timers on most sports watches count down 20 seconds, but then they stop. You need a timer that can count down 20 seconds, beep, count down 20 seconds again, beep, and so on. Radio Shack carries a small compass/watch/timer that has this countdown and repeat function; it sells for about $20.

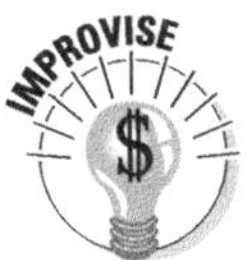

If you can't find any timers like this one, record a tape or CD of yourself that you can play while you do circuits. If you want to spend 20 seconds at each station, for example (and that's a great time interval to start off), set a clock in plain view and record yourself saying, "start" at the beginning, "next station" at the end of 20 seconds, "next station" at the end of the next 20 seconds, and maybe even "good job" and "keep it up" in between. Record as many 20-second intervals as you think you need for the number of exercises you want to do.

Understanding the procedure

Ready to start? When the stations are set up, you've decided what exercises you want to do and have written a note to yourself at each station, and your timer is ready, here's what you do:

1. **Warm up with a walk, bike ride, or other cardiovascular activity for 5 to 15 minutes, depending on how long you take to warm up and how long you want this entire workout to last.**

   You can also use the warm-up portion of an aerobics videotape to get you started.

2. **When you finish your warm up, *immediately* go to the first station.**

   Don't stop for anything but a quick drink of water. Don't sit down or chitchat with neighbors or anything like that. Do your warm up, and then go right to the first station.

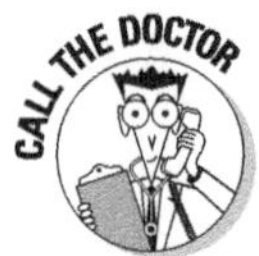

If you feel any of the signs and symptoms listed in Chapter 3, of course disregard the preceding advice to not dillydally. Always keep your pregnancy and the health of your baby in your foremost thoughts as you work out, and if something's not right, stop your activity and call your healthcare provider.

3. **Start the timer and begin the first activity (see the following sections for details).**

   Do as many repetitions of the activity as you can do in the allotted time, which you want to start at 20 seconds. (This 20-second allotment includes the time you're walking briskly from station to station, so you'll actually be doing each activity for 10 to 16 seconds, depending on how close together you put your stations. As you get more comfortable with circuit training — and if you're still feeling great, you're gaining weight normally, and your baby is growing appropriately — increase in 5-second intervals to 25 seconds, and 30 seconds, and so on.

4. **When the watch beeps, walk briskly from your station to the next one and immediately begin doing the next exercise.**

5. **When the timer beeps again, walk briskly to the next station.**

   Repeat this process until you've done all the exercises you want to do.

   When you've done a full circuit of all the stations and exercises (to understand one *circuit,* think of a circuit-riding preacher who rode around from church to church until he completed one circuit of all the churches), do another full circuit. Repeat circuits until you've worked out for your number of goal minutes, including the warm-up and cool-down.

6. **When the time beeps at your last station, immediately begin a 5- to 10-minute cool-down.**

   Walk, take a bike ride, or use the cool-down portion of an aerobics video.

Part V

The Tenth Month and Later: Staying Fit for Life

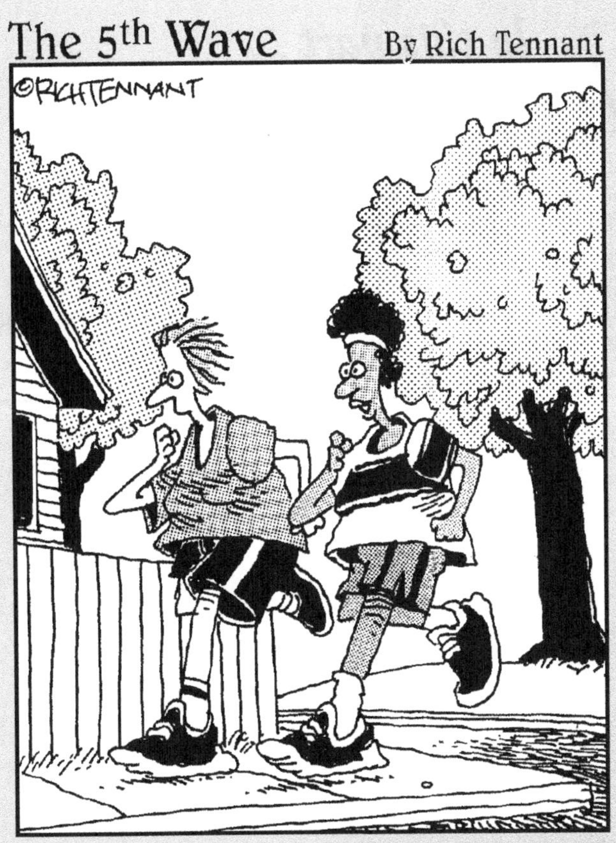

"I used to think, 'running for the endorphins' was a charity race for an endangered sea mammal."

In this part . . .

You discover that as much as your body is changing now, it's going to change all over again after you deliver your baby. When you're recovering from labor (and, potentially, from surgery), you need to know how and when to pursue physical activity again, and this part helps you sort through your options. You also discover how to blend new motherhood with a consistent workout routine, and you get some tips and techniques for keeping your child healthy and fit.

Chapter 18

Recovering from the Labor Marathon and Getting Up and at 'Em

In This Chapter

- Giving yourself a break after delivery
- Getting back on your feet
- Lifting and carrying your baby without injuring yourself
- Easing back into your fitness routine

Wheeew! You made it through that marathon called labor and delivery, and you now hold in your arms a beautiful baby boy or girl. Thanks to all the stretching and exercising you did throughout your pregnancy, your body was in good shape for this event, and you can expect it to heal more quickly than if you hadn't stayed fit and active. However, right after you deliver your baby, you need to allow some time for your body to recover.

In this chapter, we focus on the first days and weeks after you deliver your baby, a time when you need to be especially gentle with yourself. We also show you how to keep from injuring yourself as you lift and carry your baby, who will gain weight rapidly in the coming weeks.

All that bending, lifting, and carrying is definitely exercise, but sometime in the days and weeks after you deliver and as you begin to develop a daily routine with your new bundle of joy, you may begin to miss your old workout routine. You may not miss the discomfort and the sweat, but certainly the extra energy and natural high that come from exercising and the wonderful sense of accomplishment that you get when you complete a workout. The question is, when should you return to physical activity — and at what level? And if you take several weeks off, how do you start up again? This chapter dishes the dirt.

Resting Up First

The first few days after you deliver your baby is not the time to be thinking about your workout routine. After all, you've just been through the mother of all workouts — labor and delivery — and now's the time to rest. But you may have trouble getting the rest you need while meeting your baby's many needs during this time. Here are some tips for getting rest with a new baby in the house:

- **Always nap when your baby naps.** For the first few weeks of your baby's life, don't try to use your baby's nap times to catch up on housework, call your office, exercise, or do anything else except sleep. Keep a baby monitor by your side when sleeping in your own bed, or if your baby sleeps in a separate room, set up a comfortable chair or daybed in the nursery.
- **Take as much time away from work as you can afford.** Even if you're the very definition of a workaholic and can't imagine being away from your office for more than a few hours, you have to let your work go for a few weeks, for your own health and the health of your baby. You desperately need sleep right now, and trying to sneak in a few hours of work each day takes away potential nap times.
- **Get someone to help you with housework.** Don't let housework interfere with your rest time — whether your partner does your share of the chores, you enlist a family member or friend to help with laundry and cleaning, or you hire outside help, get as much help as you need so that you can take care of yourself and your baby. If friends and family ask how they can help, ask them to bring over some premade meals and to do a couple of loads of laundry while they visit. They'll be thrilled to be of service, and you'll get the rest you need. Also, don't stress about having a messy house during these first few weeks. Having a June Cleaver house isn't nearly as important as caring for your baby!
- **Arrange to do an activity you fully enjoy at least once or twice per week.** Whether you go to a movie, quietly read a book, spend a few hours surfing the Internet, take a bubble bath, go shopping, or whatever else interests you, spend some time pampering yourself. Take advantage of the time your partner is bonding with your baby, take up friends and family on offers to babysit, or hire a babysitter who's experienced with infants for a few hours. Spending time by yourself doing activities you love makes you better able to relax and actively participate in your child's care.
- **Limit visits from well-meaning friends and family.** Establish set hours during which friends and family can visit, times when you and your baby are awake. Ask your partner to enforce these boundaries during your baby's first few weeks of life.

- **Continue taking your prenatal vitamins, eat well, and drink plenty of fluids.** If you aren't getting the proper nutrients and drinking enough fluids, you may become malnourished and/or dehydrated — both add to fatigue. Research shows that including plenty of protein (such as that in lean meats, lean dairy products, beans, nuts, and so on) and vitamin C (most notably in orange juice, citrus fruits, and many green vegetables) in your diet helps your body recover quickly. Also drink eight to ten glasses of water and other fluids every day.
- **Take care when getting out of bed or getting up from lying down.** As you're healing from your delivery — especially if you had a cesarean section — be careful as you get out of bed or rise from a lying position. Rising straight up from lying on your back puts tremendous stress on your low back and abdomen, especially when your muscles are weak from the physical changes of pregnancy. Getting up that way also stresses any incisions and stitches you may have. Here's a better way to get off your back and onto your feet:

  1. **To get up from a lying position, roll over to one side and push yourself up slowly with your arms. See Figure 18-1.**
  2. **Press up to a sitting position and drop your legs down in front of you.**
  3. **Use your arms to help press up your body as you stand.**

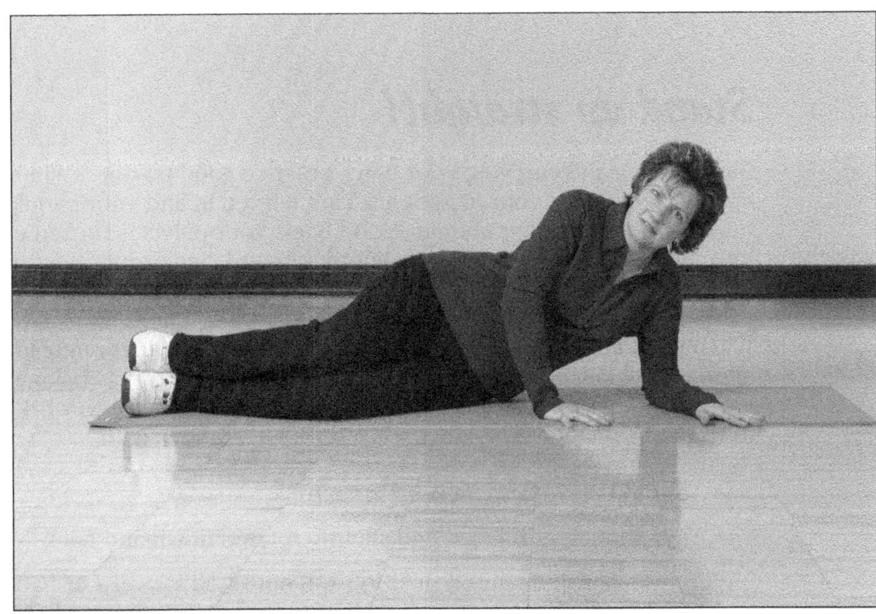

Figure 18-1: Rolling up properly from a lying position.

Caring for Your Baby without Stressing Your Body

It goes without saying that you want your time with your new bundle of joy to be pleasant, not a pain in the neck, back, or arms! Just as you have to master proper lifting technique when you go to work for UPS or FedEx and carry those heavy boxes around, as a new mother, you need to be trained in your new job of hoisting and carrying your baby. The fact is, new mothers who are instructed in proper lifting techniques suffer fewer back injuries and other aches and pains, so this section gives you the lowdown on how to stand properly when lifting any object (not just your baby), how to lift your baby from various positions, and how to carry him without straining yourself.

The source of most chronic back and neck pain after pregnancy is doing repetitive motions: lifting, carrying, and feeding your baby in the same positions every day. Try to find several positions in which to lift, carry, and feed your baby, and vary them throughout the day. Doing so helps to avoid stress on the same muscles and helps reduce fatigue.

A great book on lifting and carrying your baby is *How to Raise Children Without Breaking Your Back* by Hollis Herman, MS, PT, OCS and Alex Pirie (Ibis Publications). You can also check out the authors' Web site at `www.hherman.com`.

Stand up straight!

Before lifting and carrying your baby, practice good posture. When you're standing correctly, your lower back isn't curved in and your shoulders aren't hunched. Instead, your shoulders are back, your pelvis is tucked under your hips, and your chest is pressed slightly forward. See proper posture in Figure 18-2a and contrast it with poor posture in Figure 18-2b.

When you think of good posture, envision your body functioning in a way that allows for balanced, relaxed movement. When your body is balanced with all parts working together normally, your muscles don't have to work overtime to maintain balance. The most relaxed way to stand is with

- Your eyes level and focused forward.
- Your shoulders relaxed and slightly rotated down and back.
- Your pelvis in a neutral position and not tilted forward or back, and your weight balanced over the center of your foot. (To find the neutral position of your pelvis, tilt it forward and back several times until you find a comfortable spot in the middle.)

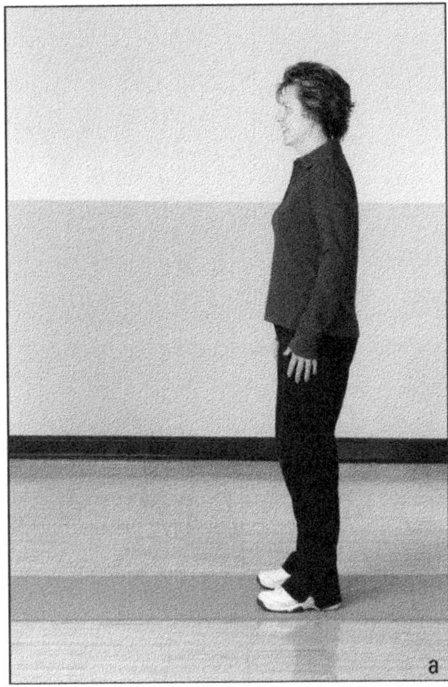

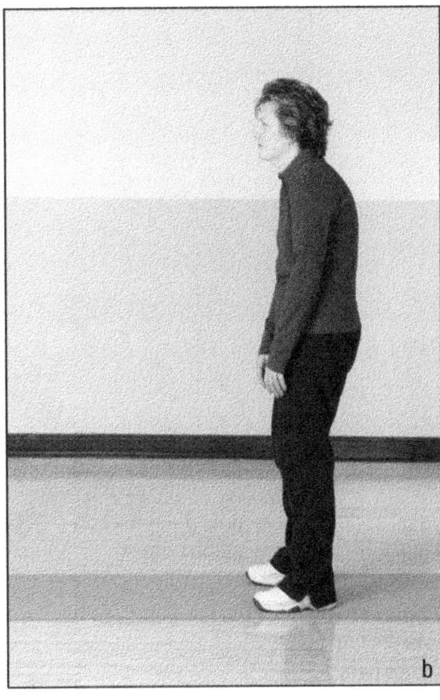

Figure 18-2: Proper posture versus poor posture.

If you drew a line from your head to your feet while standing with proper posture, the line would run straight down, in between your ears, shoulders, hips, knees, and ankles. When your posture is poor, your neck may lean forward, you may hunch your shoulders and hump your upper back, and your low back may sway. All these awkward positions can lead to headaches, neck and back stiffness and pain, and weakness and discomfort in your hands and legs.

Lifting your baby from the floor or a stroller

To pick your baby up off the floor or out of a stroller, do the following:

1. **Kneel down with one knee on the floor and the other foot planted flat on the floor.**

   You can also squat, keeping both feet flat and both knees deeply bent.

2. **Move in as close as possible to your baby (or to the stroller) so you don't have to reach out very far, as shown in Figure 18-3.**
3. **Bring your baby close to your body *before* you lift.**
4. **Breathe in, and then exhale, contracting your tummy. Take another breath and exhale as you lift.**

   This breath supports your low back.

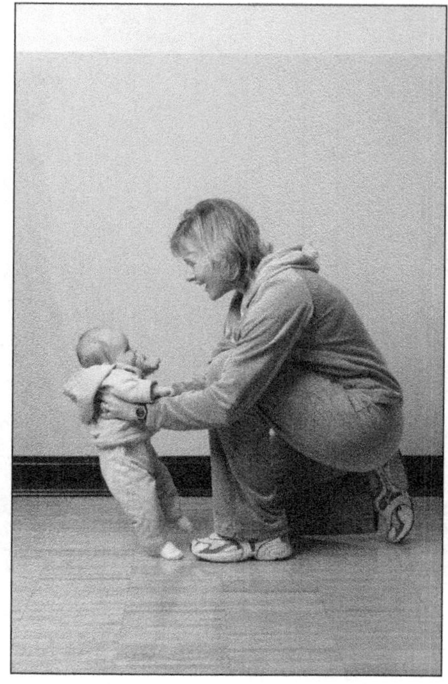

Figure 18-3: Bending down to pick up your baby.

5. **Lift your baby, holding her tight and using your leg muscles, not your back, to gradually rise to a standing position, as shown in Figure 18-4.**

Using a baby carrier is just like using a stroller. To lift a baby from a baby carrier, whether on the floor or on a car seat, follow the same steps as those just outlined: Kneel or squat in front of the carrier, position the handle up and out of your way, and slide your baby out. Keep your baby straight, as shown in Figure 18-5, while you pull the baby toward you to release her from the carrier. Reverse these steps to put your baby into a carrier.

Putting your baby down

To put your baby down (on the floor or into a stroller), reverse the process outlined in the preceding section.

1. **Hold your baby close to your body.**
2. **Squat or kneel (see the preceding section for proper form), and then set your baby on the floor or into the stroller.**

   Avoid hunching your back and/or lifting or setting your baby down while bending from your hips — doing so puts too much stress on your low back. Do all your lifting and lowering with your legs, keeping your back fairly straight and your abdominal muscles contracted.

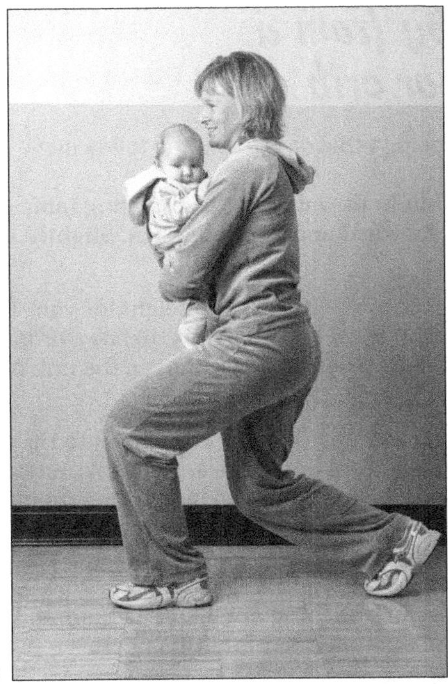

Figure 18-4: Lifting with your legs as you pick up your baby.

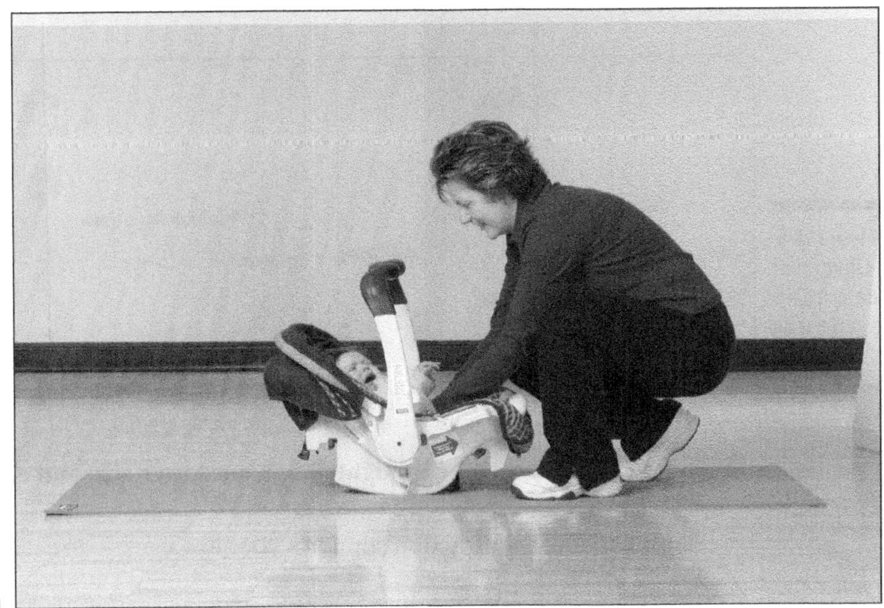

Figure 18-5: Lifting your baby from a carrier.

Lifting your baby from a changing table or crib

To lift your baby from a changing table or crib, do the following:

1. **Stand as close as possible to the edge of the changing table or side of the crib, with one foot forward and one foot back. Slightly bend both of your knees.**

   Be sure that the table or crib is at the proper height for you. The top of the table should be at about waist height. If the crib has a drop-down side, be sure to drop it down before putting your baby in the crib or getting him out.

   If you're a shorter woman and have trouble reaching into the crib, don't buy a crib that doesn't have drop-down sides. Test drive a few models before you buy by reaching down into them in the showroom.

2. **Slide your baby toward you by pulling his bottom blanket until he is at the edge of the crib.**
3. **Prepare to lift your baby by reaching one hand around and under his back and the other hand around and under his neck.**
4. **Sit your baby up and slide him toward you so that he's as close to you as possible, as shown in Figure 18-6a.**

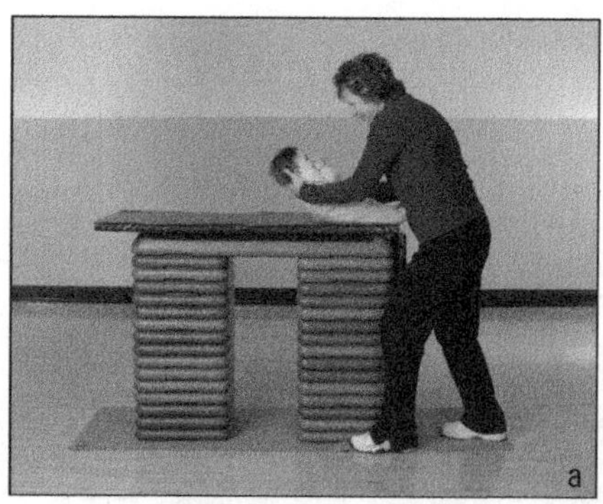

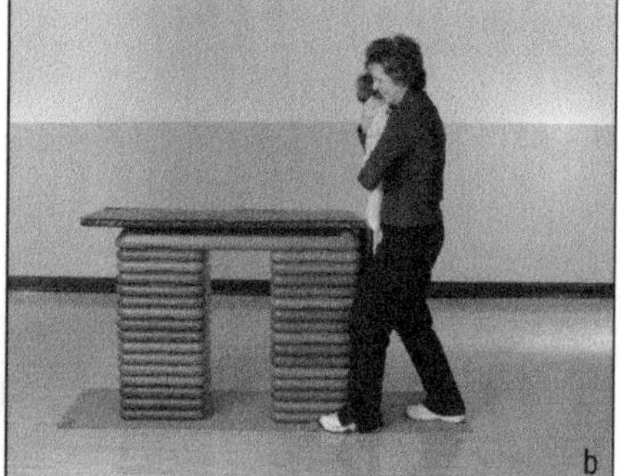

Figure 18-6: Lifting your baby from a changing table.

5. **Before you lift, breathe in, tightening your lower abs, and exhale as you lift.**

   This abdominal contraction supports your low back — use it anytime you're lifting.

6. **Lift your baby up into your arms, shifting your weight to your back leg and keeping your back straight as you lift. Refer to Figure 18-6b.**

   Never twist and lift your baby or twist and set him down — doing so puts tremendous stress on your low back.

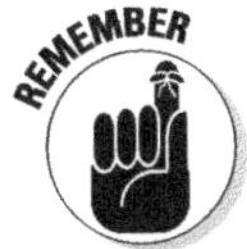

To set your baby down into a crib, reverse this process, setting your baby down into the crib as close to the side as possible, without twisting your back as you set him down and bending your knees slightly.

When lifting your baby from a crib that doesn't have a collapsible side (which means that you have to reach down in to lift your baby), always first slide the baby near the side of the crib closest to you. (To slide your baby closer to you, always place him on a blanket, which you can slide toward you when you're lifting him up.) Prepare to lift him by placing your hands under his back and neck. Then, keeping your back straight and bending your knees, breathe in, tighten your lower abs, and exhale as you hold and lift your baby, letting your legs do as much of the lifting work as possible.

Exercise and breast milk production

Studies show that exercise doesn't interfere with your ability to produce breast milk, but some physicians still believe that working out can have that impact. In order to ease your healthcare provider's fears about the effect of exercise on your breast milk production, keep a close eye on the number of wet diapers your baby produces and compare that number to the La Leche League's guidelines.

The *La Leche League* is an organization of women who help other new mothers successfully breast-feed. The league is famous for its breast-feeding guidelines, which help you monitor whether your baby is getting enough breast milk. The following is a sampling of the League's guidelines that let you know you're breast-feeding successfully:

- Your baby nurses 8 to 12 times per day, whenever she is hungry and until she is satisfied.
- Beginning her fourth day, your baby wets five to eight diapers per day and has two to five bowel movements per day.
- Beginning her fourth day, your baby gains four to seven ounces of weight per week.
- You can hear your baby swallowing as she breast-feeds.
- Your baby is growing normally.

If your baby doesn't feed this often, wet this number of diapers, gain this amount of weight, or appear to be growing normally, contact your healthcare provider immediately. And visit the League's Web site at `www.lalecheleague.org` for breastfeeding information and local contacts in your area.

Carrying your baby

As you probably already know, you're going to be carrying your baby a lot, and you're not always going to want or be able to carry her in the same way. Following are a few ways to carry your baby safely and comfortably.

The football carry

Carrying your baby like a football (see Figure 18-7), in the crook of your arm and resting on your forearm and wrist, is convenient when she's still a newborn. You may feel pressure on your wrists, however, so alternate arms frequently. As she grows, however, this method becomes too difficult.

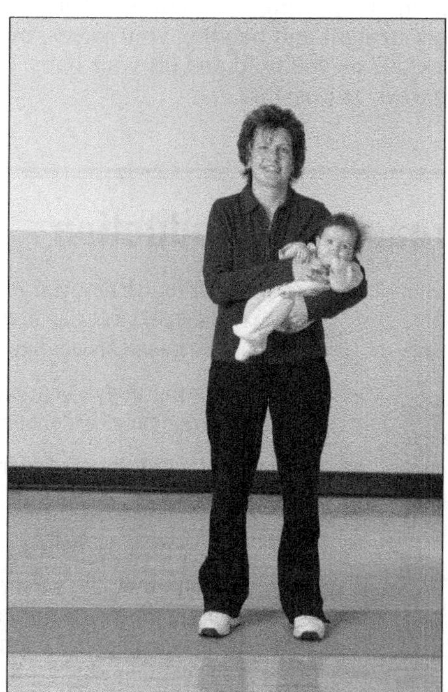

Figure 18-7: The football carry.

The hip carry

When you're preparing a meal, doing laundry, talking on the phone, or negotiating any other task that takes up one hand, use the hip carry, shown in Figure 18-8. Without thrusting out your hip, simply straddle your baby over one hipbone, alternating hips from time to time.

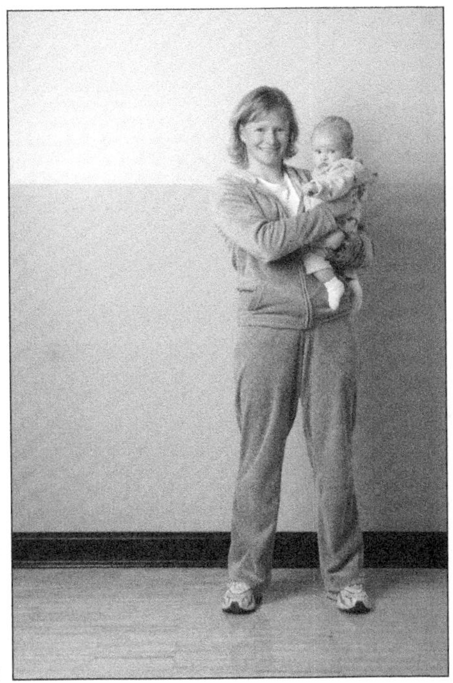

Figure 18-8: The hip carry.

The front carry

When you need to carry your baby for long periods and don't need your hands for any other activity, use the front carry (see Figure 18-9). Keep your baby tight to your body as you walk. As your baby becomes too heavy for you to lift even in a front carry, put her in a stroller or other carrying device. Try to keep your shoulder blades pulled back to avoid slouching.

The hands-free carry

If you use a *baby backpack* (in which your baby sits in a sling attached to your back), a *baby front pack* (same idea, but your baby sits on your front side), or a *baby sling* (a device that goes over one shoulder and under the opposite armpit so that your baby can lie down in front of you), be sure to set your baby in the pack or sling on a table, and then strap the pack or sling to your body. If the back or sling has a waist strap, use it to keep some of the weight off your back. Keep the pack securely fastened to your body to avoid having the weight pull away from you and cause added muscle strain.

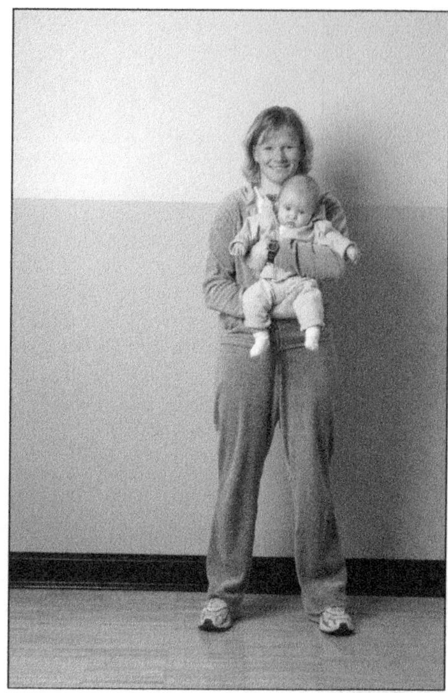

Figure 18-9: The front carry.

If you're having a lot of discomfort from a backpack or front pack, head back to the store where you purchased it and have them help you fit it properly to your body.

Pushing your baby in a stroller

When taking your baby with you on a walk, keep a straight back as you push and use your legs and buttock muscles to do the work (see Figure 18-10). Make sure that the handle height of the stroller fits you well so you don't have to bend forward or raise your hands into an uncomfortable position to push. If the handgrips are too hard, purchase some foam and tape it securely to the grips to add cushioning.

If you plan to fitness walk or run with your baby in a stroller, invest in a *running stroller,* which is made specifically for those activities. The wheels on a running stroller move easily through rough terrain, and the stroller is easy to propel. Running strollers cost more than standard strollers, but you won't regret your decision to buy one. Talk with other moms who walk or run with a stroller to find out which brands work well and hold up to consistent use.

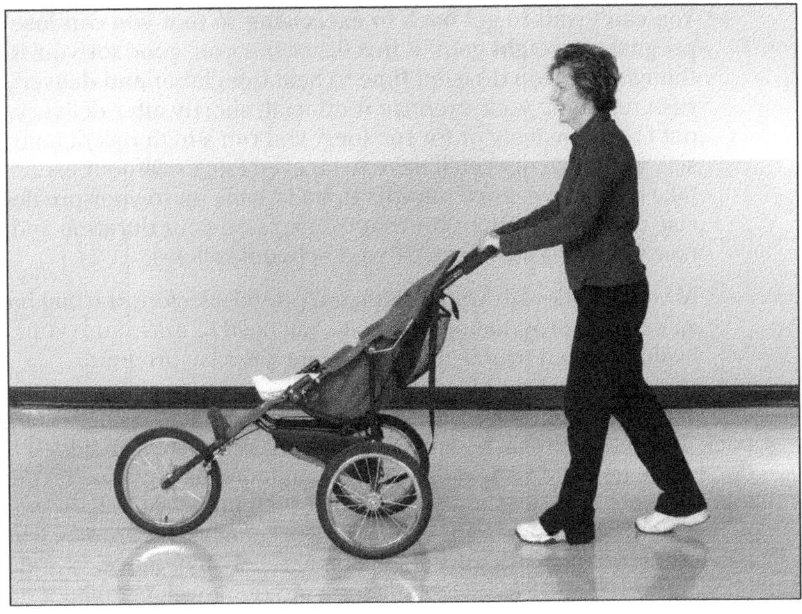

Figure 18-10: Pushing a stroller.

Deciding When to Exercise and What Activities to Do

Women generally have one of two reactions to exercise after delivering a baby:

- **You see exercise as an utter impossibility.** If you fall into this category, start with the stretches in Chapter 8, some easy pelvic floor exercises and basic core-strengthening exercises (see Chapter 11), and easy, short walks (see Chapter 12). Keep in mind that a ten-minute walk is far better than no walk at all, and any exercise tends to ease constipation and hemorrhoids (which many moms are all-too-familiar with right after delivery).

  Gradually build up your walks or other exercises to your pre-delivery routine, following the guidelines in Chapter 5, and even consider exercising more than you did when you were pregnant. You'll speed weight loss and quickly get your body back to its pre-pregnancy shape.

  Chapter 19 is all about finding the time and energy to work out as you balance all the other demands of motherhood. Flip to that chapter if you're having trouble seeing how you can possibly blend a daily exercise routine and caring for a baby.

- **You can't wait to get back to exercising so that you can lose your pregnancy weight gain.** If this describes you, good for you! Remember, though, that you do need time to heal from labor and delivery, so don't rush resuming your exercise routine. If, shortly after delivery, you work out too intensively or for too long, you run a high risk of injuring yourself, which means you'll have to go even longer without exercise. Instead, take several weeks or months to build back up to your pre-delivery exercise routine, and then continue to increase your duration and frequency (see Chapter 3) as much as your schedule allows.

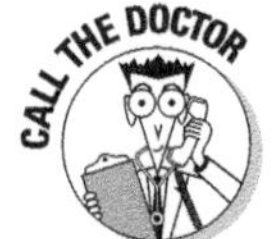

Always check with your healthcare provider before starting back into an exercise program postpartum. You need to make sure your body has healed enough to start back into your exercise program.

You can use any of the workout ideas throughout this book to get yourself back into shape after you deliver your baby. And here's an added bonus: You don't have to avoid lying on your back anymore, as you did starting in your fourth month of pregnancy, so you have even more options for working out. As you get back into a routine, aim for workouts at the 12 to 14 levels of perceived exertion (see Chapter 3). Listen carefully to your body and take a day off when you feel excessively fatigued. And don't weigh yourself too often, focusing instead on exercising consistently in a way that fits your schedule and makes you feel invigorated. Stop any exercise routine that causes excess pain or a consistent increase in bright red vaginal bleeding, and consult with your healthcare provider as soon as possible.

To get back to your exercise routine after delivering your baby, make sure you fit all the following guidelines:

- Your healthcare provider has given you the go-ahead to get started.
- Any incisions or tears have healed.
- You feel ready to get back to exercise.
- Your postpartum recovery is progressing normally, and you're healthy.
- You feel good after exercise, you don't experience any increase in vaginal bleeding, and you don't feel any other physical discomfort.

If you've had a cesarean section, don't forget that it's major surgery. You must give yourself time to recover. This means avoiding excess exertion (including going up and down stairs and lifting your baby from the floor or over your head), limiting your activities (you'll need to wait at least until your six-week checkup before working out again), and taking good care of your incision. Keep an eye on the wound and call your healthcare provider if the area becomes increasingly redder, feels warm, or starts to drain fluid, and also if you run a fever. And be sure to check with your healthcare provider before returning to your exercise program, just to make sure that you're fully healed from your surgery.

Making a slush pack

If you've had an *episiotomy,* a cut that your physician may make to enlarge your vaginal opening and minimize the risk of tearing during delivery, exercise may increase the bleeding. You may be able to reduce discomfort in your vaginal area by applying a slush pack to the affected area several times a day. A slush pack can also reduce the discomfort of hemorrhoids, a common side effect of delivery that can interfere with your desire to work out.

To make a slush pack, just fill a small bag with a little water, ice, and a few drops of rubbing alcohol. Tie the bag securely and wrap it in a thin towel. Place the pack on your incision and allow the area to cool for 10 to 15 minutes. The slush pack doesn't get as cold as an ice pack, but even so, don't leave the pack on for more than 15 minutes.

You've probably increased one bra size (from your pre-pregnancy size) after having your baby, so you may need to junk your pre-pregnancy sports bras and get larger ones. You may also find that wearing two sports bras at once feels comfortable and provides much needed support. As far as your other workout clothing goes, keep wearing your maternity gear as long as it fits and is comfortable. If your maternity clothes are too large and your pre-pregnancy workout gear doesn't fit yet, try pulling a few pieces from your pre-pregnancy wardrobe, your maternity wardrobe, and your partner's wardrobe to create a few workout outfits that fit comfortably.

Returning to Your Pre-Pregnancy Weight and Strengthening Your Abs

The good news about your postpregnancy weight is that you'll lose about 12 pounds shortly after delivering your baby. However, you gained more than 12 pounds during your pregnancy, which means you have some work to do. Instead of trying in one or two weeks to lose weight that you gained over a period of nine months, give yourself time to gradually lose the weight you need to lose — no more than ½ pound per week. With diet and exercise, you can get back to your pre-pregnancy condition. For an entire book full of dieting techniques, tips, and tricks, check out *Dieting For Dummies,* 2nd Edition, by Jane Kirby, RD, and the American Dietetic Association (Wiley).

If you're breast-feeding, you shouldn't be dieting. In order to produce enough breast milk for your baby, you need an extra 500 calories per day, which is more than you needed to eat while you were pregnant (see Chapter 10). For most mothers, this means from 2,000 to 2,200 calories per day, preferably with foods that are rich in protein (lean meats, lean dairy products, beans, peanuts, and so on) and vitamins (calcium, vitamin D, vitamin C, and so on). In fact, breast-feeding is demanding enough that it may actually help you lose weight in the weeks and months following delivery.

To firm your abdominal muscles and regain strength, begin gentle abdominal exercises as soon as you feel ready. Traditional sit-ups put too much stress on your abdomen and back, so avoid those for the next few weeks and months. A better way to safely strengthen your abdominal muscles is through a series of exercises developed by physical therapist Shirley Sahrmann. (Note that these same exercises are modified and included in the core strengthening exercises in Chapter 11.) These exercises, which we describe in the following sections, are designed to strengthen the muscles below your belly button — the ones that you rely on most for low-back support but that are most weakened during pregnancy. As you do these exercises, progress slowly and be patient with your body. Your abdominal muscles and the skin around your abdomen need time to firm up.

The Sahrmann abdominal exercise series contains five levels of exercises, all developed to progressively strengthen the lower abdominal muscles without putting stress on your low back. You can find the entire five levels of this technique in *How to Raise Children Without Breaking Your Back* by Hollis Herman, MS, PT, OCS and Alex Pirie (Ibis Publications).

If you've had a cesarean section or experienced *diastasis recti,* the separation of the abdominal muscles that we discuss in Chapter 11, check with your healthcare provider before starting any abdominal exercises.

Basic breath

The first exercise, the basic breath, shows you how to isolate and control your abdominal muscles.

1. **Lie on your back with your arms at your sides, your knees bent and together, and your feet resting on the floor.**
2. **Inhale and exhale a few times to get yourself ready.**

   Don't flatten your back or tilt your pelvis, just let the natural curve in your back remain. Breathe in and out slowly and deeply.

3. **Exhale and tighten your tummy muscles, pulling your navel toward your spine.**

   Concentrate on contracting the muscles below your belly button without flattening your back. Put one hand under the small of your back and the other hand on your belly, as shown in Figure 18-11, if that helps you maintain the proper position.

4. **Hold the contraction for a count of 5 (keep breathing normally as you hold), and then relax. Repeat 5 to 10 times.**

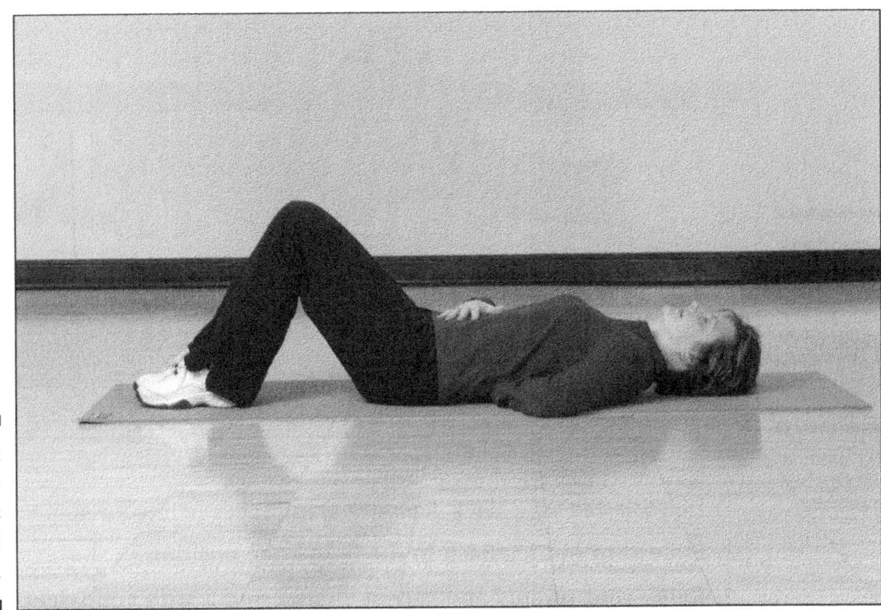

Figure 18-11: The basic breath helps you control your abs.

Leg slides (Sahrmann exercise #1)

When you're able to contract, hold, and relax your abdominal muscles without moving your back or losing the contraction in your tummy, you've mastered the basic breath, which means that you can move on to leg slides, which work the lower abdominal muscles.

1. **Lie on the floor with your knees bent and your arms at your sides. Hold your tummy in by doing the basic breath contraction.**

   Place your right hand on your belly, if needed.

2. **While continuing to breathe and holding the abdominal contraction, keep your right leg bent and slowly slide your left leg forward until it's straight and resting on the floor, as shown in Figure 18-12.**

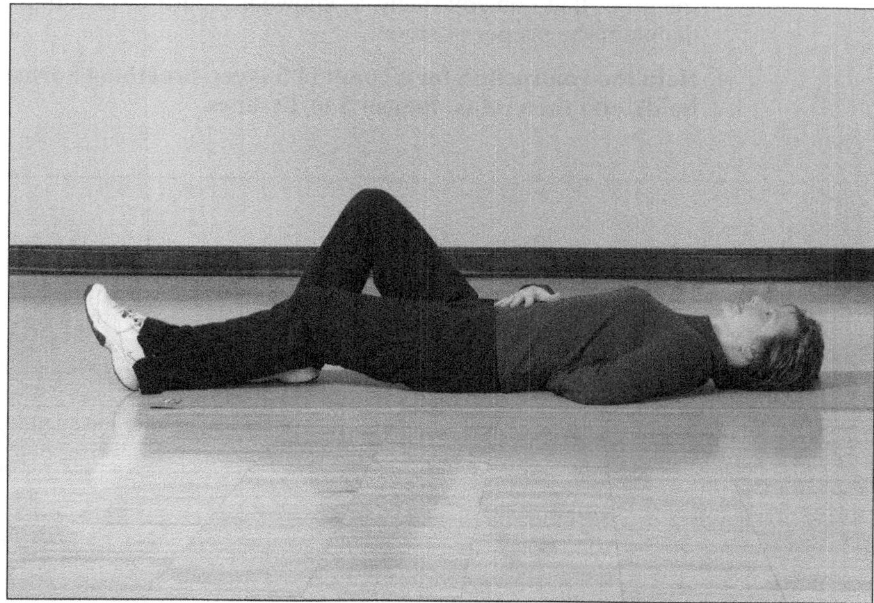

Figure 18-12: The leg slide strengthens your lower abdominal muscles.

   Don't flatten your back; keep the natural curve in your spine.

3. **Slide your left leg back to the bent-knee position.**
4. **Relax your tummy and repeat Steps 2 and 3 with your right leg.**

   Start with 5 repetitions on each leg. With time, build up to 20 leg slides on each leg.

Leg raises (Sahrmann exercise #2)

Leg raises are more difficult lower abdominal exercises; do these only when you can master 20 repetitions of leg slides. If your back keeps coming up off the floor or your tummy pops up while doing this exercise, go back to doing leg slides until your abdomen strengthens.

1. **Lie on the floor with your knees bent and your arms at your sides. Hold your tummy in by doing the basic breath contraction.**

   Place your right hand on your belly, if needed.

2. **Raise your left knee toward your chest, as shown in Figure 18-13a.**

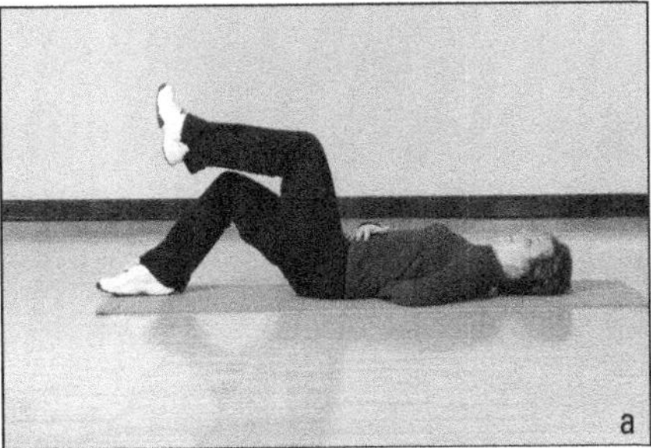

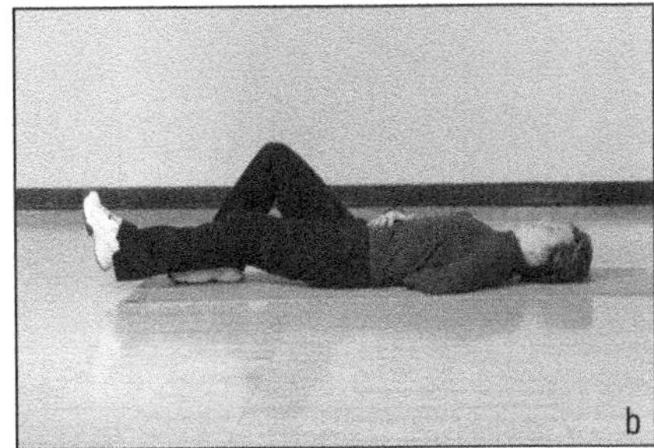

Figure 18-13: Leg raises strengthen your lower abdominal muscles even more.

3. **Slowly straighten and lower your left leg until it's parallel to and about 2 to 3 inches above the floor, as shown in Figure 18-13b.**

   Be sure to keep your left leg just barely off the floor.

4. **Return your left leg to its starting position and relax your tummy. Repeat with your right leg.**

   Start with 5 repetitions on each leg. With time, build up to 20 leg raises on each leg.

Chapter 19

Finding Time for Fitness and Motherhood

In This Chapter

- Keeping your workout routine alive
- Getting help from your partner
- Staying fit for the rest of your life

As your baby grows and you recover from labor and delivery, you may find that the demands of motherhood put a crimp in your ability to work out and stay fit. You may be so exhausted from weeks or months of sleep deprivation and from every-two-hour feedings (breast- or bottle-feeding) that you just don't think working out is an option right now. Or, you may feel that you don't have a lot of options for baby care while you work out.

In this chapter, you find tips on how to continue the work you began during pregnancy, from carving out time for your workouts to finding a safe place for your little one while you get your body back to your pre-pregnancy shape. You also discover tricks for exercising throughout the rest of your life.

Deciding Where and How to Work Out

During pregnancy, your biggest stumbling blocks to regular workouts may have involved getting motivated to work out, finding energy to exercise when pregnancy sapped all you had, and finding time to work out on long days that included visits to your healthcare provider. Now, however, your biggest challenge may be what in the world to do with your new baby as you work out and how to find time between all those feedings, changings, and your baby's other needs — in addition to still being short on sleep and time.

Working out in the comfort of your home

If you have workout equipment in your home, finding time and making sure your baby's safe may not be as big of a headache as it can otherwise be. When your child is very young, you can plan to exercise during one of his normal nap times, using a baby monitor or setting up a crib or playpen right near your workout equipment. If you're using a loud machine, however, such as a treadmill, rowing machine, or indoor bicycle, he may not sleep very long amidst all that ruckus. Likewise, the music and instructions on an aerobics tape may wake a sleeping baby. But quieter workouts do exist — from weightlifting to some elliptical trainers to yoga — and working out with your baby couldn't be much simpler.

If you're planning to leave your baby in his crib and to use his baby monitor to warn you if he awakes or needs you for other reasons, you may want to select a baby monitor that lights up when your baby cries. This way, you don't have to worry about not hearing the monitor over your workout video or treadmill.

If you're not able to find a quiet enough indoor activity that you enjoy or you just don't have room in your home for workout equipment, you can still keep your baby with you.

Taking your baby along for the ride (or run)

If she's properly dressed for the weather and not exposed to extreme temperatures, you may be able to take your baby with you on your workout. When she's very young and still lightweight enough to carry, you can keep her in a hands-free, front-mounted *baby sack* (also called a *baby pouch* or *baby sling*) or in a hands-free, back-mounted *baby backpack* while you walk or hike. Just be sure that she isn't getting jostled around, isn't too hot or cold, and isn't exposed to a draft.

When your baby can hold her head up and wear a helmet, you can bring her along in a bike trailer (such as those made by Burley; check out the Web site at `www.burley.com`) or an easy-to-maneuver running stroller (a stroller with a lightweight frame and large, all-terrain wheels — see Chapter 23). Most kids love to whiz down a bike path or sidewalk while in the protective custody of their mothers, and you don't have to hire a sitter for your daily exercise session. (Keep in mind that mountain biking on rutty trails isn't a great idea when your baby is in tow.)

Don't try to save money by fitness walking or running with a traditional stroller, because you'll be tuckered out before you've gone very far. Running strollers are lightweight and are designed to glide along smoothly, so you don't have to exert much additional effort to push your tyke along on the run. If you're just out for a stroll, a traditional stroller is fine, but for any sort of workout, get a running stroller.

Here's an added bonus: Taking your baby with you on your workouts exposes her to your regular exercise routine even before she's old enough to walk. With you as a role model, she'll quickly incorporate the idea of daily exercise into her view of the world.

Joining a gym or pool that offers childcare

Another option when you want to leave your house for a workout and still take your child along is to join a gym or pool that offers in-house childcare. Make sure that you check the credentials of the sitter(s) the gym or pool has hired and that you understand the childcare's policies. And talk with other moms who exercise at that facility to get the lowdown on the quality of childcare there.

Starting a mothers' exercise club

Do you know other newish mothers at work or in your neighborhood who want to work out? Consider starting a mothers' exercise club in your area. The club can work in three ways:

- You all work out together, and you all bring your babies with you in slings, packs, or running strollers. This is generally a walking club and can tend to have more of an emphasis on socializing than on getting an intense workout, which may be perfect for you.
- You hire one or more sitters to watch the children of all the club members, and then you all head out for a workout together, whether it's a walk, run, bike ride, swim, class, or other routine. Or, the sitter stays in one part of one club member's house, while club members work out in another area of the house.
- You take turns watching each others' kids, swapping babysitting times. If you have three or four members, and each one takes two days off of exercise to watch the kids, everyone in the club gets two days of babysitting and five days of great exercise with club members.

Before starting your own club, check to see whether one exists in your area by searching Google, Yahoo!, or some other Internet search engine for terms such as **mother's walking club** or **mother's exercise club**, followed by the name of your city or other area.

After you find an arrangement you're comfortable with, be sure to bring the following items with you so that your baby is content while you work out. Then you can plunge into your class or other workout while your baby naps, plays games, and eats with the sitter.

- Blanket
- Car seat carrier
- Change of clothes
- Diapers and wipe; diaper cream, if needed
- Formula or expressed milk
- Medical information, as appropriate
- Pacifier
- Soothing item or favorite toy
- Written information about your baby's likes and dislikes
- Your name and the location where you'll be exercising (for example, pool, track, weight room, and so on)

If you're nursing, feed your baby before heading to the gym or pool so that he doesn't get hungry during your workout.

Getting Your Partner Involved

If your partner has been involved in your pregnancy fitness routine and enjoys it, chances are, he wants to continue this routine after your baby is born. If you work out together in early morning, after work, or on weekends, you may want to take the baby with you, using the ideas described in the preceding section.

Another way to involve your partner is to alternate workout times: He watches the baby in the morning while you work out, and you watch the baby after work, when he works out. Or, he watches the baby from 5:30 to 6:30 in the morning, and you take over from 6:30 to 7:30 that morning.

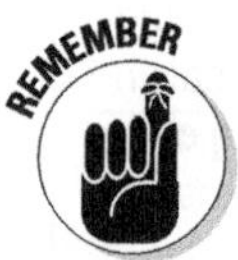

Your partner isn't "babysitting" your baby any more than you're babysitting your baby. When the child is yours, it's not called babysitting — it's called *parenting!* In this day and age, women shouldn't need to remind men that they have an equal responsibility in looking after a child, but patterns of behavior die hard, so you may need to remind him now and then. And don't fall into the trap of previous generations, thinking that the dad is less capable of watching a baby than you are. You're both cut out to be parents, and you have to trust each other to take care of and raise your child effectively.

Chapter 22 is chock full of ideas for making your significant other a partner in your fitness routine, either through his support of your solo workout routine or by working out with you.

If you and your partner are using a day-care center while you work, consider trying to find one with either early drop-offs (for example, 6:30 a.m.) or late pick-ups (say, 6:00 p.m.). Then you and your partner can use that extra time for your workouts. For example, perhaps you can drop your baby off at 6:30, get out for your walk by 6:45, complete your workout at 7:45, and still shower and get to work by 9:00.

Making Fitness Last a Lifetime

If you find yourself out of shape when you're in your 20s, 30s, or 40s, you may be all too familiar with several barriers that kept you from including fitness in your life:

- When you were a child, your family was never into sports or other physical activities, so you never developed the habit of regular exercise.
- You were a relatively fit kid (or even a very fit kid), probably participated in middle- and high-school sports, but you stopped exercising in college or during your first job and never found the time to start again.
- You worked out pretty regularly (or experienced periods of regular workouts and some periods of inactivity) until or through your first pregnancy, but during pregnancy and/or early motherhood, you stopped and never started up again.

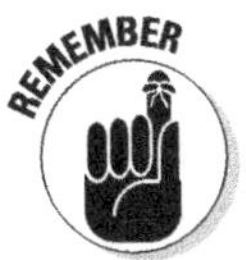

When a woman continues to exercise during and after her pregnancies, chances are good that she'll continue exercising on some level until very late in life. So, given that you've made it to your childbearing years and into this pregnancy and still have the desire to work out, you're on your way there!

To continue your consistent fitness routine throughout the rest of your life, make working out a part of your everyday life, periodically assess your fitness level, and set challenging goals that are important enough to encourage you to reach new fitness levels.

Making exercise a habit

You brush your teeth every day, even when you're busy, when you're on vacation, when you're tired and just want to go to bed, or when you just don't feel like it. You may even floss, too. And why do you this? Because you know that if you don't, your teeth won't be as healthy as they could be — and that can take a toll on your overall health and your appearance. (Not to mention that offensive breath may affect your social life.) Sounds a bit like the same reasons you exercise, doesn't it (except the funky breath part, of course)?

Just as you got yourself into the habit of brushing your teeth a couple of times per day, you can also get yourself into the habit of spending time working out every day of your life. You don't have a "goal" of brushing that you sometimes don't meet; you just do it, no matter what. You set aside a certain time each day to maintain your teeth, and you make it nonnegotiable. So it is with working out: You set aside a certain workout time, and you do some sort of physical activity at that time, no matter what. You don't let fatigue, a big deadline, the weather, or anything else take that time away from you (unless, of course, you're pregnant and aren't feeling well). The time you set aside is your grown-up recess time to run, skip, jump, and play, and you hold it dear.

Suppose you decide to work out for 30 minutes every Monday, Wednesday, and Friday. Monday can look one of two ways:

- **Do your workout all at one time, and never think about it the rest of the day.** If you like to work out at a gym, in a pool, or in a class, this pattern may fit you best, because with one drive to your workout facility, you reach your workout goal for the day. You may also benefit from morning workouts, because you can exercise, shower, get to where you need to be, and not think about working out the entire rest of the day.
- **Work out in spurts throughout the day, adding up the minutes to reach your daily goal.** For example, you may take a 15-minute walk with the dog in the morning, do several sets of sit-ups during your lunch break, and play a 10-minute game of kickball with your child before dinner.

You can get tremendous health benefits from working out 3 to 5 days per week for 30 to 40 minutes each time. That means that, if you choose to, you can take two to four days off every week and still keep your body fit and healthy. Brushing your teeth doesn't have a perk like that!

Monitoring your weight and size

In order to maintain a healthy weight and fitness level throughout your lifetime, you need to measure your weight and overall fitness from time to time.

Decide now how often you're going to review your physical condition, and then tie your review to specific dates, like the first of day of each month or every other payday. On your appointed days, do the following:

- **Weigh yourself.** Keep in mind that only children and pregnant women are supposed to gain weight every month or year; fully grown adults should establish a healthy weight for their frame and maintain that weight throughout a lifetime. However, weight can fluctuate by as much as six pounds throughout the day and from other factors, such as where you are in your menstrual cycle, so try to weigh yourself at the same time of day and under the same conditions each time. If you find that you've gained weight, reduce the number of calories you eat every day until the weight is gone. (See Chapter 10 for more on calories.) Two extra pounds may seem like nothing, but creeping up just 2 pounds per year means that, at the end of just 10 years, you'll be 20 pounds overweight. You're always going to have an easier time dealing with two pounds of extra weight rather than trying to lose ten pounds that gradually snuck up on you.

  If you aren't comfortable weighing yourself or don't have an accurate scale, you can also use other measurements, such as the way your favorite pair of pants fits (try them on every month or two). If they're tight, you've probably gained a bit of weight. In the same way, you can use a tape measure to measure around your waist, midthigh, or bicep.

- **Evaluate yourself in the mirror, without clothing.** (***Warning:*** Don't do this until several months after you deliver your baby. It's an effective habit throughout your life, but not right after pregnancy.) How do you look? Do you have areas that you want to improve, like cellulite on your thighs or sagging muscles under your arms? Or do you look strong and fit all over? If you want to tighten or strengthen certain areas of your body, adjust your workout routine to better target those areas. Consistent workouts will eventually pay off with a strong, healthy body.

  Try to look at your body with some gratitude for all it does for you, without being overly critical. Make your goal a healthy, fit body, not the body of a Victoria's Secret model.

Setting and resetting fitness goals

In order to continue working out for a lifetime, many people need to establish challenging fitness goals that give greater purpose to their fitness routines. Whether you begin to grow complacent about your need to exercise or just get bored with the same old routine, setting goals helps restart any fitness routine and makes it last a lifetime.

An ideal fitness goal has the following five components:

- **The goal is reasonable for you.** You don't want your goal to be so easy that you can reach it in two days or so difficult that you can never reach it.
- **The goal is measurable.** An unspecific goal, such as "I want to get fitter," is difficult to measure, so you really won't know when you've reached it. A specific goal is "I will able to walk three miles in 42 minutes by April 1," because you can easily determine when you've met your goal.
- **The goal is reachable over a short period of time.** If the time frame for your goal is too long — say six months, a year, or longer — you probably won't be able to use your goal as a motivating factor, because it'll just seem like it's too far in the future. Having a long-term goal, whether it's finishing a ten-mile bike race or someday hiking the entire Appalachian Trail, is terrific, but break down your long-term goal into several short-term ones (cycling 5 miles at 17 miles per hour, for example, or hiking 15 miles in one day) that you can reach within a few weeks or, at the longest, a couple of months.
- **You have a specific reward in mind for reaching your goal.** When you reach a fitness goal, treat yourself to a reward that you really want. Sure, being fitter may seem like enough of a reward, but a more tangible, fun way to congratulate yourself will likely make your goal that much more important to you.

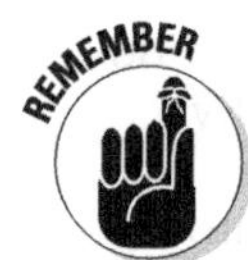

  Try not to make your reward food related, like a box of chocolate or a day of pigging out. Food is only one of many ways to reward yourself, so, instead, consider buying a new pair of biking shorts (or whatever fitness clothing you've had your eye on), ordering a subscription to your favorite fitness or other magazine, buying a book or CD, getting a massage or other spa treatment, or taking a half day off work and spending it with your baby at the beach or on a hike and picnic.
- **After reaching a fitness goal, you immediately set another.** Try not to let more than a day go by without setting a new fitness goal, especially if you tend to quickly lose interest in activities. Try to always have a fitness goal — one long term and one short term that helps you reach the longer goal — and think consciously about reaching it every time you work out.

If you're looking for other ways to stay motivated to work out (besides setting fitness goals), check out Chapter 22.

Rethinking how mothers "should" look

Sadly, a lot of people believe that, for mothers, being lean and fit just isn't physically possible. Many people believe that because most of the people they know have gained weight after having children (and just can't seem to lose it), permanent weight gain for mothers in inevitable.

We're here to tell you that it's not. If you eat the same number of calories that you're burning (see Chapter 10), you're not going to gain weight. And if you eat less than you burn, you'll lose weight. One of the major reasons so many people gain and have trouble losing weight in middle age is that they get busy, and in the midst of that busyness, they eat too much of unhealthy foods and don't take time to exercise.

So ask yourself these questions: What do you think a mother in her 30s, 40s, and beyond should look like? And how do you want to look at those ages? You're not overreaching if you want to be lean and fit during the second two-thirds or second half of your life. (Consider Priscilla Welch, who *started* running at age 34 and won the New York City Marathon in 1987 at age 42.) If you work out regularly and eat very healthfully, you can transform yourself into one fit woman! If being super-fit isn't your goal, that's great, but we just want to remind you that being really fit after your early to mid-20s is very, very possible. And doing so can help you live life more fully.

Considering competition: Something to shoot for

One of the best ways to stay interested in and focused on your fitness program is to sign up for a competition. Although some activities don't lend themselves to competitive events — yoga, aerobics, stair-stepping, and elliptical training immediately come to mind — many do. No matter what your age and whether you aim to win the event or simply finish it, you won't be out of place at a walking or running road race, cycling race, adult swim competition, cross-country ski event, weightlifting competition, rowing event, golf tournament, and so on. And keep in mind that many sports offer a separate *master's* (translated as "older athletes") category starting at age 40. These events may offer excellent prizes to master's athletes who score well against other master's competitors.

Chapter 20

Starting Your Kids Off on the Right Fitness Foot

In This Chapter

- Beating the odds by helping your kids grow up fit and healthy
- Merging playtime and fitness
- Eating well from day one

Kids love to exercise, they just call it something else — playtime! This chapter gives you an idea of the fitness challenges kids face today, but it doesn't dwell on the negative. Instead, we show you how to retain your child's natural love of activity and how to turn him or her on to healthy foods and habits from an early age.

Understanding the Impact of Low Activity and Excess Calories on Kids

Get this: More than one out of every seven kids in the United States is overweight or obese. One in seven! And the percentage of overweight and obese kids climbs every year. Those children now develop diseases that were previously thought to exist only in adult populations — adult-onset diabetes, high blood pressure, arthritis, and so on.

The culprit isn't hard to pinpoint, because it's the same reason that nearly one in three adults are overweight or obese: too little exercise and too many calories.

With so many kids (and adults) struggling with obesity, what's a new mom (or a mom who already has a few little ones) to do? Keeping your kids fit and healthy takes time and energy, but combining two approaches works:

- **Keep your kids active every day.** From the time they're old enough to walk, kids love to dance, skip, run, climb, and play games. Interaction with less-active adults and other kids may turn off this natural spigot of energy, but daily encouragement from you keeps your child's desire to run and play intact for a lifetime. The following section gives you loads of ideas for keeping your child active without forcing boring exercise routines on him.
- **Start your child on healthy foods as early as possible.** Fats and sugars are an acquired taste that can override your child's natural desire for healthy foods. Of course you want to be a cool mom and get your kids the latest snack food fad, but having unhealthy kids isn't cool. As soon as your child is eating whole foods, have only healthy snacks and meal ingredients on hand. The "Making Healthy Eating Your Family's Hallmark" section helps you stock your healthy pantry and train your child's appetite toward nutritious foods.

Helping Children Nurture Their Natural Love of Activity

The statistics in the preceding section may lead you to believe that kids don't like exercise. But nothing could be further from the truth. Babies and toddlers love to crawl, kick, push themselves up off the ground, roll over, do forward and backward rolls, play hand games (like Patty Cake), throw soft objects, walk, and run. Older kids are naturally drawn to any sort of play — you name it!

- Climbing trees, monkey bars, and jungle gyms
- Dancing
- Flying kites
- Hiking and exploring nature
- Ice-skating and rollerblading
- Jumping rope
- Playing any sort of ball sport (Wiffle ball, kickball, soccer, hockey, golf)
- Playing games of all sorts (Tag; Red Rover; Duck, Duck, Goose; Kick the Can; Capture the Flag; Hide 'n' Seek)
- Riding bikes

- Setting up and playing hopscotch
- Sledding
- Sliding on the playground slide
- Swimming and running on the beach
- Swinging

The trick is to retain that natural love so that it lasts a lifetime. This section gives you some tips.

"Working out" with your kids

Your workout routine doesn't have to be a casualty of your growing family. Babies love to go along with you as you walk, run, bike, or do any number of activities (see Chapter 19), and you'll be more motivated to work out if you take your new little workout buddy with you.

But what about after that first year? As your kids become old enough to walk, skip, jump, dance, or bike on their own, make a point of playing together every day, and you'll get a great workout in the process. Whether you're searching for turtles during a walk in the park, skipping around on a hopscotch board, dancing to funky music, making snow angels, or playing Kick the Can, you can stay active, encourage your child's healthy instincts, and have a great time. Although these so-called workouts aren't the most conventional way to exercise, as long as you and your child are moving and having fun, you're not only getting a workout, but you're also encouraging a love of activity in your child that will last a lifetime.

Introducing your child to all sorts of activities

Activities during childhood should be like a Whitman's Sampler chocolate box: a little taste of many different varieties. Now is the time for your child to try all sorts of activities and sports, no matter what your favorite is. Most kids like a variety, and if this is the case with your child, let him take the lead in deciding which activity to pursue each day. Or, if he struggles with too many options, have him choose one of two options, changing the two options tomorrow, the next day, and the next. You may take an adventure walk one day, play soccer the next, jump rope the next, then bike, and then play on the monkey bars. Keep up the activity as long as your child is enjoying himself and isn't getting overly fatigued.

Children understand even the subtlest clues, so if your child clamors every day to do the activity *you* love best, be sure he isn't responding to your reinforcement of that activity as the best one. If you light up when he suggests a certain activity and look tired or bored when he suggests any other, he'll soon begin trying to please you by asking for your favorite.

Limiting TV and video games

Kids who don't like to play often observe the people around them living a sedentary life. If your family spends any spare time in the morning, after work, in the evenings, and on weekends watching hours of television, playing video games, or doing other sedentary activities, your child will quickly lose interest in physical activity. After all, watching TV and playing video games are much easier than running around trying to capture the flag or find the tree behind which your mom or dad is hiding. When a child grows up in a family that spends its time on nonactive pursuits, she soon comes to despise any sort of physical activity. Limit TV and video games for the entire family to an occasional video rental or a once-a-week excellent TV show.

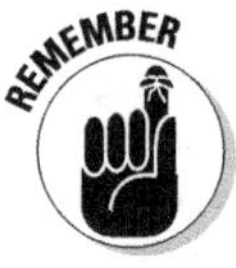

All play and no time for quiet nonphysical activities makes Jack unable to handle silence and quiet contemplation! We're not suggesting that kids have to be active 24/7; rather, a balance of physical activity, quiet time reading or studying, and lively family discussions help form a child who's fit and healthy, able to concentrate, and able to socialize.

Taking your baby along

If you walk or run outdoors, consider investing in a running stroller. A *running stroller* (commonly called a Baby Jogger after the first company to design and sell them) is a stroller that has a lightweight frame and large wheels so that it rolls easily over uneven terrain. A running stroller is easy to maneuver and offers your baby a smooth ride, so you can take him or her on every workout. Instead of having to hire a sitter for each day's exercise session, you take your tyke with you and get to work out.

Running strollers are expensive and often available only through serious fitness stores, such as specialty running and outdoor-adventure stores. You may also be able to find some running strollers online, but the shipping costs can be prohibitive. Plan to spend $250 to $300 for a high-quality running stroller — better yet, test out a few models and put a specific one on your baby registry.

If you exercise indoors and you're watching a baby or toddler, consider investing in a playpen (also called a play yard), which is a small, often fold-up area in which your baby can play and sleep, or in a baby swing. You get to do your workout, keep your baby safe and happy, and spend time in the same room with your child. A playpen is also a great way to watch your baby while your hands are full, such as when you're cooking, doing laundry, or catching up on paperwork.

Walking or biking instead of driving

If you're heading out to school, the park, the library, or other nearby location, get in the habit early in your child's life of walking or riding a bike instead of driving. And, when you're in a building with stairs and an elevator, take the stairs (walking or running) so that your child begins to do the same without even thinking twice about it. If you have to take an elevator, skip or run to the elevator with your child, and then hop up and down in the elevator until you reach your floor.

Whenever you're around your child and you have an opportunity to be active instead of inactive, do so. Not only will your child benefit from the activity, but he'll also come to think of a car (or an elevator) as an interesting option, not a necessity. That means he'll spend his life being more active than his peers.

Doing it every day

Plan your day around the chance to play with your kids. Sure, taking a bike ride on a Saturday afternoon is easier than trying to squeeze in a ride between the time you get home from work and the time the sun goes down, but no matter how busy you are, chances are, you can find time for daily physical activity with your child.

If you're tired from your day and aren't feeling motivated to go outside for your child's version of a workout, just ask your child what activity he wants to do that day. Kids are great motivators, and you may go from thinking you're way too tired to work out to climbing trees in no time.

Starting new traditions

The word *tradition* just makes you think of the holidays, doesn't it? A family's Thanksgiving Day tradition may be to sleep in, watch the parades on TV, watch football games while eating plenty of snacks, eat a big meal, take a nap, snack on leftover turkey, go to a movie, and so on. And although a tradition of that sort isn't wrong or bad, it tends to focus on food and inactivity, and you may feel that you can't change the tradition because that's how Thanksgiving is supposed to be.

Well, says who? Why can't Thanksgiving start out with a morning walk in the brisk November air? Or why can't the smaller, lighter meal be followed by a ping-pong tournament in the basement?

Holding back: Don't push your child

If you're encouraging your child to be active because you're hoping she'll be the next Mia Hamm, Michelle Kwan, Cheryl Swoops, or Marian Jones, stop. That's right: Stop! No matter how badly you want this sort of athletic success for your child nor how pure your motives, you can't "make" an athlete out of your child. Your task as a parent is to introduce her to a variety of activities — as well as the sports etiquette that goes along with them — and love her dearly regardless of whether she chooses to pursue one of those sports with vigor, play on a local athletic team, or simply be a fit, healthy child (which is far harder — and far less simple in this age of obesity and inactivity — than it may first appear to be).

Your child will let you know whether he has any interest in throwing himself into one sport and attempting that nearly impossible goal of being one of the best in the world at it. If that day occurs, be prepared to spend an almost unthinkable amount of time and money supporting him (equipment, coaching, and travel costs can be staggering), but never, ever push him to be a professional at a time when he's supposed to be a kid. Nearly all children who are forced into training rigorously for one sport grow to resent — and almost always quit — that sport before their athletic potential is tapped.

If your child wants to play on local athletic teams, also be prepared to dole out quite of bit of time and money for proper equipment and team fees. Show your support by attending all her games, meets, or matches (assuming she's indicated that she wants you there), and by providing rides to and from practices and events. Respect her coach's experience and allow your child to develop on her own schedule.

And if your child doesn't choose to participate in organized sports, you get the biggest benefit of all — time spent with him walking, hiking, cycling, dancing, doing yoga, skating, rollerblading, or doing whatever activity you both enjoy together. Don't skimp on his equipment, and start emphasizing the fun of daily exercise from the moment he's old enough as an infant to accompany you on your exercise routine.

Think about how you celebrate the major holidays in your family — birthdays, summer picnics, winter religious holidays, and even weekends. If your family tends to focus on food and inactivity, consider throwing out that tradition and replacing it with a new tradition, like the first annual Walk Three Miles While the Turkey's Cooking or Sled During Halftime event.

Keeping it fun

Kids don't think of playing as exercise. Playing is fun, even in structured games with rules. But often, exercise isn't fun. If you ask the students in a second-grade gym class to choose between running laps for 15 minutes and playing soccer for 15 minutes, they'll choose soccer, even though both activities involve running for 15 minutes. Why? Because soccer is a game — it's fun — and running laps is boring.

A definition of fun is, of course, unique to every child, but you can use Table 20-1 as a general set of fun and not-so-fun guidelines.

Table 20-1 The Kid's Guide to Fun Activities

Not Fun	*Fun*
Running laps; running on a treadmill	Running on a trail with (or behind) the dog; running while playing games, such as Tag, Kick the Can, or soccer
Power-walking down the sidewalk	Walking down the sidewalk searching for loose change while not stepping on any cracks; taking an adventure hike on a trail
Taking an aerobics class	Dancing wildly to "Rock Lobster" by the B-52s; learning to tap dance; doing gymnastics
Swimming laps	Playing Marco Polo or Sharks and Minnows in a pool

Not really rocket science, is it? To nurture your child's love of activity, being active has to be fun and not the drudgery that you may have begun to see your exercise routine as. You can get a great workout, too, as long as you keep moving. Don't worry too much about your pace, duration, or whatever else may take the fun out of being active.

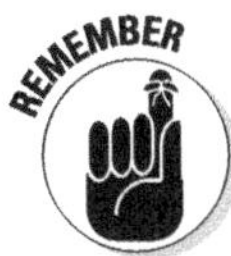

One of the fastest ways to take the fun out of an activity is to force your child to take lessons she doesn't want or join a team that she isn't interested in. Let your child — not you — be the judge of what teams or lessons are appropriate. If you were hoping your child would join Little League, but she asks to take ballet lessons instead, go with her instinct and encourage the ballet, even if you think baseball's better (and more fun). If you think developing skating skills at Saturday-morning lessons is important, but your child is dying to play hockey with her friends on Saturday mornings, don't insist on the lessons, or you may make exercise seem a lot less fun. Any time you force your expectations onto your child's fitness routine, you're going to risk snuffing out her natural love of activity.

If your child does join a team, keep the focus on having fun while being active. Wins and losses shouldn't be the focus for kids; fun and exercise are the goals.

Making Healthy Eating Your Family's Hallmark

When you have kids, encouraging healthy eating takes a two-pronged approach:

- **Make meals more meaningful than just the food.** If meals focus on just eating food — that is, when the food is gone, the meal is done — you encourage your child to eat quickly and not savor the taste of the food, and you miss the opportunity to have conversation during the meal and know each other more deeply. Instead, make meals an event that puts the food in the background and puts conversation, fellowship, and love at the center of the meal.
- **Master snacks.** The word *snack* has come to mean food that's not so good for you, like chips or cookies, but a snack is really just a way to curb your hunger between meals and can be incredibly healthy. If you keep only healthy snacks in the house from the time your child is a baby, your child will come to think of snacks in a whole different light than his "Twinkies and soda pop" peers.

Just one word of warning: Avoid going overboard. You don't want kids who don't know how to fit in and you don't want a too-tough stance to backfire and have your child rebel by eating junk. A hot dog once in a while never killed anyone, so if that's what's served at a party, that's okay. The idea is to limit the amount of unhealthy food your child eats, so if you reduce unhealthy foods by 50 percent, you've done a great job. Children can go through phases when they're unbelievably choosy — you know, they'll eat only brown foods and they have to be drenched in mustard — so in order to get your child to eat anything at all, you'll have to compromise a bit on the healthfulness of that food. So just set the stage for a healthy diet for your family and then relax and watch them grow up healthy and strong.

Avoid talking about dieting or negative body images around your children. Instead, provide a positive example through your actions and words.

Starting with healthy snacks from the beginning

Before he knows what sugary, fatty snacks are, get him hooked on good foods. Yes, he'll find out all about snacks that aren't good for him from the cool mom down the street and from the vending machines at school, but for now, get him excited about the following:

- Fresh fruit of all varieties, like grapes, apple chunks, orange sections, bananas, peaches, pears, plums, and so on
- Dried raisins, prunes, and any other dried fruit without added sugar
- Carrot and celery sticks, broccoli crowns, cherry tomatoes, and any other veggies you can think of. Consider serving with fat-free or low-fat ranch dressing.
- Popcorn without hydrogenated oil (see Chapter 9), rice cakes, crackers low in fat and salt and high in fiber
- 100 percent juice (not sugary *juice drinks* that are mostly sugar — look for a label that says "100 percent juice") and chilled water

If you're researching daycare centers for your child, make healthy snacks and plenty of playtime high priorities. If you're stocking healthy snacks and encouraging daily activity, but eight or ten hours per day he's eating cookies at the daycare, his taste buds will be turned on by sugar and fat at a young age.

Keeping good food on hand at all times

In order to encourage healthy snacking, you have to keep the good stuff around the house. Keep your pantry and refrigerator stocked with the foods listed in the preceding section (and add to that list as your child develops her own healthy tastes), and get rid of everything else. That's right — purge your house of unhealthy snacks so that your child isn't exposed to them at an early age. A child who grows up thinking that grapes are the best snack in the world is going to have a much easier time maintaining her weight as an adult than someone who grows up thinking fried chicken wings are the best snack in the world.

If you find that you just can't live without certain snacks, try low-fat, low-sugar varieties of traditionally unhealthy snacks: low-fat chips; low-sugar cookies (or experiment with recipes and make your own!); pizza made with low-fat cheese, veggies, and ground turkey breast; and so on.

Packing your child's lunch

Packing your child's lunch is always going to give him a healthier meal than having him buy a hot lunch at school, especially if the school allows him to choose his own hot lunch. Although schools know they have a responsibility to feed kids healthy foods, they have to prepare low-cost meals that can feed an army of children, so you're not going to see low-fat cheese pizza or fresh peaches on the menu. Instead, you'll see high-fat meats and cheeses (they're the cheapest and are often the only kind available in bulk quantities), canned vegetables that may be overcooked and unappealing, and fried foods (also inexpensive and easy to obtain). Cookies and other high-fat, high-sugar snacks are another inexpensive way to fill kids up, so you're likely to find those on the menu, too. Keep your child healthy and save money in the process by having him bring lunch from home.

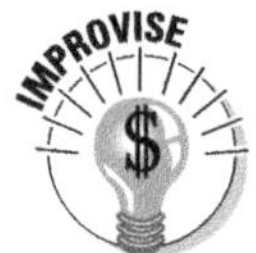

The easiest, cheapest lunches to prepare are those made with leftovers from your dinner. Simply make more dinner than your family needs and, before serving the meal (this is important to discourage overeating and to actually have leftovers at all!), fill plastic containers for the next day's lunches.

Most children can help prepare their own lunches by about second grade, so get your child involved early in deciding what he'll eat for lunch. Within a year or two of making decisions with you and watching you pack the lunch, he'll be able to prepare his lunches on his own with just a quick peek from you to make sure he didn't pack a triple-decker peanut-butter-and-chocolate-frosting sandwich.

Lobbying your child's school

The Los Angeles and New York City school districts have opted for vending machines that offer only healthy foods: bottled water, low-fat milk, and sugar-free juices. And if the two largest school districts in the United States can take this healthy stance, so can your school district. The next time you're in your child's school, ask to see all the school's vending machines. If your child doesn't have healthy choices available in those vending machines, attend the next school board meeting and lobby for healthier products in those machines. If you're overruled, start a petition that gets other parents involved.

Vending machine profits often fund some of the most important projects at your child's school, from field trips to extracurricular activities. As such, school leaders need to feel confident that changing to healthier vending-machine options won't lower their profits from those machines. With permission from the school principal, take surveys of students to find out whether and how their buying habits may change if different food choices are offered.

Steering clear of fast food

Recent studies at Children's Hospital in Boston found that among children who eat fast food, kids ate enough extra calories during those fast-food meals to add six *extra* pounds per year — that is, six pounds above and beyond the calories they need for normal growth. And these kids consuming fast food eat more fats, sugars, and other carbs, and fewer fruits and vegetables, than kids who don't eat fast food.

The study of over 6,000 children indicates that about a third eat fast food every day. The good news, though, is that about two-thirds of kids don't regularly eat fast food, and that's the category in which you want your child. Don't make fast food a treat for your family — it isn't nearly as tasty or nutritious as meals you can prepare at home. If you're looking for an occasional family treat, eat out at a restaurant that offers more nutritious options, such as many types of pasta dishes, made-to-order veggie or cheese pizza, yummy soups, salads made with a variety of ingredients, and so on.

Even on vacation, you don't have to eat fast food. Bring a cooler with you for the first day, eat at sit-down restaurants, or stop by a grocery store and buy picnic fixings, such as whole-grain bread, low-fat lunch meats, baby carrots and other easy-to-eat vegetables, fruits, and sugar-free gelatin packs. If you do find yourself in a situation where fast food is your only option, choose from among healthier options, such as the low-fat sandwiches at Subway, grilled chicken sandwiches at several fast-food restaurants, and other choices that are available from time to time. Avoid fried foods, sugary sodas, and high-fat sandwiches for your kids and never order supersized anything — getting all that extra food for just a few pennies isn't a good deal if your child eats more than his body needs.

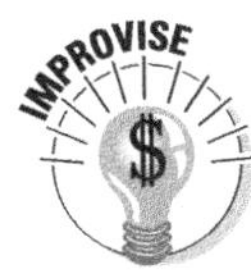

And if you tend to think of fast food as a great last-minute meal when you and your partner are too busy to cook, consider some alternatives:

- One weekend day per month, cook big batches of dishes and freeze them for use throughout the month. Thaw them in the fridge throughout the day and have delicious meals ready in no time. One easy meal is stir-fry veggies and meat: cut up chicken breast or lean beef and freeze in packets just the right size for your family's stir-fry; cut up veggies and freeze in their own packets. Another is low-fat lasagna, made with fat-free ricotta and cottage cheese, low-fat cheese, and whole-wheat lasagna noodles.
- Whip up a pasta dinner, using whole-wheat pasta and jars of low-fat pasta sauce. You can cook pasta in less than 20 minutes (a great time for fun workout games with your child) and have plenty left over for lunch the next day. Add a pan of steamed broccoli or zucchini (five minutes to cut up; five minutes to cook), some fresh fruit, and low-fat milk to drink, and you have yourself a great meal.
- If you absolutely, positively can't cook, consider getting Chinese takeout and opting for dishes with lean, unfried meats and plenty of vegetables. Or stop by the grocery store on your way home and pick up a rotisserie chicken breast and salad fixings for a ten-minute meal.

Most kids love to prepare foods and cook, so let your child prepare easy snacks and dishes under your supervision. After he masters the basics, try making foods from different cultures so that he combines a fun lesson about other parts of the country or world with healthy eating.

Eating dinner at the table

Have you and your partner gotten in the habit of eating dinner while watching TV? Although no one's forcing you to change that habit — and it may work perfectly well for adults who've developed healthy habits and can make good choices — you may want to consider whether this is a healthy eating environment for your child.

We're not suggesting that you become Donna Reed and slave in the kitchen for hours, preparing a gourmet sit-down dinner. Instead, consider whether you and your partner can create fast, simple, healthy meals that your family can eat while sitting at a table, discussing the events of the day. A recent study at the Baylor College of Medicine shows that when kids eat dinner together at a table with conversation and family time as the focus of the meal, they eat less fat and more fruits and vegetables than when they eat on the run or in front of the TV, so trying this approach may reap rewards for you and your kids.

Taking your kids grocery shopping

Does taking kids shopping seem impossible? Perhaps for some parents, but if you start your child out early with some basic ground rules, taking your child shopping is a great teaching opportunity. Here are a few tips to keep in mind:

- **Stick to a shopping list.** When your child sees that you don't give in to impulse (Read that: unhealthy) temptations, he understands your commitment to healthy eating.
- **Make choices together.** If you're looking at several varieties of an item on your list, talk about which makes the best choice and why. Ask for your child's opinion and buy the one he recommends whenever possible. If you don't think his choice is the best one for your family, talk about why.
- **Limit the options.** If you want to buy your child one item at the store (and no one says you have to), before you go, make a list of some healthier food snacks and let her choose one from the list. That way, your child gets to choose an item for herself but isn't immediately drawn to candy bars or cookies.

You can't eliminate all junk food from your child's life, but you can subtly encourage other types of food. If a treat is a bowl of cherries or grapes as often as it's a brownie, kids come to think of healthier foods as treats, too. But if brownies are absolutely your child's favorite food, allow him that pleasure one or two days per week after a meal.

Part VI
The Part of Tens

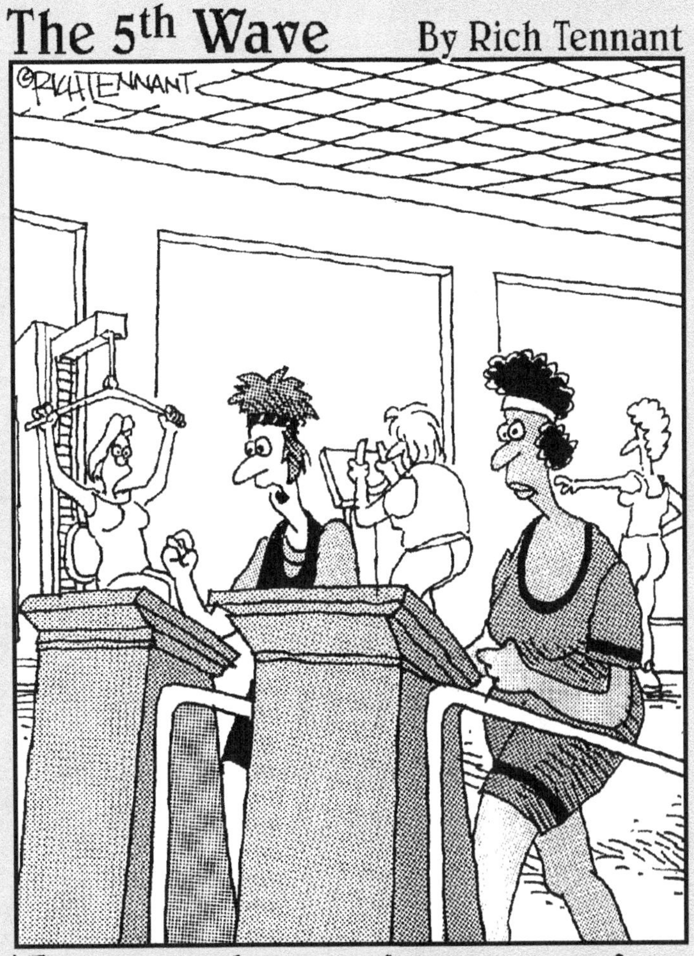

"I exercised so much during my first pregnancy that the baby was born with athlete's foot."

In this part . . .

You get three separate lists of ten tips, including ten ways to work out indoors, ten inventive ways to include your family in your workout routine, and ten helpful ways to find pregnancy workout gear.

Chapter 21

Ten Ideas for Staying Fit without Leaving the House

In This Chapter

- Finding ten ways to work out indoors
- Discovering unique ways to get fit within the comfort of your own home

Is it too cold, hot, rainy, dusty, snowy, icy, or otherwise uncomfortable outside? Do you have to work out before the sun comes up or after it goes down? Or are you concerned that you may start labor while you're away from home? This chapter discusses ten great indoor activities that make the weather, time of day, and your delivery date moot (at least as they relate to exercise!).

Pop in an Exercise Video

Hands down, this is one of the simplest ways to work out indoors. All you need is a TV, a VCR or DVD player, an exercise video or DVD, and an area in front of the TV where you can work out. The video provides all the enthusiasm and instruction you need; you just follow along and sweat a lot. See Chapter 14 for a listing of the top-rated pregnancy workout videos.

If you're working out on any hard surface — such as hardwood floor or the concrete in your basement — consider getting a workout mat or other cushy surface. Because a concrete floor is a hard surface, working out on it can lead to discomfort or injury. See Chapter 14 for more information on choosing exercise mats. If you're working out on carpeting, you may prefer a mat just to keep your sweat off the carpet, but it isn't necessary.

If you're trying hard not to wake someone in your house (for example, if you're working out early in the morning), make sure you're exercising on floor boards that won't shake the house and are far from the sleeper's bedroom. A bouncy surface — like the floors in many older homes — can shake the whole house, and that factor combined with the noise from your video and your heavy breathing can wake someone sleeping close by.

Set up a Low-Impact Circuit Routine

A *circuit routine* is a series of strength-building exercises that you set up in your own home. (You can also set up circuit stations in your backyard in nice weather.) The idea is that you start at one station (say, doing curls with hand weights — see Chapter 11) and do that exercise for a predetermined amount of time (for example, 30 seconds), and then briskly walk to the next station (say, lunges — also in Chapter 11) that's set up 10 or 15 feet away. You then do that exercise for the preset amount of time, walk briskly to the next station, do the next exercise, and so on.

You set up your stations based on the exercises that you want to do, including anywhere from 5 to 20 stations, based on how much space you have (and remember that you can use several rooms or even your backyard for circuit stations), how long you want your workout to be, and what sort of exercises you're interested in. Chapter 17 explains in further detail how to set up a circuit workout.

Along with using an exercise video, doing a circuit routine beats the indoor exercise boredom blues better than any other activity.

Take Up Yoga

Yoga is a gentle, relaxing way to tone up. If you know a yoga routine, all you need is a yoga mat. If you're new to yoga and haven't taken a class or had any other instruction, consider getting a copy of *Yoga For Dummies* by Georg Feuerstein and Larry Payne (Wiley), either from your library or your local bookstore. Also, see whether you can borrow or rent a beginner's yoga video from your library or local video store for a week or so — that's about all you need until you're ready for a more advanced tape, which you can buy and use over and over again. Chapter 14 has the lowdown on yoga videos.

The gentle moves of yoga are wonderful ways to relax, gain flexibility, and tone muscles, but yoga isn't much of a calorie burner. Consider alternating yoga with walking or another cardiovascular activity — see Chapter 17 for more on cross-training (alternating exercises every day or so).

Purchase a Treadmill, Stationary Bike, Stair-Stepper, and So On

Granted, this is one of the most expensive ways to work out indoors, although a well-built piece of equipment purchased today may still be working in 15 or 20 years, and that's probably more than you can say about your car! And these pieces start at around $200, which, when compared to a gym membership, is a pretty good deal. Plus, by shopping the classified ads in your area, you can probably get an expensive piece of equipment for pennies on the dollar.

Treadmills, discussed in Chapter 12, give you the option to run or walk indoors, at varying speeds, for as long a workout as you're ready to take on. Some treadmills even simulate hills, which adds some interest (not to mention intensity) to your workout. If you're short on space, look for one that folds up when not in use, but be wary of fold-up models that are so heavy that you need someone's help to unfold them.

Walking, running, cycling, and rowing indoors can be *much* more boring than doing these same activities outside, where you have constantly changing scenery in front of you. You may be okay if you work out for 20 minutes or less; more than that, though, and you're going to need a radio, TV, or TV/VCR combination to chase away boredom. (Keep in mind that on some of the louder pieces of equipment, you have to be able to turn the volume on your radio or TV up very loud to hear it over the sound of the machine. You may need to purchase some external speakers to pump up the sound.) Don't get so tuned in to the TV, however, that you're not aware of what you're doing — you don't want to misstep and fall on a treadmill, for example. Some people also read while working out by buying an attachment that holds an open book in place. The same caution as watching TV applies here: Don't get so wrapped up in the book that you aren't watching what you're doing.

Accept Offers of Exercise Equipment from Anyone

If you have the space for a weight bench, cross-country ski machine, stair-stepper, elliptical machine, stationary bike, or other indoor exercise equipment, put the word out to family, friends, and co-workers that you'll accept whatever they want to get rid of (for free or for a very low price — like $25), as long as they're in good working condition, without any problems that would affect the safety of the equipment. Tell them you'll also take any hand weights, resistance bands, and exercise balls. The sad truth is that a lot of people invest in exercise equipment and either tire of it within a few days or never even use it after taking it out of the box. You can help them clean up and help yourself get fit at the same time by taking this equipment off their hands. In fact, if you have a fairly large area (such as a basement), you may want to accept more than one piece of equipment — it'll be much more convenient than traipsing over to a gym, and you can cross-train (see Chapter 17), using a different machine every day.

Don't know of anyone who's giving away exercise equipment, but you still want to get your hands on cheap stuff? Visit garage sales and watch the classified ads in your local paper. Even in most small towns, ads for ski machines, stair-steppers, and stationary bikes appear every few weeks.

Don't put off exercising while you're waiting for second-hand exercise equipment to come your way. While you're waiting for your aunt to get tired of her elliptical machine, try some of the other low-cost suggestions in this chapter.

Keep Hand Weights or Resistance Bands by the TV

An extraordinarily simple way to burn calories and build strength while inside is to keep a pair of hand weights (three pounds, five pounds, or ten pounds, depending on your strength and experience) or resistance bands by the TV. Whether you're watching the news or some hotties on prime-time TV, just pick up the hand weights and do any of the exercises described in Chapter 11.

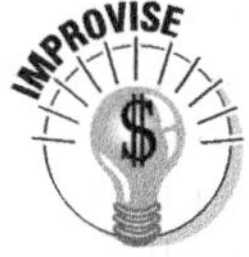

If you don't own hand weights, consider using soup cans, old milk jugs filled with sand, and other homemade weights.

If you think that lifting weights will be too distracting during your favorite show, try lifting only during commercials. Doing this gives you starting and stopping points (start lifting when the commercials begin; stop when your show comes back on), lets you rest between sets (while your show is on), and doesn't distract you or anyone else in the room from the program you're watching.

Dance Around

No doubt about it: Dancing is exercise. In fact, aerobics is essentially doing a choreographed dance that works out specific muscles. (In fact, a dancer who recognized the advantages of working out to pumped-up music invented jazzercise.) But you don't need choreography to get a good workout. If you enjoyed dancing before you got pregnant, pop in some music and get a groove on, right there in your living room (blinds closed, of course!).

Don't do any crazy kicks or jumps from your punk-rock days, but move to the music with your arms, legs, shoulders, butt, and so on. Try to dance for 10 minutes starting out, taking a break between songs, if you need to, and work up to 30 or 40 minutes nonstop.

Treat dancing just like any other workout and warm up before you really get moving (see Chapter 5). And after you're done, be sure to stretch (visit Chapter 8).

Garden with a Purpose

Okay, we admit that gardening isn't something you can do without leaving the house (except for watering those indoor blooms), but you certainly don't have to go far, and you can light your garden area for early-morning or late-night workouts. And it is a workout: Gardening (like dancing) is recognized as a way to exercise, especially if you do it daily. Gardening burns 270 calories per hour and can build strength in both your upper and lower body. You find more about calories in Chapter 10.

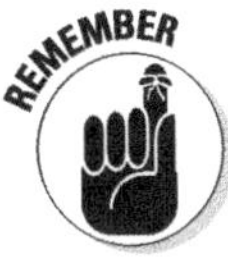

In order for gardening to be a workout, you have to think of it like a walk: Don't pause too often (unless something doesn't feel right — see Chapter 3), try to keep up a certain pace, and move continuously for 20 minutes or more. Ease into gardening (giving your body time to warm up), use good posture as you lift and move objects, and stretch a bit when you're finished. Avoid carrying heavy buckets, pushing a too-full wheelbarrow, and tossing large shovels full of dirt from place to place. And when you're down on your hands and knees, really tugging on those weeds, use a kneeling mat to help cushion the impact on your knee joints.

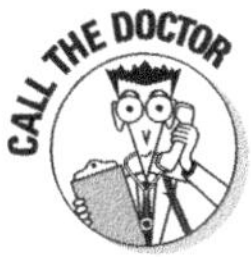

If you have a cat, or if a neighbor's cat prowls around your yard, talk to your doctor before gardening during your pregnancy. Cat feces may contain a parasite that causes *toxoplasmosis,* an infection that can cause serious problems in pregnant women. (This is also why you don't want to change cat litter while you're pregnant.)

Clean the House Vigorously

If you're still doing any housecleaning (and frankly, having your partner do all the housework while you go through pregnancy is a more-than-fair tradeoff), think of it like a workout, and you can burn calories and strengthen muscles. Whether you vacuum with vigor or clean windows with relish, put your whole body into the activity to make this a workout. Always use good posture and stretch at least a little when you're finished.

Exercise in Unusual Ways in Usual Places

Standing in the shower, making dinner, washing dishes, watching TV — what do these activities have in common? They're all times when you can be exercising certain isolated muscles while still soaping up, making a stew, getting the last bit of gunk off the plates, and watching the news.

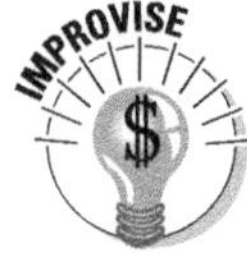

Here are some suggestions for ways to sneak in some exercise during the most mundane tasks, while standing or sitting.

- Do the pelvic floor (or Kegel) exercises discussed in Chapter 11.
- Contract your buttocks for one second, release, and repeat, doing 10 to 30 contractions.
- Do 1 or 2 sets of 10 to 12 shoulder shrugs or shoulder circles (see Chapter 11) anytime you're not using your arms.
- Squeeze your shoulder blades together (you'll feel this in your upper back) for 2 to 3 sets of 5 to 10 repetitions.

Chapter 22

Ten or So Ways to Get Family and Friends Involved in Your Quest for Fitness

In This Chapter

- Getting your family and friends to support you in your workouts
- Motivating your family to work out, too!

Your family and/or your friends can be involved in your workouts in one of two ways:

- They can support you in your fit pregnancy and not work out themselves.
- They can support you in your fit pregnancy and work out with you.

Notice that, in either case, you need the support of your family or friends as you get or stay fit during pregnancy. If your partner, kids, closest friends, parents, or other support people are against your fitness routine, we can give you a nearly 100 percent guarantee that you'll soon give it up. You absolutely must get support from a few key people in your life, or they'll make working out so difficult that all the benefits won't be worthwhile.

As a result, this chapter shares two types of advice: how to get your family or friends to support you and how to get your family or friends to work out with you.

Gathering Support While You Work Out

In order to work out consistently, you need the support of the people you live and socialize with. If, for example, you work out every day after work — and your friends and family all know this — but three days a week, they ask you to go out to dinner immediately after work, encouraging you to bag your workouts, they're not supporting your workout routine. They may or may not be intentionally sabotaging your efforts to get and stay fit, but regardless of their intention, they're making your fitness routine harder to maintain than it has to be. So, how do you get your friends and family on board? Consider the following tips.

Stick to a schedule they can count on and that fits their lives

First, choose a workout time that doesn't interfere with long-held rituals or other important activities. If your family always eats breakfast together, for example, and this is important family time, don't work out in the morning during breakfast time.

After finding a time that works for you and the people who are most important to you (and this may take some experimentation), stick to it. Suppose you plan to work out every morning so that you and your partner can eat dinner at 5:30 like you always have. But three days this week, you get up too late to exercise, so you decide to exercise after work instead and don't get home until 6:30 those nights. Do you think he's going to be gung-ho about your workouts? Probably not. But if he's also encouraging you to stay up until 11:00 and that's why you have trouble getting up so early, you may need to talk to him about your need to set aside time to exercise in a way that's convenient for both of you.

The purpose of exercise is to enhance your life, not complicate and detract from it. Although finding a time to work out that fits your schedule and the schedules of the people most important to you isn't easy, stay at it until you find something that works.

Plan vacations/weekends with exercise in mind

One of the world's great mysteries to people who don't exercise is why people would want to "spoil" their weekends and vacations with workouts. After all, it's supposed to be a vacation, not a carbon copy of the rest of life.

You may find that you don't want to work out on the weekends or while you're on vacation and that's fine, but more than likely, if you've been exercising regularly, you probably enjoy the feeling you get during and after a workout and don't want to give that up, even on the days you're otherwise relaxing. If that's the case, before you go on vacation or before Saturday morning rolls around, be sure the important people in your life understand that you will be continuing your workouts and plan to work out at a time that works for everyone.

To get the full support of the people you spend time with during the weekends and while on vacation, keep your exercise routine as unobtrusive as possible. If, for example, you can get up 45 minutes before everyone else and have your workout done just as they're getting out of bed, they not only won't mind your routine, but they may also be inspired by what you've accomplished while they were snoozing!

Meet up at the end of a workout

If you're concerned about exercise taking time away from your partner or close friends, arrange to meet them at the end of a workout for a quick bite to eat or other casual gathering. For example, if your partner always heads to the coffee shop on Saturday mornings, leave a little earlier than he does and walk to the coffee shop while he drives. He can even bring you a sweat shirt or complete change of clothes. After you arrive, do a few quick stand-up stretches (see Chapter 8), get into comfortable clothes, and continue with the Saturday morning coffee routine. Sure, you'll be a little sweaty and smelly, but you'll be getting fitter *and* spending time with your partner.

Get help with chores to free up time for exercise

If you're so busy right now with commitments at work and at home that you don't see how you can possibly find time to exercise (or if you've been exercising but are finding that important tasks are being left undone), have a heart-to-heart with your partner or other roommate and see which tasks can be done less frequently (can you change the sheets every other week, for example?), taken off your plate (that is, taken over by your partner), or hired out (hiring a cleaning person or eating ready-made food so that you don't have to cook).

If your partner takes over a chore for you so that you can exercise, take it back over on any days you don't exercise. That way, you reinforce that he's doing the chore to help you with your fitness, not just because you were able to wheedle him into it.

Getting Your Family or Friends to Exercise with You

If you've gone beyond simply needing support from family and friends and are, instead, determined to have them join you, this section shares three tips.

As your baby gets older, involve him or her in a consistent exercise routine, keeping the following in mind.

Make exercise a game

Even if you're a serious exerciser who doesn't need exercise to be fun in order to enjoy and appreciate it, don't expect others to share that way of thinking. Instead, you have to entice others by making activities as fun as possible. Is bike riding a fun family activity or a serious, difficult workout? Is walking down a beautiful, quiet road "exercise," or is it just a great way to spend an afternoon? (Hint: If your family and friends can't tell the difference between a workout and a fun time outdoors, you're on the right track.)

Keep everything you do as a group fun and happy. And avoid the words "exercise" and "workout" at all costs.

Vary the activities

Cross-training could've been invented for reluctant beginning exercisers, because it takes all sense of drudgery out of workouts. If you *cross-train* with your family or friends (that is, do one activity one day and a different one the next — see Chapter 17), you're never giving newcomers a chance to get bored with the whole idea of exercise. It also helps to give them a say-so in what you do from one day to the next.

Use bribery

Just as you reward yourself as a form of motivation (see Chapter 5), you can also reward others. Talk about what forms of rewards would inspire your friends/partner/kids, and then, together, set up a goal to reach in exchange for that reward. Goals may include working out for a certain number of days (such as 4 or 5 days in one week), working out in one session for a certain number of minutes (that is, gradually building up to a 40-minute walk), losing a certain amount of weight (not for you while you're pregnant, of course, but for others), and so on.

Chapter 23

Ten (Plus One) Resources for Pregnancy Workout Gear

In This Chapter

- Finding weights, exercise balls, indoor machines, and other equipment
- Locating great-fitting, great-looking workout clothing

In this chapter, you get the inside scoop on where to purchase the workout gear (clothing and small, inexpensive pieces of equipment) discussed throughout this book. See Chapter 7 for the ins and outs of choosing workout gear.

Your Local Discount or Sporting Goods Store

Target, Walmart, Kmart, ShopKo, TJ Maxx, Dunham's, and other large discount stores and sporting goods stores often carry the following products:

- Aerobics and yoga videos
- Yoga mats
- Exercise balls
- Resistance bands
- Hand weights and weight sticks/bars

- Socks, loose-fitting sweat pants, large T-shirts (short sleeved and long sleeved)
- Some types of maternity workout clothing (although many stores don't have any)
- Limited supply of stationary bikes, elliptical trainers, stair-stepping machines, and weight benches (also check Sears, Sam's Club, and Costco)
- Treadmills (also check Sears, Sam's Club, and Costco for good prices on limited quantities of treadmills)

You probably won't have much luck finding maternity workout wear at nationwide discount stores. If the store carries any workout clothing for pregnant women, the selection and range of sizes may be so limited that you're better off going with a mail-order company (see the "Maternity Clothing Shops" section later in this chapter).

At sporting goods stores, you also find exercise equipment (discussed in Chapter 7 and in the Part IV chapters, which talk about individual activities) that discount stores may not have:

- Water aerobics equipment, including floatation vests, weights, and shoes
- Bike helmets and biking gloves, which are handy if you're planning to bike outdoors during your first trimester (and your healthcare provider hasn't asked you to bike indoors)
- Aerobics shoes and walking shoes; also running shoes, but you're better off going to a running specialty shop to get fitted for those

Athletic Specialty Shops

Stores that specialize in cycling, running and walking, yoga, and other sports dot the country and may be located in your area.

- **Cycle shop:** Go to a cycling specialty store for outdoor bikes, indoor traditional and recumbent bikes, helmets, biking gloves, biking shoes, odometers, and all sorts of other cycling gear and gadgets. Prices will be high, but so will the quality of the equipment, so if you plan to cycle for years to come, these types of stores are where you want to go.

- **Outdoor-adventure store:** Here's where you find hiking equipment, and in colder climates, everything for winter workouts, including equipment for cross-country skiing and snowshoeing.
- **Running store:** Go to the running store for running shoes. Many, although not all, running stores also sell a wide variety of walking shoes. Don't expect to see much maternity fitness clothing at most specialty shops — plan to get those items via mail order, instead (see the following section).
- **Yoga shop:** Yoga shops sell mats, pregnancy yoga outfits, videos, and all sorts of relaxation tapes, scents, and accessories. Some yoga shops also offer classes; many even offer special pregnancy yoga classes.

Maternity Clothing Shops

Stop by your local sporting goods store or even a sports specialty store (like a bike shop), and you're likely to be disappointed in their selection of maternity workout clothing — as in, they won't have any! In spite of the growing popularity of working out during pregnancy, store buyers just haven't caught wind of this trend. Thank goodness for Internet technology, though, because new Web sites that offer maternity workout clothes in a variety of styles and sizes pop up every month.

Given the fluid nature of the Internet, some of the Web sites listed in the following sections may no longer exist by the time you read this chapter. If you can't find a site listed here and a search on Google or some other search engine for the company name doesn't yield any results, search for **maternity workout clothing** and see what pops up.

See Chapter 7 for an explanation of what the clothing in this section is used for and what it looks like.

Fit Maternity and Beyond

Laurie Bagley founded Fit Maternity and Beyond to share the benefits of her fit pregnancy with other women. The company (`www.fitmaternity.com`; 888-961-9100; 530-926-6208) features Adidas and Reebok maternity workout clothes, plus a host of other brands to facilitate one-stop shopping, all at moderate to high prices (watch for sales).

The selection of maternity workout wear is the best you'll see anywhere, including

- Baby carriers (including running strollers)
- Belly braces and other supports
- Biking shorts
- Hats
- Jackets
- Pants and tights
- Running and walking shorts
- Special creams for stretch marks
- Sports bras
- Swimsuits
- Tank tops
- Tennis outfits
- T-shirts
- Unitards
- Yoga mats

The company's innovation, the Nine Month Club allows you to sign up (or, better yet, your partner, friends, or relatives to sign you up) for a monthly delivery of a new workout outfit that's appropriate for the season and the proper size for you. Gift certificates are also available.

Mothers in Motion

When Bess Hilpert was pregnant with each of her four children, she continued to run but couldn't get her pre-pregnancy running clothes to fit or support her in any way. As a result, she experienced quite a bit of discomfort in her training and knew that she could create a product that was better designed and more comfortable than anything she'd tried.

Enter Mothers in Motion, a line of maternity products sold through the company's Web site (`www.mothersinmotion.com`), via telephone (877-512-8800; 512-733-7637), and in some Nordstrom stores. The basic design of the clothing is really unique, and researchers have tested it to verify the company's claims. Each piece of clothing provides specially designed belly support that acts like an internal belly brace, gives back support to reduce back pain, and offers thigh support to relieve sciatic nerve pain. All fabrics are also designed to draw moisture away from your body as you work out.

Look for the following products, all in several colors and styles:

- Biking and running shorts
- Jackets
- Leggings and pants
- Sports bras
- T-shirts and tank tops
- Unitards

Prices are surprisingly low, and occasional sales make them even more appealing. You won't find any products at this site beyond those designed by Hilpert, so you won't see books, yoga mats, and so on, but the comfort, durability, and quality of the products make this company a winner.

Title 9 Sports

Title 9 Sports sells workout gear exclusively for women — the company is named for the 1972 federal law that called for parity in men's and women's athletic programs at public universities and other schools. The company's catalogs showcase fit women who are neither professional athletes nor models, and that makes for an inspiring read!

The company (`www.title9sports.com`; 800-342-4448) sells mostly non-maternity wear (stuff to dream about for after you deliver your baby), but the company makes an ultracomfortable, pleated maternity short and maternity pant, both crafted of 90 percent cotton and 10 percent spandex with a wide waistband that doesn't bind but rather gently supports your abdomen. Title 9 tends to be a little pricey, but you get high-quality workout wear that lasts for years — so if you plan to be pregnant more than once, this clothing is a good investment.

Baby Style

In addition to maternity clothing, Baby Style offers baby clothes, toys, and gear, so if you're in the mood to shop for everything related to babies, you can stock up on adorable clothing and workout gear at the same time. Go to www.babystyle.com and click on Maternity and then Workout & Swim Wear and you see a small but complete selection of clothing, including

- Jackets
- Pants and leggings
- Shorts
- Sports bras
- Swimsuits
- T-shirts and tank tops
- Unitards

You can also call the company directly at 877-378-9537.

Motherhood Maternity

Motherhood Maternity (www.motherhood.com; 800-466-6223) sells an excellent selection of colorful, comfortable, flattering, inexpensive swimwear. You'll also find some jackets, leggings, and pants, but just about everything else in this company's line is nonworkout clothing. Look for occasional sales that make good prices even better.

Motherhood Maternity also sells some workout clothing through its 800 stores across the United States and Canada. Check the Web site for the store nearest you, but call before you visit the store to make sure that it offers a selection of workout wear.

Anna Cris Maternity

The Anna Cris Maternity boutique (www.annacris.com; 800-281-2662; 201-337-8940) is a maternity fashion store that sells select workout wear. Although the company mostly offers hip everyday clothing, you find a nice selection of yoga apparel, mats, and videos and a few pieces of maternity swimwear. Prices are on the high side, which you probably expect from a fashion company.

Japanese Weekend Maternity

Japanese Weekend, a company that specializes in fashion maternity clothing, also sells several workout items, including shorts, pants, and jackets, at its Web site (www.japaneseweekend.com), catalog (800-808-0555), and stores in California, Texas, and Florida.

The product that you really want to try is the during-and-after pant, which fits you while you're pregnant and — through the magic of elastic and darts — looks great after you get back to your pre-pregnancy size. The price is a little high, but this product should last for years. Best of all, Japanese Weekend offers free shipping on all returns, so you have little risk in ordering these pants and giving them a try.

Mom Shop

The Mom Shop (`www.momshop.com`; 800-854-1213) is another store that offers mostly nonworkout maternity clothing, but the company offers a line of beautifully designed swimwear in dazzling colors. If you want to wow the pool crowd, check out these suits.

Your Partner's Closet

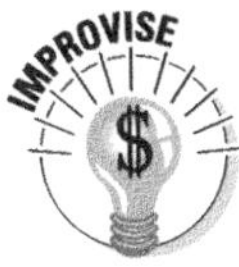

Although your partner may not like having his closet raided, consider whether you can use some of his clothing for these 40 weeks:

- Drawstring shorts
- Jackets
- Large, baggy sweat shirts
- Long T-shirts

Index

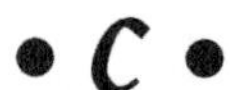

• D •

• E •

• F •

• G •

• H •

• I •

• J •

• K •

• O •

• P •

• Q •

• R •

• S •

• T •

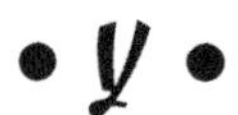

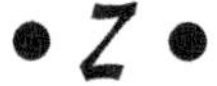